Practice Nurse Handbook

Fifth edition

Gillian Hampson
RGN, RCNT, DN, PN/Dip HE in Community Health Care
Independent Practice Nurse

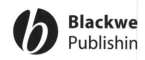 **Blackwe**
Publishin

Editorial offices:
Blackwell Publishing Ltd, 9600 Garsington Road, Oxford OX4 2DQ, UK
    Tel: +44 (0)1865 776868
Blackwell Publishing Inc., 350 Main Street, Malden, MA 02148-5020, USA
    Tel: +1 781 388 8250
Blackwell Publishing Asia Pty Ltd, 550 Swanston Street, Carlton, Victoria 3053, Australia
    Tel: +61 (0)3 8359 1011

First published 1984
Second edition published 1989
Reprinted 1989
Third edition published 1994
Fourth edition published 2002

ISBN-10: 1-4051-4421-1
ISBN-13: 978-1-4051-4421-6

Library of Congress Cataloging-in-Publication Data
Hampson, Gillian D.
    Practice nurse handbook.—5th ed. / Gillian Hampson.
      p. ; cm.
    Includes bibliographical references and index.
    ISBN-13: 978-1-4051-4421-6 (pbk. : alk. paper)
    ISBN-10: 1-4051-4421-1 (pbk. : alk. paper)   1. Nurse practitioners.   2. Primary care (Medicine)
    3. Nurse practitioners—Great Britain.
    [DNLM: 1. Nursing Care.   2. Family Practice. WY 101 H2312p 2006]   I. Title.

RT82.8.H35 2006
610.7306′92—dc22

                                                                                    2006006002

A catalogue record for this title is available from the British Library

Set in 10/12.5pt Palatino
by Graphicraft Ltd, Hong Kong
Printed and bound in Singapore
by Fabulous Printers Pte Ltd

The publisher's policy is to use permanent paper from mills that operate a sustainable forestry policy, and which has been manufactured from pulp processed using acid-free and elementary chlorine-free practices. Furthermore, the publisher ensures that the text paper and cover board used have met acceptable environmental accreditation standards.

For further information on Blackwell Publishing, visit our website:
www.blackwellnursing.com

Contents

Preface to the Fifth Edition   vii
Acknowledgements   viii

1 Teamwork in General Practice   1
The National Health Service   1
Teamwork   7

2 General Practice Nursing   16
Historical background   16
Nurse employment in general practice   20
Networking for support   22
Practice nurse education   24
Identifying good practice   25

3 Practice Organisation   31
Information about patients   31
Protocols, guidelines and clinical pathways   36
Policies and procedures   37
Meetings   39
Public involvement   39

4 Management of the Nurses' Rooms   42
Design and furnishing   43
Health and safety   44
Control of infection   47
Supplies and equipment   54
Training in emergency procedures   55

5 Nursing Treatments and Procedures   59
Injections   59
Wound care   60
Wound healing   60
Eye treatment   68
Ear care   68
Assisting with minor surgery   72

6	**Diagnostic and Screening Tests**	79
	Laboratory tests	81
	Investigations and tests within the practice	91
7	**Emergency Situations**	104
	General principles	104
	Collapse	105
	Asphyxia	109
	Management of other emergency situations	112
	Respiratory problems	119
	Haemorrhage	120
	Poisoning	123
	Pain	124
	Trauma and minor injuries	124
	Stings and bites	127
	Eye problems	129
	Foreign bodies	130
	Emergency midwifery	131
8	**Common Medical Conditions**	134
	Medication	135
	Upper respiratory tract infections	136
	Ear conditions	138
	Headache	139
	Insomnia	140
	Gastrointestinal disorders	140
	Urinary problems	144
	Vaginal discharge	145
	Infectious diseases	147
	Human parasites	150
	Other skin conditions	151
9	**Health Promotion**	160
	National Service Frameworks and Quality and Outcomes Framework	160
	Inequalities in health	160
	Cultural diversity	161
	Education for practice nurses	161
	Terminology	161
	Health promotion and the primary healthcare team	163
	Health promotion in general practice	164
	Dietary advice and monitoring	170
	Smoking cessation	175
10	**Child Health, Childhood and Adult Immunisation**	180
	Child health promotion	180

Safety   183
Child abuse   184
The Children Acts (1989 and 2004)   185
Childhood immunisation   185
Adult immunisation   191
Conclusion   196

11 Travel Health   200
Nurse education   200
Advice for travellers   202
Immunisation for travellers   211

12 Sexual Health   219
Sexual identity   219
Relationships   220
Education for nurses   220
Fertility and fertility control   221
Termination of pregnancy   233
Sexually transmitted diseases   234

13 Women's Health   239
Menstruation   239
Cervical cytology   241
Breast awareness   243
Preconceptual care   244
Infertility   245
Pregnancy   246
Hysterectomy   249
The menopause   249
Osteoporosis   251
Bladder problems   252
Information for patients   254

14 Men's Health   258
Morbidity and mortality   258
Male patients in general practice   261
Well-man checks   262
Testicular cancer   263
Prostate disease   264
Erectile dysfunction   269
Conclusion   271

15 Mental Health   275
The historical background to the development of mental
health services   275

Mental healthcare in general practice   277
Self-awareness in the caring professions   289

16 Supporting Patients with Chronic Diseases   292
The expert patient   292
Clinics in general practice   293
Asthma   294
Chronic obstructive pulmonary disease   300
Diabetes mellitus   304
Hypertension   312
Coronary heart disease   316
Conclusion   317

Appendix 1   Examples of the clinical equipment needed in the nurses' rooms   321
Appendix 2   Emergency equipment   325

Index   327

Preface to the Fifth Edition

Throughout this new edition I have aimed to provide the type of information I really needed as a new practice nurse and have used the same format that I used in the previous edition. I have included practical information and emphasised the legal aspects of the work. I have also stressed the need for education and have provided information about useful courses and qualifications. I have spent long periods each day searching the internet and have recommended some of the more reliable websites.

At times, I have felt overwhelmed by the need to make sense of all the changes in the National Health Service. Hardly a day goes by without some new target or directive from above. I have not included details of the health service structures and legislation of the other countries in the United Kingdom in the interests of brevity. Many of the documents produced by the English Department of Health have their equivalents in Scotland, Wales and Northern Ireland. I apologise to readers in those countries for supplying mainly English references.

Gillian Hampson

Acknowledgements

Thanks are due to colleagues at Richmond and Twickenham Primary Care Trust for their helpful comments on some of these chapters. Particular thanks are given to Shona Henderson, Infection Control Lead, and Angela Versey, Family Planning Lead, for their very constructive comments.

Chapter 1
Teamwork in General Practice

This chapter outlines the background to the work of practice nurses so that the role can be considered within the context of the whole primary healthcare team.

THE NATIONAL HEALTH SERVICE (NHS)

In 1948 the National Health Service was established on the basis that everybody should have free access to medical care irrespective of financial status. At that time, it was assumed that the demand for care would decrease once the unresolved 'pool' of illness in the population had been treated. In the light of experience, it has become clear that the amount of treatable illness is small compared with both chronic conditions, which cannot be cured, and problems created by environmental and personal stress, the underlying reasons for many consultations in general practice.

Developments in general practice

Prior to 1948 most general practitioners worked independently, usually from their own homes. Patients who were unable to afford private medical care belonged to a doctor's panel. The cost was supported by various insurance schemes and hospital beds were endowed especially for 'the poor'. The hospitals were nationalised in 1948 but general practitioners, dentists, retail pharmacists and opticians stayed as independent businesses with contracts to supply specific services to NHS patients. Executive councils were set up to administer these arrangements. The local authorities employed the district nurses and health visitors.

The early days of the NHS were a catalogue of disasters, with neither doctors nor patients really knowing what to expect of the new system. Patients had been led to believe that everything was free so extra demands were made upon doctors, who were themselves unprepared for the organisational and practical difficulties created by the new system. Between 1948 and 1956, expenditure in the NHS had risen by 70%.[1]

The Family Doctors' Charter

The British Medical Association, through its General Medical Services Committee, has always been responsible for the political aspects of general practice, including terms of service and remuneration. The College of General Practitioners, established in 1953 (to become the Royal College in 1966), was mainly concerned with educational issues. The effects of these two bodies on government policies brought about the so-called *GPs' Charter* in 1966, in response to the threat of resignation by disillusioned doctors.[2] The Charter radically altered the way in which GPs were paid and gave them incentives for having better premises and reimbursement for ancillary staff salaries. Nurses were included among these ancillary staff.

NHS reorganisation

The structure of the NHS was reorganised in 1974, when management first assumed a specialist function. Executive councils became family practitioner committees (FPCs) and community nurse employment was transferred from local authorities to the health service. Area health authorities were abolished in 1982 and their powers devolved to district health authorities. However, 1990 saw a more radical change to the NHS. The introduction of the internal market created a separation between the purchasers and the providers of services. Hospitals were invited to become self-governing trusts and GPs in group practices were encouraged to become fundholders to purchase secondary services on behalf of their patients. FPCs were changed to family health service authorities (FHSAs) with greater managerial responsibilities in relation to general practice.[3] FHSAs later merged with health authorities and some of their functions were devolved to primary care agencies.

The GPs' Contract of 1990 required them to provide a range of screening and health promotion services. Many practice nurses were employed at that time to undertake the extra work.[4] In that same year, the government introduced targets for reducing disease and disability through its *Health of the Nation* strategy for England. The Labour government replaced this with 1997's strategy on saving lives.[5] Similar strategies were produced in the other countries of the United Kingdom.

The change of government in 1997 led to the development of *The New NHS*.[6] Fundholding was abolished and instead of being in competition, all the practices in a locality became part of a primary care organisation. These were subcommittees of health authorities, with a devolved budget to purchase services on behalf of the local community and a remit to monitor and improve the quality of services (clinical governance) and promote improvements in health (health improvement programmes). The pace of change became relentless, with a stream of targets to reduce waiting lists and National Service Frameworks (NSFs) to specify the standards for services for the common diseases and patient groups.

The National Institute for Clinical Excellence was established to make recommendations on the use of new drugs and treatments in order to end the 'postcode lottery', whereby patients in one health authority area could be denied treatments available elsewhere. The Commission for Health Improvement (rebranded as the Healthcare Commission in 2004) was established to inspect health authorities and trusts (including general practices) and to monitor performance. In 2001 a special health authority, the National Clinical Assessment Authority, was set up, in the wake of several medical scandals, to provide a rapid investigation into the performance of certain doctors and dentists.[7-9] The functions of the NCAA were transferred in April 2005 to the National Clinical Assessment Service, a division of the National Patient Safety Agency.

The NHS Plans

In the year 2000 the government published an ambitious plan for investment and reform of the NHS to take place over ten years.[10] The plan outlined the intention to provide extra beds, hospitals and staff, as well as modernisation of general practice, new doctors' contracts and a greater role for nurses. The role of patients in the modernisation process was also stressed. The 2004 *NHS Improvement Plan* contained even more ambitious promises, with less emphasis on reducing waiting times and more on improving the care of people with chronic conditions and the local control of services.[11] The involvement of the independent sector was included and the full extent of such proposals became clear in the contracting guide produced by the NHS Confederation on alternative providers of medical services.[12] Community nurses began to feel concern about their future employment status.

Primary care organisations (PCOs)

Enlarged PCOs became autonomous providers of general practice and community nursing services and commissioners of secondary care. As many of the functions of the health authorities were devolved to PCOs, health authorities were merged into larger strategic regional bodies. Proposals were also contained in *The NHS Plan* for PCOs to merge with social service departments to form care trusts, with budgets to provide integrated health and social services.

Care in the community

Other changes accelerated within the community from April 1993 as a result of the NHS and Community Care Act (1990). Social service departments assumed new responsibilities for assessing the needs of and providing tailor-made services for vulnerable people. Hospitals had to ensure that the appropriate services were in place before such patients could be discharged home. More resources were needed to provide effective community care and plans were made to modernise mental health services.[13] The National Service Framework for Mental Health, published in 1999, was intended to address some of the failings of care in the community (see Chapter 15).

Health service structures

Although politics can seem remote from direct patient care, it is essential to keep abreast of developments in the NHS, which is a highly politicised organisation. The endless change can seem daunting but nurses have a key role to play in the changing NHS and in developing innovative services and ways of promoting health for the public.

The NHS structures for Scotland, Wales and Northern Ireland have always been slightly different but space does not allow for more than a general overview. All nurses should be aware of their own country's health service management structure and policies.

General practice as a business

Unlike hospital doctors, who are salaried, the majority of GPs have always been independent contractors, with the same contract with the NHS for providing general medical services (GMS). This had a very complicated system of remuneration and *The Statement of Fees and Allowances* (known as the Red Book) provided details of all the payments which GPs could receive from the NHS. Some practices employ salaried GPs but this is still uncommon.

Personal medical services (PMS)

The Primary Care Act of 1997 permitted a departure from the national GMS contract.[14] PMS practices (the first pilots started in 1998) demonstrated new ways of providing general practice services, through local contracts with health authorities (later with primary care organisations). Nurses who employ salaried GPs to provide medical services to their practice populations have led some pilots. The majority of nurse-led schemes have tended to provide services for specific population groups, such as the homeless, refugees and asylum seekers or people in underdoctored areas.

New general medical services (nGMS)

From April 2004, GPs not covered by PMS accepted a new standard GMS contract, administered by local primary care organisations. *The Statement of*

Financial Entitlements, a 250-page document which specifies how payments to practices should be calculated, superseded the Red Book.[15] Practices are paid a global sum to cover the provision of services to patients, staff costs and locum payments. The nGMS Contract (known as the Blue Book) specifies how services should be provided in general practice.[16] Three types of services are identified.

- *Essential services* – the diagnosis and treatment of illness, including terminal illness, and the management of chronic diseases.
- *Additional services* – including cervical screening, contraception, some immunisations, child health surveillance, maternity services excluding interpartum care, basic minor surgery such as curettage, cautery and cryocautery of warts and other skin lesions.
- *Enhanced services* – are commissioned by the PCO and might not be provided by all practices. These services could consist of higher standards of essential or additional services, e.g. advanced minor surgery, or deal with specific health needs, provided by practitioners with special interests and expertise. There are three forms of enhanced services.
  1. **Directed enhanced services** – specified and priced nationally. They include childhood and influenza immunisations, improved access, services to support staff dealing with violent patients, quality information preparation and advanced minor surgery.
  2. **National enhanced services** – specified and priced nationally but not directed. These include anticoagulant care, insertion of IUDs, intrapartum care, specialised care of patients with depression, enhanced care of the homeless, services for drug and/or alcohol misusers, immediate and first response care, minor injury services or more specialised sexual healthcare.
  3. **Local enhanced services** – agreed locally between the practice and the PCO.

Quality and Outcomes Framework (QOF)

This part of the contract deals with the quality of services provided in general practice and is voluntary. Payment is made for the achievement of specified quality indicators on a points system in four domains: clinical, organisational, patient experience and additional services. The clinical domain consists of: CHD, stroke/TIA, hypertension, diabetes mellitus, COPD, epilepsy, mental health and asthma. Each of these has a number of quality indicators, which have to be achieved in order to receive payment. The contract specifies several principles regarding the QOF.

- Indicators should, where possible, be based on the best available evidence.
- The number of indicators in each clinical condition should be kept to a minimum number compatible with patient care.
- Data should not be collected purely for audit purposes.
- Only data useful to patient care should be collected. A consultation should not be distorted by an overemphasis on data collection.

- Data should never be collected twice, i.e. data required for audit purposes should be data routinely collected for patient care and obtained from existing practice clinical systems.[17]

Education for general practitioners

Qualified GP trainers provide placements in approved training practices for doctors who wish to become GPs. Consultations are sometimes video-recorded, with the consent of the patient, for teaching and assessment purposes. Postgraduate training was introduced on a more formal basis in the 1970s, followed by various parliamentary regulations. Legislation allowing the free movement of doctors within Europe has been in place since 1986. New regulations came into force in 1998, outlining the training required for all doctors working in general practice in the NHS.[18] Vocational training is overseen by the Joint Committee on Postgraduate Training for General Practice, the body which sets the standards of general practice training, approves GP trainers and training practices, as well as issuing the certificates required for doctors to work unsupervised in general practice.

Revalidation and appraisal

The GMC plans for revalidation have been in existence for several years, in order to demonstrate a doctor's fitness to practise. However, the plans are undergoing further consideration in the light of the Shipman Inquiry.[19] Doctors currently keep folders about their professional practice for use at annual appraisals, which may form part of their revalidation procedures. Nurses are already accustomed to keeping professional profiles and to re-registering every three years. All staff are required to have personal development plans and to undertake an annual appraisal.

Practice population profiles

The changes within the NHS necessitate the identification of the particular health and social needs of local populations in order to provide appropriate services. Such profiles should cover: age/sex ratios, ethnic groups, family structures, numbers on the child protection register, social class, poverty levels, employment, housing, vulnerable groups, morbidity and mortality, environmental hazards and amenities. Since April 2000 practices have also been required to identify all informal carers registered with them, whether or not the person for whom they care is registered at the same practice.[20] Practices have a duty to ensure that carers are offered the support and help to which they are entitled.

TEAMWORK

The explosion of work within general practice highlights the need for good teamwork but just being together in one place will not create a team. All teams share certain characteristics, whatever their functions:

- A shared purpose or goal
- A sense of team identity
- An understanding of the role and valuing of the contribution of individual team members.

Teamwork needs some committed hard work to succeed. It can be hindered by ineffective leadership, divided loyalties, when members belong to more than one team, or sabotage by disaffected members.

The historical background to the different professions means that modern-day, independent-minded nurses and GPs accustomed to assume authority may have very different perceptions of the same situation, which can lead to conflict. The importance of team building has been recognised for many years in the commercial world and many of their methods are being adopted in the health service.

Primary healthcare

Primary healthcare refers to health promotion, treatment and care within general practice and the community, as compared with secondary care provided by hospitals and specialist services. The government is keen to promote primary care services.

Primary healthcare teams have been around since the 1960s in one guise or another but in reality, there are often two types of team involved with general practice.

The practice team

A practice team tends to incorporate all those people based within the practice, most of whom are either partners or employees of the GP. Apart from the doctors, practice teams include the following.

The practice nurse(s) (see Chapter 2)

The title *practice nurse* has always been generally understood to apply to a qualified nurse employed by a GP or GP partnership. However, it is becoming more common for practice nurses to be employed directly by primary care organisations. Some practice nurses are partners in their practices, while others are self-employed as independent nurses. A practice may also include a nurse practitioner in the team, although the Nursing and Midwifery Council does not yet protect the qualification and title and the work undertaken is subject to wide variations. Healthcare assistants are being employed by many practices to undertake basic tasks, in order to allow time for practice nurses to utilise their skills more effectively.

The practice manager

A practice manager has responsibility for organising the systems which allow the practice to run smoothly, as well as for financial and personnel management, staff development and liaison with all the staff and the PCO. A modern practice manager will usually have had the specific management training needed to cope with the demands of running a busy practice, which can include a university degree in business management. The specific role may differ from practice to practice but the success of each organisation can depend on the effectiveness of the manager. Many practice managers are members of the Association of Medical Secretaries and Practice Managers, Administrators and Receptionists (AMSPAR).

The receptionists

The receptionists are the first point of contact with the public. They must be able to stay calm in the face of conflicting demands from patients, other staff and the telephone. Receptionists frequently act as gatekeepers to the doctors and nurses by prioritising appointments or controlling the number of telephone calls put through. A very fine line exists between efficient organisation and the denial of a patient's right to consult a doctor or nurse.

Apart from running the appointment system and taking telephone messages, there is plenty of administrative work. Most practices are computerised and registration data have to be processed. Data entry clerks type data into the computers. Some receptionists organise repeat prescriptions. Training for receptionists often takes place in-house but recognised courses are also available. Practice receptionist training, organised by some PCOs and colleges of further education, leads to a qualification from AMSPAR.

The medical secretary

A medical secretary needs office skills and knowledge of the terminology used in medical correspondence. In smaller practices, secretarial duties may be combined with reception or administrative work but large practices usually employ a qualified medical secretary to deal specifically with referral letters, reports, office administration and the practice correspondence.

Paramedical staff

Larger practices may employ or facilitate access to other professional staff – dietitians, physiotherapists, counsellors and chiropodists – to increase the range of services available for patients. Pharmacists are joining many practices to help with more effective prescribing. Alternative therapists such as acupuncturists, aromatherapists and masseurs are also being welcomed into some teams.

Phlebotomists

Larger practices often employ a phlebotomist to take routine blood tests. In some areas, a member of the clerical staff will be trained in phlebotomy in order to free up valuable nursing time. This potentially risky work calls for adequate training and assessment as well as immunisation against hepatitis B (see Chapter 10).

The primary healthcare team (PHCT)

When group attachment was introduced, it was thought to allow better communication between the professional groups than when nurses work in geographical patches. District nurses, health visitors, community midwives and community mental health nurses also relate to teams in their own specialities, which may have different aims and priorities from those of the practice. Practice nurses have traditionally been unique among NHS nurses in being employed by a GP and not by a community or hospital trust. However, sometimes practice nurses, district nurses and health visitors are all employed by the same local primary care organisation.

Integrated nursing teams

The idea that community nurse attachment to GP practices would lead to integrated primary care teams has only rarely been fully realised. There have been a number of teams created in recent years consisting of district nurses, public health nurses and practice nurses.[21] The success of such teams often seems to rely on the degree of self-direction and budget control permitted, as well as on the personalities of the team members themselves. The need to avoid duplication or gaps in the service is leading to a radical rethink of the way nursing services are delivered. The Department of Health has spelled out how nurses can help to deliver *The NHS Plan*.[22]

Specialist community nurses

In 1994 eight branches of community nursing were accorded equal recognition by the United Kingdom Central Council, now the Nursing and Midwifery Council (NMC). Modules in common core subjects as well as discipline-specific modules in each of the specialities lead to a BSc or Honours degree in one of the eight specialist fields:

- General practice nursing
- Community mental health nursing
- Community learning disabilities nursing
- Community children's nursing

- Public health nursing/health visiting
- School nursing
- Community nursing in the home/district nursing
- Occupational health nursing.

The expansion of specialist nursing and the roles of autonomous practitioners and nurse consultants resulted in a consultation exercise by the NMC on establishing a standard of proficiency for advanced nursing practice.[23]

District nurses

A district nurse is responsible for providing skilled nursing services in the community by:

- Assessing the care needs of patients and their families
- Formulating individualised care plans and revising them as necessary
- Implementing the care or delegating to other members of the district nursing team
- Monitoring patients' progress and reassessing care needs
- Supervising the care given by other members of the district nursing team.

Liaison with other PHCT members, social services and voluntary agencies is often as important as direct care giving. The role also includes providing support to carers and teaching patients, other nurses and medical students. District nursing teams work in a similar way to hospital ward teams, with mixed skills and grades. Most district nursing care takes place within the patients' homes, although some district nurses also run clinics within health centres or general practices, e.g. leg ulcer clinics.

Health visitors (specialist community public health nurses)

Despite the new title, the term 'health visitor' still tends to be used and understood. The role of health visitors is in a state of change. Health visiting evolved in the Victorian era to promote the welfare of mothers and children. Many health visitors still devote a high proportion of their time to work with the under-fives and to child protection work. However, the role can encompass health promotion with people of all ages and the importance of the public health role has also been reasserted in recent years.[24]

Community midwives

Midwives have statutory responsibilities for the care of women during pregnancy, confinement and post partum. Community midwives organise antenatal and postnatal care and run antenatal and parentcraft classes. A community midwife will attend a home confinement and be responsible for a DOMINO scheme or delivery within a GP hospital maternity unit. The midwife will care for a mother and baby in the postnatal period and notify the health visitor when they are discharged. A wider public health role has been proposed for midwives in recent years.[25]

Other community nurses

Other nurses may be considered as peripheral members of the PHCT. Each has a specific contribution to make but the links with general practice are often more tenuous.

Community mental health nurses (CMHNs), previously called community psychiatric nurses (CPNs), are registered mental health nurses who have undertaken postregistration studies in their field of expertise. The service developed out of hospital-based psychiatric nursing and most CMHNs continue to be based in hospitals within community mental health teams. CMHNs carry out mental health assessments, support patients and their families within the community, and offer a range of therapeutic strategies (see Chapter 15).

School nurses have a major role in health promotion for school children, as well as in dealing with their health problems at school. The role has expanded significantly since the days of the 'nit nurse' and school nurses are expected to have expertise in all aspects of child health and wellbeing.[26] School nurses carry out wide-ranging immunisation programmes for school-age children and play a key role in helping to reduce the number of teenage pregnancies through sex education and the provision of practical advice. Practice nurses may have most contact with school nurses through the care of children with asthma or other chronic conditions.

Community children's nurses care for children with acute and chronic illnesses in their homes and provide valuable support for families. The children's nurse role ranges from teaching wet wrapping for eczema to managing a terminal illness at home. Their degree of contact with the practice nurse can depend on local arrangements.

Community learning disability nurses help people with learning disabilities to maximise their potential for independent living within the community. They help clients and carers to deal with physical, mental and social problems, including challenging behaviour, and liaise with a range of support services.

Hospital and community-based specialist nurses are a valuable resource for advice and teaching on their individual subjects, e.g. diabetes, continence, stoma care, HIV/AIDS and infection control. Macmillan nurses provide a palliative care service for patients with cancer and support them and their families.

Community matrons

This new breed of nurse was mentioned in the *NHS Improvement Plan* and it is proposed that by 2008, the NHS will have 3000 community matrons using case management techniques to care for patients with complex needs.[27]

Social services

Referrals can be made on behalf of patients who require home care, meals-on-wheels, occupational therapy or other social service support. However, relatively few practices have an attached social worker and referrals for social services are usually made by telephone or letter. Social workers are expected to make a full needs assessment of the patients referred to them, although the National Service Framework for Older People requires health and social services to work together to ensure that single assessments of needs are carried out.[28]

Public health nurses and GPs are sometimes involved with social workers on child protection issues. Also, an approved social worker is needed when a patient is compulsorily detained under the Mental Health Act (see Chapter 15).

Voluntary services

A huge number of voluntary services, self-help groups and charities exist. They provide financial and practical assistance, as well as information, advice and research funding. Some are organised locally to help people in need in that community, while others are organised nationally to help sufferers of a specific illness or disability. Patients and their carers can benefit from the knowledge of a practice nurse who can tell them whom to approach for help. A database of contact addresses and websites can be useful but it needs to be regularly updated. The internet is a good way of finding out about support groups and there may be a directory produced by the local Council for Voluntary Service.

Some larger practices have a League of Friends, who organise voluntary transport, collect prescriptions, visit elderly or bereaved patients and even raise funds to buy special equipment for the practice. This type of voluntary work can provide significant help in both urban and rural communities.

Involvement of the public is one of the key elements of the plan for modernising the NHS. PCO boards have several lay non-executive members and practices are expected to seek the opinions of patients about the quality of their services. Patient participation is a key factor in the government's plan for the NHS.[29]

Suggestions for reflection on practice

- How much do you know about the way your local NHS is run? Who are the nurse leaders?
- What sort of contract does your practice have? What services does your practice provide? Could they be improved?
- How integrated is your primary healthcare nursing team? What changes could be made to improve the service to patients?
- What statutory and voluntary services are available locally? How do you find out?
- How much involvement do patients have in the organisation of your practice? What changes could be made?

REFERENCES

1. Allsop, J. (1984) *Health Policy and the National Health Service*. Longman, Harlow.
2. Ministry of Health (Gillie, A., Chairman) (1963) *The Field of Work of the Family Doctor*. HMSO, London.
3. Parliament (1990) *The National Health Service and Community Care Act 1990*. HMSO, London.
4. Atkin, A., Lunt, K., Parker, G. & Hurst, M. (1993) *Nurses Count: a national census of practice nurses*. Social Policy Research Unit, University of York.
5. Department of Health (1999) *Saving Lives: our healthier nation*. Stationery Office, London.
6. Department of Health (1997) *The New NHS: modern, dependable*. HMSO, London.
7. Department of Health (2001) *Harold Shipman's Clinical Practice 1974–97: a clinical audit commissioned by the Chief Medical Officer*. Department of Health, London.
8. Command Paper: Om5207 (2001) *Learning from Bristol: the report of the public enquiry into children's heart surgery at Bristol Royal Infirmary 1984–95*. Department of Health, London.
9. Department of Health (2001) *Assuring the Quality of Medical Practice – implementing 'Supporting doctors, protecting patients'*. Department of Health, London.
10. Department of Health (2000) *The NHS Plan. A plan for investment, a plan for reform*. Department of Health, London.
11. HM Government (2004) *The NHS Improvement Plan: putting people at the heart of public services*. Stationery Office, London.
12. NHS Confederation (2005) *Alternative Providers of Medical Services: a contracting guide for primary care trusts*. www.nhsconfed.org/publications (accessed 2/9/05).
13. Department of Health (1998) *Modernising Mental Health: safe, sound and supportive*. Department of Health, London.
14. Parliament (1997) *National Health Service (Primary Care) Act 1997*. HMSO, London.
15. Department of Health (2005) *GMS Statement of Financial Entitlements (SFE) 2005 Onwards*. www.dh.gov.uk (accessed 09/07/2005).
16. Statutory Instrument 2004 No. 291 (2004) *The National Health Service (General Medical Services Contracts) Regulations 2004*. Stationery Office, London.
17. Department of Health (2004) *Quality and Outcome Framework – updated 2004*. www.dh.gov.uk (accessed 27/7/2005).
18. Parliament (1997) *National Health Service (Vocational Training for General Medical Practice) Regulations 1997*. Stationery Office, London.
19. Dame Janet Smith DBE (Chairman) (2004) *The Shipman Inquiry. Fifth Report: safeguarding patients: lessons from the past – proposals for the future*. Stationery Office, London.
20. Department of Health (1999) *Caring about Carers: a national strategy for carers*. www.dh.gov.uk/publicationsandstatistics/ (accessed 27/07/05).
21. Edmonstone, J., Hamer, S. & Smith, S. (2003) Integrated community nursing teams: an evaluation study. *Community Practitioner*, **76**(10), 386–9.
22. Department of Health (2002) *Liberating the Talents: helping primary care trusts and nurses to deliver the NHS Plan*. Department of Health, London.

23. Nursing and Midwifery Council (2004) *Consultation on a Framework for the Standard for Post-registration Nursing.* Circular 41/2004. Nursing and Midwifery Council, London.

24. Department of Health (2001) *Health Visitor Development Resource Pack.* www.dh.gov.uk (accessed 22/7/05).

25. Department of Health (2004) *The Chief Nursing Officer's Review of the Nursing, Midwifery and Health Visiting Contribution to Vulnerable Children and Young People.* Department of Health, London.

26. Department of Health (2001) *School Nurse Development Resource Pack.* www.dh.gov.uk (accessed 22/7/05).

27. Department of Health (2004) *Community Matrons.* CNO Bulletin 31. Department of Health, London, p.5. www.dh.gov.uk/publicationsandstatistics/chiefnursingofficerbulletin/ (accessed 3/9/05).

28. Department of Health (2001) *National Service Framework for Older People.* Department of Health, London.

29. Farrell, C. (2004) *Patient and Public Involvement: the evidence for policy implementation.* Department of Health, London.

FURTHER READING

Department of Health (2003) *Delivering Investment in General Practice: implementing the new GMS contract.* Department of Health Publications, London.

Department of Health (2005) *Creating a Patient-led NHS: delivering the NHS Improvement Plan.* Department of Health Publications, London.

National Association of Primary Care (2004) *PMS Agreement Framework – version 3.1.* www.napc.co.uk

Peckham, S. & Exworthy, M. (2002) *Primary Care in the UK: policy, organisation and management.* Palgrave Macmillan, Basingstoke.

Pollock, A.M. (2004) *NHS plc: the privatisation of our healthcare.* Verso, London.

Sines, D., Appleby, F. and Frost, M. (eds) (2005) *Community Health Care Nursing*, 3rd edn. Blackwell Publishing, Oxford.

Webster, C. (2002) *The National Health Service: a political history*, 2nd edn. Oxford University Press, Oxford.

West, M. (2003) *Effective Teamwork: practical lessons from organizational research.* Blackwell Publishing, Oxford.

USEFUL ADDRESSES AND WEBSITES

Department of Health
Richmond House, 79 Whitehall, London SW1A 2NS
Website: www.dh.gov.uk

NHS Institute for Innovation and Improvement
University of Warwick Campus

Coventry CV4 7AL
Telephone: 0800 555 550
E-mail: enquiries@institute.nhs.uk
Website: www.institute.nhs.uk

National Primary Care Development Team
Gateway House
Piccadilly South
Manchester M60 7LP
Telephone: 0161 236 1566
Website: www.npdt.org

Healthcare Commission
www.chi.gov.uk

Chapter 2
General Practice Nursing

One of the attractions of practice nursing is the flexibility it allows. Progressive nurses have blossomed in the atmosphere of general practice and some have become nursing celebrities through their innovations in health promotion and chronic disease management. However, herein lies a dilemma, because that same flexibility can also lead to a diversity of standards. Clinical governance is intended to iron out variations in quality. It is the modern term for the framework covering all the activities which contribute to a high-quality service. This includes: education, risk assessment, evidence-based practice and audit, as well as patient feedback and the analysis of critical incidents and mistakes. The Healthcare Commission has a statutory responsibility for assessing the performance of healthcare organisations.[1]

HISTORICAL BACKGROUND

Practice nursing evolved over time, partly from the work of those GPs' wives who were nurses and partly from district nurse attachment to general practice. More practice nurses began to be employed by doctors in the early 1970s when it became apparent that district nurses were unable to spend as long in the surgery, undertaking tasks such as dressings and injections, as the doctors wanted them to do. One solution to this was for doctors to employ nurses directly. After 1966, when salaries could be partially reimbursed, practice nurses were classified with secretaries and receptionists as ancillary staff on the Family Practitioner Committee returns. Even as late as 1992, when asked by the Social Policy Research Unit to furnish the names of practice nurses for the National Census, some family health service authorities could not identify all the nurses in post.[2]

Neighbourhood nursing

The Cumberlege Report in 1986 caused outrage among many practice nurses when it was suggested that all community nurses should be employed in neighbourhood nursing teams.[3] Practice nurses did not receive this concept of integrated nursing with great joy. The proposal led to a new sense of group identity as practice nurses came together to fight for the right to continue being employed within general practice. The apparently illogical preference for members of one profession to be employed by members of another owed more than a little to the negative attitudes of many practice nurses towards inflexible management in the NHS at that time.

Practice nurse education

The 1990 GP Contract led to a huge increase in the number of practice nurses employed. This phenomenon caused a stir in nursing circles and concern at the lack of professional control over such a large group of nurses. Practice nurse education finally began to receive serious attention. Practice nurses were suddenly overwhelmed by educational opportunities from a variety of sources but there was no simple way of assessing the quality of the education. The amount of study leave granted to practice nurses varied from one practice to another.

Project 2000 changed the traditional nurse training into a higher education system comparable with that of other disciplines.[4] Initially it was expected that this would equip nurses to work in any setting but it became obvious that more education would be needed for work in the community. From 1996, the United Kingdom Central Council decision on community education gave qualified practice nurses and other community nurses equality with district nurses and health visitors as specialist practitioners. Future postregistration qualifications are currently being debated by the Nursing and Midwifery Council, which replaced the UKCC in 2002.

Nursing in general practice

The diversity of work undertaken by practice nurses makes a precise description of the role very difficult. A study in Sheffield found both a seasonal variation and a wide range in the nursing activities and the time spent on them by individual nurses.[5]

Treatment room nurses to healthcare assistants

Treatment room nurses were originally employed by the NHS for nursing work within health centres. They were not employed directly by the general practitioners. Few treatment room nurse posts exist nowadays but healthcare assistants (HCAs) are being employed in many practices. They perform some of the basic administrative, organisational and treatment room work previously undertaken by practice nurses. HCAs are able to study for national vocational qualifications (NVQs) to equip them for the role. They allow a practice to make the best use of the time and expertise of all its nurses.

Practice nurses

Practice nurses usually have a wide remit, although some practice nursing still contains an element of treatment room work. Practice nursing can be considered under several headings.

1. *Management*, which could include:
   - Organising the nurses' rooms and work, including call/recall for health promotion
   - Supervision of subordinate staff
   - Ensuring clinical stocks and supplies are maintained
   - Collaboration on organisational and professional issues, including policies, protocols, quality standards and educational needs.
2. *Clinical*, which could include:
   - Assessing patients' care needs
   - Nursing procedures
   - Performing tests and health screening
   - Immunisation
   - Assisting with minor surgery
   - Chronic disease management.
3. *Specialist services*, such as family planning.
4. *Communication*, which could include:
   - Giving information, support and advice to patients and carers
   - Counselling
   - Health promotion
   - Teaching patients, other nurses and students
   - Liaison with other members of the practice team, the primary healthcare team, social services and other agencies
   - Telephone consultations.
5. *Audit and research*, which could include:
   - Evaluation of care given
   - Compiling statistics and reports on nursing activities
   - Identifying ways to improve nursing practice.

The need for up-to-date knowledge is increased because the work of practice nurses is so varied and challenging. Many practices have a practice library, which should include a nursing section. There are journals relevant to practice nursing and the internet provides an easy way of accessing information. Many websites provide links to support for practice nurses.[6,7] The NMC, Department of Health and nursing organisations, such as the RCN and CPHVA, are all accessible on-line.

Nurse practitioners

Nurse practitioners are experienced nurses who have undertaken further specialised education at degree level to be able to work autonomously in a variety of settings. Examination skills and the management of injury or diseases, traditionally the prerogative of doctors, are among the subjects taught on nurse practitioner courses. However, because the title is not yet protected by the NMC, there is nothing to stop a nurse calling her/himself a nurse practitioner by virtue of experience, without having undergone a recognised course and examination. Consultation is in progress to establish a recordable qualification of Advanced Nurse Practitioner, possibly at Master's degree level.[8]

Nurse practitioners originated in the United States. The first one in the UK, whose background was in health visiting, took up her post in Birmingham in 1982. Since then the numbers have grown considerably. Some nurse practitioners undertake work with neglected, underprivileged groups in the community; others work in hospitals, general practice or walk-in centres. There can be an overlap with some of the work of practice nurses and the titles may still be used rather indiscriminately. It is not unusual to see job advertisements specifying the experience required, which could apply to either type of nurse. Conflict can arise in a practice which employs a nurse practitioner and a practice nurse, both of whom have qualified at degree level and expect to be accorded the same level of respect. It is essential that a clear understanding be reached, so that the patients benefit from the expertise of all the nurses.

Skill-mix

Skill-mix is the system for identifying the knowledge and expertise needed to perform any job, so that the most appropriate person can do it. The reform of services in general practice has made delegation inevitable.[9] Any practitioner who wishes to review her/his role can consider each activity in turn and list the knowledge, skills and education needed to perform it effectively. It will become apparent which activities could be delegated and a case can then be made, on economic grounds, for utilising nursing skills most effectively. Phlebotomy is a case in point, for while it can reasonably be argued that practice nurses may deal with other important issues while taking blood, it would be hard to justify the routine use of a highly trained nurse in such a role.

The nurse practitioner, healthcare assistant and nurse triage roles could be considered as examples of skill-mix, using nursing expertise most effectively. Nurse prescribing has also increased the autonomy of nurses in general practice (see Chapter 8).

Triage

Historically, this term arose from the assessment of trauma victims in order to prioritise treatment. Nurse triage was introduced in general practice as a way of managing requests for urgent appointments. Triage could be by telephone or in face-to-face consultations and be carried out by an experienced practice nurse. NHS Direct nurses deal with telephone encounters by using computerised algorithms to assess patients but they may take longer and cost more than practice-based triage.[10]

NURSE EMPLOYMENT IN GENERAL PRACTICE

Medical training has traditionally been concerned with the diagnosis and treatment of patients, with little time left over for management and issues of human resources. It follows that while some GPs are excellent employers, there are others who are less so. This can leave an inexperienced nurse vulnerable to exploitation. The terms and conditions agreed at the job interview are binding but employees are entitled to receive a written contract of employment within two months of starting work.[11] Employees' rights were enhanced by employment legislation in 1999, which established new rules for fair treatment of employees and the right to trade union representation.[12] A new Employment Act in 2002 introduced more family-friendly policies.[13] Part-time workers have the same rights as full-time staff.[14]

Nurses accustomed to pay and conditions being negotiated nationally may never have had to negotiate on their own behalf before. Not all nurses are naturally assertive, so it is important to know what to ask at the interview and how to present a good case when negotiating for a change in conditions or salary. The Royal College of Nursing (RCN) and other trade unions have produced guidelines on the employment of practice nurses. The following points should be considered in relation to employment.

Job description

A job description should specify the job title, the key activities and responsibilities, the conditions of employment, clinical grade/band and salary and to whom the employee is accountable. A comprehensive job description also provides a tool for appraisal at a performance review.

The RCN guidelines on employment for practice nurses specify the type of work and the responsibility suitable to each grade, although all NHS employees are currently undergoing a job evaluation exercise called Agenda for Change (AfC).[15] Practice nurses, unless directly employed by a PCO, are unlikely to be included so will have to make their own case with their employers. The RCN has published advice about AfC for members not employed by the NHS.[16]

Job descriptions can prevent misunderstandings if everyone involved knows what they are required to do. When all staff members have a job description, it will become apparent if the responsibility for those small tasks necessary to the smooth running of a practice has not been specified. Unnecessary conflict can be prevented if such issues are resolved promptly.

Contract of employment

A statement of terms of employment should cover the following:

- Salary and incremental dates, plus rates of pay for overtime hours
- The normal hours and times of work plus expectations of overtime to cover the absence of colleagues
- Holidays, study leave, sick pay, maternity/parental leave and compassionate leave entitlements
- Pension arrangements
- Period of notice for the termination of the employment.

In addition, the contract should set out the disciplinary and grievance procedures. Any health and safety hazards in the place of employment should also be included. If home visiting is part of the job description, then a mileage and car allowance should be negotiated. Practice nurses are strongly advised to seek a contract which guarantees pay and conditions of service in line with those of other NHS nurses.

Pensions

Pensions need careful consideration. Since 1997, practice employees have been entitled to contribute to the NHS pension scheme and to receive an employer's contribution. The practice manager will be able to provide advice on NHS pensions and any additional voluntary contributions, which may be paid. Many people wait until middle age before considering pension arrangements but it is worth getting independent advice as soon as possible about the best ways of maximising income after retirement.

Insurance

National Insurance contributions, deducted at source from the salary, together with contributions made by the employer, pay for sickness, maternity and unemployment benefit and for the state pension. GPs have indemnity insurance to cover vicarious liability for injury caused by their employees. However, personal indemnity insurance is essential because nurses, as individuals, could also be sued. The Royal College of Nursing, Medical Defence Union, the Community Practitioners' and Health Visitors' Association (CPHVA) and Unison provide indemnity insurance and give legal advice to members if needed.

Accountability

Accountability for one's actions is one of the hallmarks of a professional person. Ultimately, nurses are accountable to their patients, via the NMC, for the standards of nursing care provided. Among other things, the Code of Professional Conduct requires all nurses to only undertake practice and accept responsibilities for activities in which they are competent.[17] Many aspects of practice nursing go far beyond what is taught pre-registration and nurses may sometimes feel pressurised to take on work for which they are not adequately prepared. Assertiveness training can be helpful in dealing with difficult situations, but it is up to every nurse to ensure that she/he practises safely.

Professional registration

Current registration with the NMC is required in order to practise as a nurse. The registration fee and notification of the intention to practise are sent every three years. Each registered nurse is issued with a plastic card, bearing a personal identification number (PIN). Evidence of continuing professional development needs to be available in a personal professional profile as part of the requirements for re-registration. A minimum of five days (35 hours) of learning in three years must be undertaken in subjects relevant to the area of work. Many practice nurses already achieve much more than this, but arrangements are needed to help those who do not. Formal study days are not necessary, as long as the learning and its influence on nursing practice are documented. In addition, a minimum of 100 days (750 hours) of clinical practice must have been worked, or an approved return to practice course have been successfully undertaken.[18]

Appraisal and professional development

It is now common practice for staff to have a regular performance review, which should help to identify the strengths and weaknesses in their work, identify their learning needs and contribute to their professional development. All practitioners are expected to have a personal development plan and be able to demonstrate when their personal objectives have been met. Appraisal interviews should never be confused with disciplinary procedures.

NETWORKING FOR SUPPORT

Traditionally, it has been thought that practice nurses work in greater isolation than other groups of nurses but while this may be true in some instances, there is a large support network stretching out for those who look for it. The loss of public confidence in elements of the health service, as a result of various scandals in recent times, calls for all practitioners to be able to demonstrate their competence. The use of support networks is vital to achieve this aim.

Local support

Clinical supervision

Although not a new concept, clinical supervision was slow to develop among practice nurses because of their unique employment status, but is now considered to be essential as a means of support and of promoting high standards.[19] Various ways have been suggested for organising clinical supervision, either in groups or on a one-to-one basis, and every nurse should be able to access the form of clinical supervision to suit her/himself.

Practice nurse groups

Local practice nurse groups developed spontaneously across the country as practice nursing spread but as other educational and support opportunities arose, local groups sometimes became redundant. However, there is still a need for groups of nurses to meet to share ideas and listen to speakers on topics of common interest.

The valuable support of the primary care facilitator was lost in many areas as health authorities prepared to devolve responsibility to primary care organisations. So, although some practice nurses were left in limbo for a time, the new PCOs have usually appointed practice development nurses with a remit to look after the interests of practice nurses. At the present time, few of these practice development nurses have a direct managerial responsibility for practice nurses but all professional staff are required to meet agreed standards of practice as part of clinical governance.

Regional support

Some local practice nurse groups are affiliated to regional associations, which can often lobby for change more effectively than small groups and individuals. The National Practice Nurses Conference and Exhibition is planned and organised by a different regional group each year, either alone or in conjunction with other organisations or professional conference organisers. About 500 nurses attend the three-day event, which provides an opportunity for social contact with colleagues as well as topical lectures and seminars.

National support

The RCN Practice Nurse Association is active on behalf of its members and all the specialist groups within the RCN run study days and conferences. The Community Practitioners and Health Visitors' Association and Unison also offer membership to practice nurses and publish helpful literature.

The internet is an ideal way for nurses to network. Practice nurse e-groups allow nurses to contact colleagues from all areas in order to seek or provide information. Protocols can be shared and contributors often provide web addresses of other useful internet sites.

PRACTICE NURSE EDUCATION

When the UKCC policy on community nurse education came into operation in 1996 (see Chapter 1), transitional arrangements were made for experienced practice nurses to acquire a recordable qualification in line with the automatic use of the title given to district nurses and health visitors, who qualified under the previous system. Most areas have experienced practice nurses in post with teaching qualifications, who act as practice nurse teachers. Training practices are also being designated, where a practice nurse who has a nurse education qualification provides supervision and support for nurses in training. Since September 2001, a new system for educating nurse teachers has been in place. Mentors, practice educators and lecturers have become the only recordable nurse teaching qualifications.[20]

CATS, APEL and APL

Credit accumulation and transfer (CATS) is a way of evaluating the academic content of different courses so that points can be collected towards an academic award. Three levels of credit are awarded in England and Wales:

- 120 credits at level 1 = certificate level
- + 120 credits at level 2 = diploma level
- + 120 credits at level 3 = degree level.

Scotland has four levels of credits (SCOTCATS).

Assessment of prior experiential learning (APEL) is a way of awarding credits for previous learning. Life experiences, professional knowledge and skills are assessed and credited towards a relevant academic course. A professional profile needs to be prepared, which outlines previous learning experiences and how they have influenced practice. Colleges usually charge for these assessments, which are complex to administer.

Assessment of prior learning (APL) allows credits to be awarded for relevant courses and examination results.

IDENTIFYING GOOD PRACTICE

Reflection

All nurses are expected to make time to reflect on situations in their own practice and to learn from both positive outcomes and those which could have been handled differently.[21] Reflections on practice can also be an essential part of clinical supervision sessions and written reflections form part of the professional profile to demonstrate learning from experience.

Evidence-based practice

Increased public expectations and the growth of communications mean that practitioners must be able to base their practice on the best available evidence. Since no doctor or nurse could possibly read and consider all the material relevant to his/her sphere of work, ways are needed to assess the validity of evidence and disseminate information on best practice. The National Institute for Clinical Excellence (NICE) was established to make recommendations and distribute guidelines on clinical treatments. The new National Institute for Health and Clinical Excellence (also called NICE) was created in 2005.

Systematic reviews

Various groups have evolved to help practitioners to make decisions based on the best available evidence. Systematic reviews rigorously assess the research evidence available. The various databases provide information about reviews completed and in progress. Local clinical librarians will usually help anyone who needs assistance to search for evidence.

Other sources of information include:

- National Electronic Library for Health
- Cochrane Collaboration
- NHS Centre for Reviews and Dissemination, York
- NHS Health Technology Assessment Programme.

Despite the wealth of information available, some nursing practice has still not changed significantly in response to research findings and there has been a conspicuous lack of good research in the field of practice nursing. The clinical governance agenda makes it imperative for practitioners to establish strong theoretical foundations to their practice in order to give good clinical care.

Audit

Audit means measuring what is actually being done, compared to an agreed standard of practice. For example, a practice could have a policy for all diabetic patients to be reviewed annually, i.e. 100% of diabetic patients. Taking an audit would involve looking at the records of all patients with diabetes to see when they were last reviewed. As an example, it might transpire that only 85% of the patients were reviewed in the past year.

There is no point in doing this exercise unless the practice is prepared to act on the findings and take steps to remedy the deficiencies. Having done so, the audit should be repeated to see if the percentage rate has improved. The use of computers can make audit a less onerous task, providing the data being sought have actually been entered. The need to collect data for the Quality and Outcome Framework has resulted in an increase in audit activity in many practices.

Local primary care audit groups welcome nurse involvement in audit and will usually provide helpful advice and training. Nurses are also employed by some organisations to advise on nursing and medical audit.

Nursing research

Research explores the boundaries and establishes the body of knowledge required to practise in a profession. Research may be an academic and exhaustive study based in a university department but it can also simply be the questioning of routine procedures or asking the question 'why?' in relation to day-to-day work. A practice nurse could be involved with research in several ways:

- Keeping her/his own knowledge up to date by reading research reports
- Conducting a literature search on a particular topic
- Designing a study to test an idea for improving nursing practice
- Taking part in a wider research programme organised by a general practitioner, research nurse or other outside body.

The term 'hierarchy of evidence' is commonly used in relation to research, with greater credence being given to the methods considered to be most rigorous and providing the strongest evidence.[22]

Quantitative studies

Prospective randomised controlled trials (RCTs) are considered to provide the best evidence about the effectiveness of healthcare interventions.[23] Participants are randomly allocated to either an experimental group or a control group. Since all the characteristics of both groups are meant to be the same, any difference in outcome should be due to the intervention. Some of the problems of RCTs include:

- Difficulties with randomisation
- Ethical issues when using a placebo or withholding a potentially valuable treatment
- Cost
- The length of time before the outcome of the trial is known
- Generalisability – can the results of the trial be transferred to people other than those studied?

Many nursing activities, by their very nature, do not lend themselves readily to RCTs.

Cohort studies identify and measure exposure to a risk or treatment. Intervention and control groups are used and the outcomes analysed. The lack of randomisation can mean that results could be due to variations between the groups unrelated to the intervention being studied.

Case control studies are used retrospectively to compare one group with a particular condition to a similar group without the condition, in order to compare exposure to the risk factor by both groups and thus to establish a causal relationship.

Qualitative studies

Qualitative studies often attempt to explain what is happening in a given situation. Observation and interviews are methods commonly used for this type of research. The aim is to increase understanding of those particular situations. Therefore, sampling in this type of research is not randomised from the whole population but from the people likely to have the experiences being studied. Qualitative reports often contain direct quotes from participants to illustrate the study theme.[24] Much of the research into nursing tends to be qualitative in nature.

Suggestions for reflection on practice

- Analyse your job description. Are there any activities which could be delegated? Are there any activities for which you need more education?
- How is your clinical supervision organised?
- Does your professional profile provide a comprehensive account of your learning?
- What are your professional development goals?
- How would you know if your nursing practice could be improved?

REFERENCES

1. The Healthcare Commission homepage: www.healthcarecommission.org.uk (accessed 27/7/05).

2. Atkin, K., Lunt, N., Parker, G. & Hurst, M. (1993) *Nurses Count: a national census of practice nurses*. Social Policy Research Unit, University of York.
3. DHSS (1986) *Neighbourhood Nursing – a focus for care*. HMSO, London.
4. United Kingdom Central Council (1986) *Project 2000: a new preparation for practice*. United Kingdom Central Council, London.
5. Centre for Innovation in Primary Care (2000) *What Do Practice Nurses Do? A study of roles, responsibilities and patterns of work*. Centre for Innovation in Primary Care, Sheffield.
6. CNO Bulletin (2004) *Supporting Practice Nurses*. Department of Health Publications: www.dh.gov.uk (accessed 29/7/05).
7. Scottish Executive Publications (2004) *Framework for Nursing in General Practice*. www.scotland.gov.uk (accessed 29/7/05).
8. Nursing and Midwifery Council (2005) A level beyond initial registration. *NMC News*, **12**, 11.
9. Medical Practices Committee (2001) *Skill Mix In Primary Care – implications for the future*. Department of Health, London.
10. Richards, D., Godfrey, L., Tawfik, J., Ryan, M., Meakins, J., Dutton, E. & Miles, J. (2004) NHS Direct versus practice based triage for same day appointments in primary care: cluster randomised controlled trial. *British Medical Journal*, **329**(7469), 774.
11. Department of Trade and Industry (2004) *Employment Relations – contracts of employment*. www.dti.gov.uk/er/ (accessed 6/8/05).
12. Parliament (1999) *The Employment Relations Act 1999*. Stationery Office, London.
13. Parliament (2002) *Employment Act 2002*. Stationery Office, London.
14. Statutory Instrument 2000 No. 1551 (2000) *The Part-time Workers (Prevention of Less Favourable Treatment) Regulations*. Stationery Office, London.
15. Department of Health (1998) *Agenda for Change – modernising the NHS pay system*. Department of Health, London.
16. Royal College of Nursing (2005) *AfC and Nurses Employed Outside of the NHS*. www.rcn.org.uk/agendaforchange (accessed 6/8/05).
17. Nursing and Midwifery Council (2002) *Code of Professional Conduct*. Para. 6.2, p.8. Nursing and Midwifery Council, London.
18. Nursing and Midwifery Council (2004) *The PREP Handbook*. Nursing and Midwifery Council, London.
19. Nursing and Midwifery Council (2002) *Supporting Nurses and Midwives Through Lifelong Learning*. Nursing and Midwifery Council, London.
20. Nursing and Midwifery Council (2004) *Standards for the Preparation of Teachers of Nurses, Midwives and Specialist Community Public Health Nurses*. Nursing and Midwifery Council, London.
21. Bulman, C. & Schutz, S. (eds) (2004) *Reflective Practice in Nursing*, 3rd edn. Blackwell Publishing, Oxford.
22. Devereaux, P.J. & Yusuf, S. (2003) The evolution of the randomized controlled trial and its role in evidence-based decision making. *Journal of Internal Medicine*, **254**(2), 105–13.
23. Roberts, J. & DiCenso, A. (1999) Identifying the best research design to fit the question. Part 1. *Evidence-Based Nursing*, **2**(1), 4–6.
24. Ploeg, J. (1999) Identifying the best research design to fit the question. Part 2. *Evidence-Based Nursing*, **2**(2), 36–7.

FURTHER READING

Best, D. & Rose, M. (2005) *Transforming Practice Through Clinical Education, Professional Supervision and Mentoring,* Churchill Livingstone, Edinburgh.

Hopkins, S. & Young, L. (2005) *Employing Healthcare Assistants in General Practice.* Royal College of Nursing primary care and public health zone: www2.rcn.org.uk/pcph/resources/9–3_of_resources

Polit, D. & Beck, C. (2005) *Essentials of Nursing Research.* Lippincott, Williams and Wilkins, Philadelphia.

Royal College of General Practitioners (2004) *Practice Nurses.* Information Sheet No. 19. Royal College of General Practitioners, London.

Royal College of Nursing (2005) *Nurse Practitioners – an RCN guide to the nurse practitioner role, competencies and programme approval.* Royal College of Nursing, London.

Royal College of Nursing (2005) *Nurses Employed by GPs – RCN guidance on good employment practice.* Royal College of Nursing, London.

Royal College of Nursing (2005) *Agenda for Change. Making a pay claim if you work outside of the NHS.* Royal College of Nursing, London.

USEFUL ADDRESSES AND WEBSITES

Community Practitioners' and Health Visitors' Association
40 Bermondsey Street, London SE1 3UD
Telephone: 020 7939 7000 Fax: 020 7939 7034
Website: www.msfcphva.org.uk

Medical Defence Union
230 Blackfriars Road, London SE1 8PJ
Telephone: 020 7202 1500
Membership helpline: 0800 716376
Website: www.the-mdu.com

Royal College of Nursing
20 Cavendish Square, London W1G 0RN
Telephone: 020 7409 3333
Website: www.rcn.org.uk

RCN Direct
24-hour information and advice for members of RCN
Telephone: 0845 7726100

Nurses' and Midwives' Council
23 Portland Place, London WIN 3AF
Telephone: 020 7637 7181 Fax: 020 7436 2924
Website: www.nmc.org.uk

Open University
Walton Hall, Milton Keynes MK7 6YG
Telephone: 01908 274066 Fax: 01908 653744
Website: www.open.ac.uk

Practice Nurse
Elsevier Ltd, Quadrant House, The Quadrant, Sutton, Surrey SM2 5AS
Telephone: 020 8652 8879 Fax: 020 8652 8946
Website: www.elsevier.com browse Journals.

Practice Nursing
MA Healthcare Ltd, St Jude's Church, Dulwich Road, London SE24 0PB
Telephone: 020 7738 5454 Fax: 020 7733 2325
Website: www.practicenursing.com

Practice Nurse e-group
Website: http://health.groups.yahoo.com/groups/practicenurse

Practice Nursing Community
Website: www.practicenursing.co.uk/forum

NHS Centre for Reviews and Dissemination, University of York
Website: www.york.ac.uk/inst/crd

Cochrane Collaboration
Website: www.cochrane.org

NHS R & D Health Technology Assessment Programme
Website: www.hta.nhsweb.nhs.uk

RCN Research & Development Coordination Centre
Website: www.man.ac.uk/rcn

UK Department of Health Research
Website: www.dh.gov.uk/research

National Research Register
Website: www.nrr.nhs.uk

Chapter 3
Practice Organisation

INFORMATION ABOUT PATIENTS

The staff in general practice have access to a great deal of information, which raises important issues about the way that information is utilised and stored.

Confidentiality

Patients have a right to expect that any personal information about them will remain confidential. The confidential aspects of the work must be impressed on all staff members when they join the practice and the consequence of breaching confidentiality must be made explicit in the statement of terms of employment.

The NMC Code of Professional Conduct insists that nurses may only disclose confidential information: if the patient gives consent, if required by law or by order of a court or if the wider public interest justifies the disclosure. Actions with regard to child protection must be in accordance with national and local policies.[1] Unwitting breaches can occur unless careful steps are taken to prevent them. There are risks to confidentiality in any of the following situations:

- Conversations or telephone calls in the hearing of other patients
- Discussing a patient with a third party without consent
- Gossip about incidents that occur at work
- Computer screens which show other patients' details
- Records left lying open
- Personal information in the rubbish bin.

Computers with a screensaver facility will stop showing data after a few minutes but it is much better to get into the habit of clearing the screen immediately after use.

Apart from heightened staff awareness, thought given to the design of reception and waiting areas and to soundproofing consulting rooms can prevent conversations from being overheard. Manual records must be filed as soon as possible and computer systems must be secure. Any waste paper that could identify patients needs to be shredded. Investigation results must not be given to anyone other than the person who had the test, unless they have given their consent to disclosure. As a cautionary tale, picture the effect on the wife who was told by a receptionist that her husband's post-vasectomy sperm count was negative, when as it turned out, the wife herself had already had a sterilisation operation!

There should be a practice policy to cover situations when a patient does not speak English. An interpreter, who is not a family member of the patient, should be arranged whenever possible. Link workers are able to interpret and act as advocates in areas with mixed ethnic populations. We live in a multicultural society and although lip service is paid to this fact, many nurses have not been taught how to meet the health needs of people from different backgrounds. Training in cultural awareness is provided locally for health and social care workers. All practice nurses are advised to access this training.

Record systems

A good record system is vital for the efficient management of patient care. Practice nurses are major contributors to the information system and to this end, it is important to understand the records systems. The purpose of a record is to:

- Record all the relevant information about a patient
- Enable appropriate preventive care to be offered to patients
- Facilitate the management of patients with chronic diseases
- Enable all members of the PHCT to work together for the benefit of the patients
- Act as a focus for the education of GP registrars and other members of the PHCT
- Enable data to be extracted for practice audit, performance review and research purposes
- Provide evidence, if required, for medicolegal purposes.

The medical record envelope

The medical records, still known as 'Lloyd George envelopes', have been the main source of information about patients since they were introduced in 1911, the year that Lloyd George started a national health insurance scheme for working men. The fact that the envelopes have been around for so long says something about their durability but paper records are becoming obsolete. Electronic patient records are now the norm. Meanwhile, the NHS still has a cumbersome system for transferring records around the country, when patients move away. It is essential that printouts of computer records are sent with paper notes when they are recalled.

Computers

Computerised record systems are commonplace in general practice. Some practices still use manual records as well but many practices are 'paper light', relying more and more on computers. Most clinical summarising is done electronically and letters and reports are scanned into a computer. Apart from the obvious uses, such as recording registration information, clinical notes and printing prescriptions, computers can be used for many other purposes.

- Computerised appointment systems allow information to be gathered easily about waiting times, length of consultations and non-attendance. Doctors and nurses can also see on screen when patients have arrived.
- Disease registers can be accessed easily.
- Searches can be made for a variety of reasons:
  1. Call and recall of patients with specific medical conditions, e.g. asthma, diabetes, hypertension. For health promotion, e.g. children for immunisation, women due for cervical smears, patients aged over 65 for flu and pneumococcal injections. Mail merge can be used to produce standard call/recall letters
  2. Patients receiving a particular medication can be identified for research purposes, audit or drug checks
  3. Auditing of achievements towards QoF targets.
- Databases of useful information can be kept, such as voluntary services and self-help groups. Some clinical systems also provide patient information leaflets.
- The internet provides a gateway to a world of information but it is essential to check that sites accessed are reputable because anybody can post information, which might not be reliable.
- Supplies can be ordered by electronic mail.
- Hospital appointments can made electronically through the Choose and Book system.
- The NHSNet is a national, virtually private network, used by hospitals, health authorities, GP practices and others. It is protected from unauthorised access via the internet by firewalls and other security devices. As electronic recording and messaging becomes more central to the way people work in the NHS, this network is carrying increasing volumes of information.
- Health and personal information can be saved in a secure HealthSpace that one day may form the focus of an electronic health record.

At present, electronic links allow registration data to be sent directly to the primary care agency and pathology results to be received from the laboratory. In time, practices will be able to send test requests and receive more information, such as discharge summaries and x-ray results from hospitals, via the NHSNet. The transmission of pictures, for such specialities as dermatology, is being used successfully in more rural areas for remote consultations with hospital consultants.

Although computers are exciting to use, there are security, reliability and confidentiality aspects to be considered as well.

- A plan of action should be prepared in case of a computer failure and all users have a responsibility to protect the system as much as possible.
- Eating and drinking should not take place near a computer or keyboard.
- A modem and service provider allows access to the internet. However, a modem also renders a computer system vulnerable to hackers, who can invade a system for fun or to access patient information. Entry to the system should be protected by codes and passwords, which must be unique to each user, changed regularly and kept as secret as any credit card personal identification number.
- Under the terms of the Data Protection Act, computer users have to be registered as data users.[2] The practice manager usually arranges this.
- Every practice should have one person, preferably a health professional, responsible for computer security. This person is known as a Caldicott Guardian.[3]
- A power failure or a fault with the equipment could cause essential patient information to be lost. For this reason, daily copies of all the data must be made and a copy of this back-up kept off site in case of fire or theft in the practice.
- All staff have a responsibility for the security of the building. Procedures for locking windows and doors must be followed rigorously. Computer equipment can be very attractive to burglars and the loss of both the hardware and the data could be devastating.

The facilities and health protection required for staff who work with visual display units (VDUs) are laid down in Health and Safety Executive regulations.[4]

Disease register

A register of patients with specific conditions can be compiled by all of the following means:

- At registration and during registration health checks
- When records are being summarised
- When diagnosed in the practice or a letter is received from a hospital
- From repeat prescriptions.

Disease registers have assumed even greater importance since the introduction of National Service Frameworks and the Quality and Outcome Framework because practices need to be able to audit the care of specific groups of patients.

Practices are required to compile a register of all their patients who are carers, even if the person for whom they care is not registered with that practice.[5] Details must also be collected on ethnicity, in accordance with Department of Health policies.[6]

Access to records

In the past, medical records were jealously guarded from the eyes of the people most concerned – the patients themselves. As a result of this, sardonic comments in the notes, such as 'this patient enjoys very poor health', were not uncommon. Patients were not told the whole truth about their illness, especially if the prognosis was poor. So if the records later became mislaid, a patient might never know what the original diagnosis had been.

The attitude to disclosure is now quite different and most patients expect to be given factual information. In the main, patients have a legal right to see any health records held about them in computer or manual files, regardless of when they were made.[7] A charge can be made for this, as specified in the Data Protection Act 1998. A doctor can refuse to disclose information held manually or on computer in the following circumstances:

- If it is likely to cause serious mental or physical harm to the patient or another person
- Where the record relates to a third party who has not given consent for disclosure (where the third party is not a health professional who has cared for the patient).[8]

Nursing records

Most nurses write directly into the patients' NHS or computer records. Nursing records should provide a comprehensive, chronological account, which covers:

- An assessment of the patient's general health and the specific problems identified
- The type of care planned and consent for treatment
- The nursing interventions, advice or information given
- The outcomes of the care given, and further actions planned or implemented.

Good communication is essential for continuity of care, especially when more than one nurse is treating a patient. In the event of litigation, records will be used to prove or disprove a case of negligence. Without accurate records, it would not be possible to prove that satisfactory care had been given.

The guidelines for record keeping issued by the NMC clearly specify the nurse's responsibilities with regard to records.[9] Every nurse should have a copy of this document and be familiar with its contents.

Private patients

Many practices are designated Yellow Fever Centres, providing immunisation for patients who are not registered with the practice. People ineligible for NHS treatment may also be seen privately. There is no official record for private patients (unlike those for registered patients and temporary residents) but if injections or treatments are given privately, then a system must be in place for recording the relevant information for each patient.

PROTOCOLS, GUIDELINES AND CLINICAL PATHWAYS

When a nurse joins a practice, she/he will need to discuss the nursing role with colleagues. The exact scope and responsibility of each nurse will be governed by her/his previous experience and training. The limits of a nurse's freedom to act autonomously can be negotiated and then recorded in a protocol.

Protocols

This word 'protocol' is used rather freely and can be viewed as either a protection or a threat. If a protocol is too rigid then any deviation from it could possibly place a practitioner at risk of prosecution if anything should go wrong. This is a particular concern of doctors, who fear being constrained to provide medical treatment exactly as specified in a treatment protocol. On the other hand, many nurses feel they can work with greater confidence if they have agreed boundaries. Protocols tend to be prescriptive, outlining the actions required in a particular situation and the information to be given. Nurse-run clinics often follow a protocol. Patient Group Directions have replaced protocols for the administration of vaccines and drugs without prescription[10] (see Chapter 8).

Guidelines

Guidelines are generally considered to be less rigid than protocols and the term has become more commonly used. Systematic reviews and guidelines are regularly produced by the National Institute for Health and Clinical Excellence. National and European bodies such as the British Hypertension Society and European Resuscitation Council produce guidelines in their respective fields of expertise.

Clinical or care pathways

A more recent addition to the terminology is the clinical or integrated care pathway. This is intended to be used by all members of the multidisciplinary team in primary and secondary care as a template for the coordination of treatment and care of patients with specific conditions. Integrated care pathways meet the requirements of the new NHS to provide seamless care, with efficiency, effectiveness and involvement of the public. Their use has been shown to provide better quality care at a lower cost.[11] Clinical pathways tend to have a locality focus, such as a stroke pathway used by everyone in a hospital and the community in a particular area.

Whatever the terminology used, any protocol, guideline or care pathway must be reviewed regularly and updated in the light of new clinical evidence.

POLICIES AND PROCEDURES

Policies or rules are needed in any organisation so that all the staff know what is expected of them. Some policies in general practice are dictated by legal statute or public safety requirements. For example:

- Health and safety issues, in accordance with the Health and Safety at Work directives, e.g. manual handling
- Fire regulations, covering the maintenance of fire extinguishers, staff training and the procedure in the event of a fire
- Control of infection, covering the handling of specimens, dealing with body fluids, the disposal of sharps and clinical waste, methods of preventing cross-infection.

Other policies may cover more domestic issues such as: the arrangement of holidays and study leave, communicating messages, setting healthy examples for the public, avoiding waste of energy and resources.

Complaints

If there is dissatisfaction with any aspect of treatment, it is hoped that the problem could be resolved amicably by discussion, in preference to a formal complaint. Where a policy of openness already exists, patients may have no need to resort to the law. However, all practices are also legally required to have a formal policy for dealing with complaints.[12] In the first instance, this may be to the practice manager or senior partner but patients and the staff must be made aware of the practice complaints procedure. The Department of Health website gives information about how to complain and about the Independent Complaints Advocacy Service. Patient Advice and Liaison Services (PALS) have replaced the old community health councils and patients should be provided with information about their local service.

Appointments

The requirement in *The NHS Plan* for patients to see a practitioner within a specified time has resulted in some bizarre appointment systems. Practices have different ways of arranging access for patients to the GP or practice nurse.[13] Appointment systems allow the workload to be spaced out and planned in advance which, in theory, should save patients from having to wait more than a few minutes to be seen. However, patients cannot be ill by appointment, so time must always be set aside for dealing with urgent problems. If an emergency arises during surgery time, the booked appointments are likely to be delayed. Most people will accept such delays providing they are kept informed and do not feel they are being treated unfairly. With a simple queuing system, patients arrive at the beginning of surgery and are seen on a first-come, first-served basis. This can lead to long waits for patients and a lack of control by practitioners over their consulting time.

Computerised appointment systems can log the time a patient arrived, when the patient was seen, and even how long the consultation took – all valuable information for auditing the effectiveness of the organisation. If patients do not keep their appointments, this is not only a waste of professional time but it can also deprive other patients of the chance to be seen sooner. A graph in the waiting area, showing the number of hours wasted by non-attenders each week, can remind the public about their responsibilities towards the service.

Practice nurses who use appointment systems can give the receptionists a list of the times to be allowed for specific procedures and consultations. A policy of allowing patients to select times to suit themselves can increase the number of people who are able to attend for health promotion and screening.

Investigation results

A system is needed for ensuring that patients get the results of investigations. A patient must either know when to return to the surgery or when to telephone for results. Abnormal results should not be filed until the necessary steps have been taken for the patient to be followed up.

Telephone calls

A policy is needed for the handling of telephone calls. Too many interruptions during surgery time can be disruptive but patients have to be put through in urgent situations. Callers can be given a time to call back, although no patient should have to ring more than twice. Some doctors and nurses overcome this problem by having allotted telephone times for giving test results or dealing with other enquiries. Any advice given over the telephone should be recorded in the patient's records and telephone messages should be written down immediately in case they get forgotten. A record must be kept of all visit requests. It is now possible to make a recording of all incoming and outgoing telephone calls from a practice. This is not illegal but nurses are advised to ensure that patients are aware that calls are being recorded.

MEETINGS

Clinical meetings between members of the primary healthcare team are essential for exchanging information and giving feedback about patients, as well as providing learning opportunities for all concerned. Support can also be offered to individual team members who are dealing with stressful situations.

Joint staff meetings are valuable when domestic policies are being decided. Compliance will be better if everyone has been consulted and understands the need for the policy. Off-the-cuff pronouncements, which are subsequently changed, can be very damaging for morale. Team meetings need to be structured so that everyone is able to make a valid contribution and when decisions are reached, everyone who is likely to be affected must be made aware of them. Such decisions should be minuted and the minutes distributed for reference.

PUBLIC INVOLVEMENT

Involvement of patients is a key part of the NHS reforms.[14] Many patients are articulate and well informed and much less deferential than their predecessors. They expect to be involved in decision making and often arrive armed with articles relating to their individual problem. Patients are offered the chance to have copies of correspondence relating to them.

Patient satisfaction questionnaires are used frequently to obtain the views of patients about primary care services. Many practices and health centres have established consumer groups, where patient representatives can make suggestions or take practical steps for improving the service. Some patient groups are highly organised, with fund-raising committees and groups to support the housebound, bereaved patients or mothers with young children.

Suggestions for reflection on practice

- How easy is it to maintain confidentiality in your working area? How could any improvements be made?
- Are you using your computer system fully? What further training is needed?
- Does all your record keeping meet the NMC standards?
- Are the protocols/guidelines/PGDs you use up to date and comprehensive? Are changes needed?
- Would you know what to do if a patient wanted to make a complaint?

REFERENCES

1. Nursing and Midwifery Council (2002) *Code of Professional Conduct*. Para 5. Nursing and Midwifery Council, London.

2. Parliament (1998) *Data Protection Act 1998*. Stationery Office, London.
3. Department of Health (1997) *The Caldicott Committee Report on the Review of Patient-Identifiable Information*. Department of Health, London.
4. Health Service Executive (2003) *Working with VDUs*. www.hse.gov.uk (accessed 20/8/05).
5. Department of Health (1999) *Caring About Carers: a national strategy for carers*. Department of Health, London.
6. Department of Health, Health and Social Care Information Centre and NHS Employers (2005) *A Practical Guide to Ethnic Monitoring in the NHS and Social Care*. www.dh.gov.uk Publications library (accessed 30/8/05).
7. Department of Health (2003) *Guidance for Access to Health Records Requests under the Data Protection Act 1998*. Department of Health, London.
8. British Medical Association (2002) *Access to Health Records by Patients*. www.bma.org.uk/ap.nsf/Content/accesshealthrecords (accessed 20/8/05).
9. Nursing and Midwifery Council (2005) *Guidelines for Records and Record Keeping*. Nursing and Midwifery Council, London.
10. Statutory Instrument No. 1917 (2000) *The Prescription only Medicines (Human Use) Amendment Order 2000*. Stationery Office, London.
11. Bandolier Forum (2003) What is an integrated care pathway? www.jr2.ox.ac.uk/bandolier Extended essays (accessed 22/8/05).
12. Statutory Instrument No. 1768 (2004) *The National Health Service (Complaints) Regulations 2004*. Stationery Office, London.
13. Royal College of General Practitioners and NHS Alliance (2004) *The Future of Access to General Practice-based Primary Medical Care – informing the debate*. Royal College of General Practitioners, London.

FURTHER READING

Health and Safety Executive (2004) *An Introduction to Health and Safety – health and safety in small firms*. Health and Safety Executive Books, Suffolk.
Holland, K. & Hogg, C. (2001) *Cultural Awareness in Nursing and Healthcare: an introductory text*. Hodder Arnold, London.

USEFUL ADDRESSES AND WEBSITES

Health and Safety Executive
Infoline: 0845 345 0055
Book order line: 01787 881 165
Website: www.hse.gov.uk

National Association for Patient Participation (NAPP)
Website: www.napp.org.uk

National Programme for IT in the NHS
Website: www.connectingforhealth.nhs.uk

HealthSpace
Website: www.healthspace.nhs.uk

Electronic booking of hospital appointments
Website: www.chooseandbook.nhs.uk

NHS Complaints Procedure
Website: www.dh.gov.uk: Policy and Guidance A–Z complaints policy under letter C

Chapter 4
Management of the Nurses' Rooms

As the work in general practice and the number of nurses increase, the accommodation needed by the practice nurses can change. The basic requirements include:

- A treatment/consulting room
- A waiting area for patients
- An accessible toilet for patients to use, with wheelchair access
- A secure storeroom
- A safe area for storing clinical waste and sharps before collection
- Access to a changing room and refreshment area or common room.

The practice nurse(s) should be involved when new or extended buildings are planned. The extra rooms or refinements to the nurses' accommodation might then include:

- A separate consulting room
- A separate minor surgery room
- An annexe to the treatment room for dealing with used instruments and specimens, etc.
- Office space for administration
- A non-clinical room for counselling
- A room for group sessions.

The Disability Discrimination Act requires all buildings open to the public to meet designated standards of accessibility for the public and staff.[1] Some premises might never be able to meet these stringent standards, so nurses could become involved in a move to new premises. NHS guidelines on designing new premises have been published.[2] There are also Health and Safety requirements on heating, ventilation, lighting and other aspects of the workplace to be considered when designing a working environment.[3]

DESIGN AND FURNISHING

A friendly environment can be created by the imaginative use of space and colour. Suitable storage space is needed to reduce clutter. Leaflet racks on the walls make information easily accessible and pin-boards are better than adhesive tape for displaying travel charts and other reference material. Attractive decor will create a welcoming atmosphere. Many people are nervous in a clinical environment: pictures, plants and play areas for children can help to put them at ease. Concerns have been expressed about the risk of cross-infection from children's toys.[4] Nurses should be aware of the potential risk and follow the practice policy regarding the use of toys. Soft toys pose a greater hazard and should not be used. If plastic toys are allowed, they must be cleaned regularly with hot, soapy water and checked for any damage. Damaged toys must be discarded.

Well-kept noticeboards dealing with seasonal topics can have a greater impact than walls smothered with depressing posters condemning every known human weakness and telling patients how to behave.

Lighting should be chosen with care. Bright, even lighting is needed in treatment areas and, in addition, directable lamps with heat filters are needed for minor surgery and taking cervical smears. Lamps must be easily cleanable. Softer lighting from lamps or wall lights is desirable for counselling or teaching relaxation. Blinds can be used to control sunlight and to provide privacy when needed. Basic furnishings include a desk, chairs, couch, lockable cupboards and bookshelves. A screen gives extra privacy and a mirror is helpful for the patients when they are getting dressed. Curtains are not recommended in rooms where minor surgery is performed.

Treatment and minor surgery couches should be easily accessible for the practitioner and, ideally, be height-adjustable and tiltable. Couches should be washable and non-permeable and must not be torn. Cotton couch covers and blankets should not be used because of the risk of cross-infection. Disposable paper rolls should be used instead and changed after use. A secure step is needed for patients to get on and off a non-adjustable couch.

Patients will feel less intimidated if sitting at the same level as the nurse at the side of the desk, not being confronted across it. Comfortable chairs away from the desk are preferable for counselling and informal discussions. Furniture should be arranged so that the nurse's exit is not obstructed if a patient becomes aggressive. An alarm is needed for summoning help in any sort of emergency. Work surfaces and flooring in treatment areas should be hardwearing, washable and able to withstand chemical disinfectants. Ideally, flooring should have sealed edges. Surfaces near plumbing should be smooth, non-porous and water-resistant. All joints must be sealed.[5]

A dedicated sink is needed for hand washing only. It must not be used for any other purpose and must have no overflow and no plug. The water must not drain directly into the drainage aperture and it should have an elbow-/foot-operated mixer tap or one activated by a sensor. There should be a different, deep-sided sink if instruments are to be decontaminated in-house. Also a separate sink is needed for rinsing items. There should be a dirty work area designated for dealing with specimens, etc.

All emergency equipment must be easily accessible. A visible plan of the location of all the equipment stored can save a nurse from returning to a scene of devastation after a day off!

HEALTH AND SAFETY

Although work areas are planned for practicality, the overwhelming consideration should be for the safety of the public and staff. Employers are legally required to produce a safety policy and to report serious incidents to the Health and Safety Executive (HSE). All employees have a duty to take reasonable care to avoid injury to themselves or others and to cooperate with employers in meeting the statutory requirements for health and safety.[5] Manual handling training is a requirement for all staff.[6]

Control of Substances Hazardous to Health (COSHH)

Employers are required to carry out a risk assessment for any substance which could be hazardous to health and keep a record of the main findings, where five or more people are employed.[7] The assessment should cover:

- The type of substance
- The type of hazard and precautions to be taken
- The planned use of the substance
- Possible unplanned events and the action to be taken
- Training needed by staff.

Any staff member likely to be exposed to substances hazardous to health must understand the risks and the precautions to be taken to protect themselves and the public. Hazardous substances which might be found in general practice include: ethyl chloride, phenol, formaldehyde, industrial spirit, sodium hypochlorite solution, liquid nitrogen, silver nitrate, pathological specimens containing infectious agents, latex gloves, and contaminated waste and sharps.

Special precautions are needed if a mercury sphygmomanometer is broken because mercury fumes are toxic. The mercury should be contained within the apparatus, if possible, or be tipped into an airtight container, covered with water and sealed. Gloves and a mask should be worn and the window opened to increase ventilation of the room. Mercury spillage kits are available, with special absorbent sponges and containers for storing the mercury for disposal. Detector pads left in the vicinity of the spillage will change colour if mercury fumes are present. Mercury spillage kits are expensive but are essential if there is any risk of spillage. The handling of mercury waste is covered by COSHH regulations but mercury counts as hazardous waste and must be disposed of safely. It should not be put with clinical waste for incineration or poured down a sink. A vacuum cleaner must not be used to remove spilled mercury and carpets or soft furnishings will have to be replaced if contaminated.

Mercury sphygmomanometers are being phased out because of the risk to health and the environment from spilled mercury. Arrangements are needed for their safe disposal. Any new automated devices purchased should meet the recommendations of the British Hypertension Society.[8]

The storage of medicines and other substances

Controlled drugs are regulated under the Misuse of Drugs Act (1971). They must be stored in a special locked cupboard, which is out of sight of any windows and the public. A register must be kept on the premises for recording new stock, the date it was obtained and the dispensing of any of the stock to patients or to individual doctors for their emergency bags. Out-of-date or unwanted controlled drugs may only be destroyed by authorised persons.[9]

Care must be taken with all drugs, lotions, cleaning materials and vaccines. They should always be kept in locked cupboards/vaccine refrigerators but because on occasions in a busy treatment room, a cupboard might accidentally be left unlocked, extra precautions are also sensible.

- All liquids should have childproof bottle tops and be stored out of reach of children. (The case of the unfortunate child who once gained access to a treatment room and drank some phenol proved the need for such precautions.[10])
- Safety catches, available cheaply from childcare shops, on cupboard doors, drawers and fridges will help to deter inquisitive toddlers.
- All trolleys must be cleared after use. (Imagine the possible effect of a silver nitrate pencil used as a play lipstick.)

The storage of vaccines

A doctor or nurse could be held liable for vaccination failure as a result of inadequate storage if it could be shown that the cold chain was intact before the product reached the practice.[11] Vaccines must be stored at temperatures between +2° and +8°C. Domestic refrigerators are not suitable for this purpose. Special vaccine fridges have a thermostatically controlled temperature range and a built-in maximum and minimum thermometer and alarm. They must be dedicated to vaccine storage alone and must have adequate ventilation. A vaccine fridge must be lockable or be kept in a locked room when unattended. The new chapter of the 'Green Book' deals in detail with the management of vaccines.

Some vaccines have to be destroyed if the cold chain is broken. There should be a written policy for vaccine storage and the action to take if a problem occurs.

Seek advice from a community pharmacist or the vaccine manufacturers in such an event. A maximum/minimum thermometer should be used, irrespective of whether a vaccine refrigerator incorporates a temperature indicator dial. A digital thermometer has a probe attached to a wire. The display part of the digital thermometer can be fixed to the wall, so that the refrigerator temperature can be seen at all times. The flexible wire passing into the fridge will not affect the door closure.

Recommendations for vaccine storage are shown in Table 4.1.

Table 4.1   Recommendations for vaccine storage

Action	Rationale
A named person, with a designated deputy, should be responsible for vaccines	To ensure the correct procedure is followed
Check and record min./max. temperatures at least once daily and reset the monitor according to the manufacturer's instructions	To ensure the correct temperature has been maintained throughout the 24 hours and as proof of regular monitoring
Make sure the fridge is wired in or has a dedicated socket, clearly marked	So it cannot be turned off accidentally
Defrost fridge regularly if not self-defrosting	For the most efficient and cost-efficient running
Store vaccines in another fridge or wrapped in bubble wrap in an approved cool box while defrosting the vaccine fridge. Bring the fridge to the correct temperature before replacing vaccines	To maintain the cold chain
Do not store vaccines on the shelves or in compartments of the refrigerator door and make sure the door is closed properly	To maintain the correct temperature at all times
Do not load more than 50% of the fridge and allow room between batches on each shelf	Temperatures are maintained more easily if air can circulate freely
Do not stockpile vaccines and make sure that those delivered earliest are used before more recent ones	To ensure they are not kept too long or pass their expiry dates. A change in immunisation policy could result in some vaccines becoming obsolete
Do not store food or anything other than vaccines in the vaccine fridge	To reduce the need to open the fridge door unnecessarily and to comply with health and safety regulations
Ensure that a maintenance programme is in place for the vaccine fridge	To reduce the likelihood of breakdown and increase the efficiency and life of the fridge
Keep records of cleaning, defrosting and servicing of refrigerator	As proof of maintenance of refrigerator

CONTROL OF INFECTION

Every primary care organisation has a control of infection policy, which should be followed in general practice and appropriate training be provided. Practice nurses should ensure that they have had adequate training in all aspects of health and safety and control of infection. PCOs usually employ a control of infection adviser, who will provide support and information as needed.

Patients with diarrhoea and vomiting, or who are known or suspected of having an infectious disease, should be asked not to visit the surgery. A home visit should be offered in the interests of protecting other vulnerable patients and staff. Immunisation against influenza is offered annually to front-line NHS staff and take-up should be encouraged.

Hand washing

Hand-washing sinks, as described above, with liquid soap in disposable containers and paper towels in wall-mounted dispensers, are needed in all the toilets and clinical areas to encourage effective hand hygiene. Bacteria have been shown to multiply on soap bars and reusable towels. They are a possible source of cross-contamination and should not be used in clinical settings. Alcohol-based rub can be used on visibly clean hands if appropriate. It must be applied to all the skin surfaces of the hands and be allowed to dry. Antiseptic hand-wash, e.g. *Hibiscrub*, should be used prior to invasive procedures.[12] A poster demonstrating the correct hand-washing technique should be displayed near hand basins in each clinical area.

Protective clothing

Protective clothing should be used in the following circumstances.

- Disposable aprons should be worn when there is a risk of splashing or of clothing becoming wet or soiled.[13]
- Powder-free gloves are needed when there is any risk of contact with blood or bodily fluids and for the application of creams and lotions. Gloves are single-use items that must be removed and placed in the clinical waste bin as soon as the patient contact is finished.
- Non-latex gloves will be needed if a patient or staff member is sensitive to latex. They are more expensive and should be kept explicitly for this purpose. An allergic reaction to latex can be a life-threatening condition, which could affect the employment of a staff member who develops such an allergy. The Health and Safety Executive website gives information about risk assessment and the choice of gloves.[14]

- Visors should be worn when there is any risk of splashing.
- Clear guidelines must be displayed on the action to be taken in the event of an inoculation/splash injury.

All the staff must be familiar with the procedure for dealing with body fluids when accidents occur. Although HIV infection causes the most concern, the virus is less easily transmitted than hepatitis B. Much smaller amounts of hepatitis B virus are needed for infection and it is stable in organic matter outside the body for long periods.

Hepatitis B infection

The virus is spread by contact with infected body fluids through inoculation or contact with mucous membranes or broken skin. Any cuts or breaks in the skin should be covered with waterproof plaster. Clinical staff and phlebotomists need to be immunised against hepatitis B and to have their immunity checked. A record should be kept of the immunisation dates and checks of antibody levels. There should also be a practice policy on sharps injuries.

Human immunodeficiency virus (HIV) infection

This virus is particularly dangerous because it attacks the cells of the immune system and is able to evade the body's defence mechanisms by rapid mutation. The damaged immune system makes the patient susceptible to other infections. There is no cure for HIV infection but the use of antiretroviral drugs is able to prevent the progression of the condition for many years.

Three factors must apply before HIV can be transmitted.

- *Amount* – there must be enough of the virus. HIV can be found in high concentrations in blood, semen and vaginal secretions of infected people. Sweat, tears, saliva, urine and faeces contain much less concentrated amounts.
- *Condition* – HIV deteriorates rapidly outside the body and is destroyed by heat, bleach and detergents. The enzymes in saliva and gastric acid also attack the virus.
- *Route of infection* – there must be a way into the bloodstream.

The most common means of spread are by unprotected sexual intercourse, sharing unclean equipment for IV drug use or from mother to child. Infected blood inside a used needle could be injected during a needle-stick injury. Individuals with severe eczema have, on rare occasions, contracted HIV.[15] The macrophages in the exudate of the eczematous lesions are thought to have ingested the virus in infected blood in contact with the skin.

Table 4.2   Action to be taken in sharps injury

Action	Rationale
Encourage the puncture wound to bleed freely and wash under running water	To flush any organisms from the wound
Avoid squeezing or sucking of the wound	A vacuum effect may draw organisms inwards or hepatitis B virus could be ingested
Dry and apply a waterproof dressing	To cover a puncture wound
Irrigate any mucous membranes exposed with plenty of water. Do not swallow if splashed into the mouth. Irrigate eyes before and after removing contact lenses (if worn)	Microorganisms can gain entry through aerosols of blood in contact with mucous membranes
Report the injury immediately to the employer	An accident report must be completed and tests may have to be performed
Ask the patient to wait (if known)	Blood tests may be requested, after appropriate counselling and obtaining informed consent, for hepatitis B and HIV antibodies
Blood may be taken from the person injured	As a baseline against later tests for hepatitis B and HIV. Immunisation against hepatitis B may be needed

Sharps/splash injuries

A strict adherence to the procedure for the use of sharps will prevent all but the most untoward accidents. If a sharps injury occurs, action should be taken immediately (Table 4.2).

Practices now have access to occupational health services for their staff but if not available in the event of a sharps injury, the affected person should attend the local accident and emergency department.

Disinfection and sterilisation

Every practice should have a policy for the decontamination of equipment with which practitioners have a duty to comply. Central sterile supply (CSS) is the ideal way of ensuring a regular standard of sterile equipment but the service may be unavailable to some practices. The correct use of benchtop steam sterilisers is expensive in both time and running costs. Single-use disposable items should be used whenever possible and these items must never be reprocessed.[16] The practice nurse is usually responsible for the decontamination of non-disposable surgical and examination equipment. A thorough understanding of the principles is needed. The local control of infection nurse will provide training and advice if needed. Equipment may be treated according to the level of cross-infection risk.

- *Low-risk items* – not used for patient contact or for contact with intact skin only can be washed with warm water and detergent. For example, plastic injection trays and bowls used to wash feet, if they are not contaminated with blood or bodily fluids.
- *Intermediate-risk items* – in contact with intact skin or mucous membranes but possibly contaminated by pathogens. For example, aural specula used for infected ears. Careful washing and disinfection is required. Disposable specula should be used for preference. Vaginal specula must be cleaned and sterilised between uses but do not usually need to be sterile at the point of use.
- *High-risk items* – used in invasive procedures such as minor surgery and inserting IUDs. Cleansing and sterilisation are necessary.

Cleansing

The following points should be observed when items are to be decontaminated in-house.

- There should be designated 'clean' and 'dirty' areas. Instruments should be decontaminated in the dirty area and stored in suitable containers in the clean area.
- All washable equipment must be cleaned with warm water and detergent, rinsed thoroughly and dried. This should be done as soon as possible after use because any organic matter allowed to dry on the instrument's surface will be difficult to remove later. Instruments must be visibly clean or washed again before sterilisation.
- A long-handled nylon brush should be used, which should either be discarded or be cleaned and autoclaved after use, allowed to dry and be locked away. Brushes should be replaced regularly.
- Gloves, a disposal apron and eye protection should be worn and splashing should be avoided by cleaning the items in a deep-sided sink while they are submerged under water.
- Blood or debris dried on the surface of an instrument will prevent adequate sterilisation. The use of ultrasonic baths and enzyme detergent solution is recommended where possible.[17] The maker's instructions must be followed faithfully and users need to have been trained in using the equipment.

Sterilisation

Sterilisation destroys microorganisms and spores and is the only safe method of decontaminating high-risk instruments. If a CSS service is not available, autoclaving is the most effective method of sterilisation in general practice.

Table 4.3   Sterilisation times at different temperatures

Temperature	Pressure (bar)	Holding time (minutes)
134–137°C	2.25	3
126–129°C	1.50	10
121–124°C	1.15	15

Autoclaves

This process uses steam under pressure to sterilise instruments and other devices. Autoclaves can be obtained in different sizes but they are required to meet all the necessary safety standards.[18–20] Sterilisation may be achieved with a high temperature for a short period or with longer cycles at lower temperatures. In order to be effective, the appropriate temperature must be maintained for the correct length of time. The times taken to reach a temperature and to cool down afterwards are immaterial.

Sterilisation times at different temperatures are shown in Table 4.3.

Downward displacement steam sterilisers do not have a vacuum feature and cannot be used to sterilise items with a lumen or wrapped items. Items must be processed unwrapped in this type of autoclave; as such, they are best suited for the decontamination of instruments that are not required to be sterile at the point of use. If such an autoclave is used for items needed for invasive procedures, then the items must be sterilised and laid up immediately prior to use because sterility is lost once the autoclave door is opened.

The steam must be able to reach all the surfaces of an object. The blades of instruments must be open and overloading of the trays avoided. Gallipots and receivers should be placed upside down to prevent the pooling of water in them.

Vacuum steam sterilisers can be used to sterilise items with a lumen, such as a trochar for inserting HRT pellets, or for wrapped items required to be sterile at the point of use. Special racks are used to keep the pouches separate and in a vertical position. The autoclave cycle must include a drying cycle in such instances. Pouches should be completely dry when removed from the autoclave. Care is needed to avoid puncturing a pouch but instruments in correctly autoclaved pouches will remain sterile until needed. A system is required for making sure that instruments are used within a reasonable time or are re-sterilised.

The reservoir must be drained, cleaned and left dry at the end of each working day. The autoclave reservoir should be filled with sterile water for irrigation (SWFI) before use. The contents of part-used bottles of SWFI should be discarded. Nurses should be aware of all the safety recommendations for autoclave use. These include:

- Daily and weekly checks by the user. Details of these checks can be obtained from the MHRA website.

- Four-monthly servicing, with emergency repairs as necessary by a qualified engineer.
- Annual tests. It is usual to have a service contract with a competent organisation, so that quarterly and annual checks are made in accordance with the regulations for benchtop steam sterilisers.

Good record keeping is essential when an autoclave is used. A permanent log must be kept to prove that the autoclave was functioning correctly, in case of any adverse incident. Details of the temperature and holding times must be logged, ideally from a printout of the sterilisation data. Photocopying of printed data may be necessary because the printouts from thermal printers can fade. It is necessary to have a system for recording the specific instruments autoclaved and the name of the patients on whom they were used.

A system is also needed to ensure contaminated equipment is never put into the autoclave until ready to start the sterilisation process. That way, unsterile equipment cannot be taken out of the autoclave and reused by mistake. This applies particularly to unwrapped items. When pouches are used, the indicator on the back of the pouch changes colour when it has been sterilised, so a mistake is less likely to be made.

Disinfection

Chemical disinfectants and boiling water can destroy bacteria and other microorganisms but do not destroy spores.

Chemicals may be used for low-risk items and items that cannot be autoclaved.

Alcohol and chlorine-releasing products are most commonly used in general practice. Ethanol 60–80% can be used to disinfect clean, heat-sensitive items. This destroys non-spore forming bacteria, fungi and virus in ten minutes on pre-cleaned surfaces.[21] Sodium hypochlorite, as household bleach or Milton, can be used in dilution for 30 minutes to disinfect plastics and glass. Sodium dichloroisocyanurate (NaDCC) tablets, e.g. Chlor-clean, Haz Tabs or Presept, can be dissolved in water to give a more reliable dilution of chlorine. The dilutions needed depend on the brand. The instructions on the label should be followed. Once prepared, solutions must be clearly labelled. Chlorine-releasing solutions used for decontamination must be discarded after use or within 24 hours, as they lose their potency.

Each day before use, the electric ear irrigator should be cleaned with NaDCC solution as advised by the Primary Ear Care Centre.

- Fill the machine's tank with the solution prepared to the manufacturer's instructions.
- Run the machine to pump the solution through the tubing, turn off and leave to stand for ten minutes.
- Empty the tank, refill with tap water and pump it through the tubing to rinse it.

Table 4.4 Spillages

Action	Rationale
Wear household rubber gloves and an apron	To avoid contact with hands and clothing
Cover the spillage with chlorine granules or a 1% hypochlorite solution; leave for ten minutes or as directed by the manufacturer	To inactivate any organisms
Remove any broken glass with forceps	To avoid accidental cuts
Cover the spillage with paper towels or use scoop in the special spillage kit, if available, to transfer the spillage to a yellow bag	For incineration as clinical waste
Wash the area with warm water, rinse and dry it	To remove organic matter
Wash the area with hypochlorite solution 1000 ppm	To destroy bacteria and viruses
Wash the area again with warm water and detergent	To remove any traces of the hypochlorite
Use warm water and strong detergent for surfaces such as carpets	Where bleach would cause damage to the fabric
Remove apron and gloves and wash hands	Once the procedure is finished

Disinfect the machine at the end of the day, rinse with sterile water and pump it through the tubing; dry the machine well. Chlor-clean is recommended by the Primary Ear Care Centre because it contains a surfactant as well as a disinfectant.[22] Reusable jet-tips are no longer being sold, in anticipation of new legislation expected soon. Disposable jet-tips should be used.

NaDCC granules can be used to decontaminate a blood spillage. All the staff should be aware of the procedure if a spillage occurs, as outlined in Table 4.4.

The disposal of clinical waste

Dressings and other soft waste contaminated with blood or bodily fluids must go into yellow bags contained in foot-operated pedal bins. Used bags must be tied securely with a special plastic fastener.

Clinical waste is covered by the Hazardous Waste Regulations 2005. A surgery which produces more than 200 kg hazardous waste in 12 months must be registered as a hazardous waste producer. Computer monitors and fluorescent tubes are also classified as hazardous waste now. Changes to the regulations covering waste management, which may have an impact on general practice, are likely to occur very soon.

At present, everybody who produces clinical waste is required to ensure that:

- The waste is stored in a designated, secure area, inaccessible to the public until it can be collected.
- A written description of the waste is supplied. It must be possible to trace the waste back to the person responsible and so it must carry a label with the practice address and date of disposal.
- The waste is transferred by a registered carrier. The practice must have a contract for a regular collection of the clinical waste. On no account must it be put into the ordinary rubbish bins.

Blades, needles and syringes must be deposited in sharps containers which meet the British Standard BS 7320:1990. The containers should be assembled correctly and placed in a position at waist height so that sharps can be safely disposed of close to their point of use. The containers must not be stored on the floor and they must be kept out of reach of children. Sadly, accidents have been known to occur whereby children have sustained needle-stick injuries through reaching into used sharps bins.

Unwanted medicines must also be disposed of safely to comply with current legislation. Pharmacies have special arrangements for dealing with unwanted drugs under the essential services part of the new pharmacy contract.[23]

SUPPLIES AND EQUIPMENT

The amount of clinical equipment needed varies from practice to practice (see Appendix 1). The practice nurse is responsible for overseeing the proper upkeep and for knowing the correct way to use the equipment in her/his care. Instruction booklets and guarantees should be kept on file. Any faulty equipment must be withdrawn from use, labelled and reported to the practice manager or GP. Maintenance contracts are needed for essential or potentially dangerous items such as autoclaves.

Emergency equipment

Every practice must have a basic supply of emergency drugs and equipment kept easily accessible. The exact items to be kept should be agreed by the clinicians. The practice nurse is usually responsible for ensuring that emergency supplies are checked and maintained. Epinephrine (adrenaline) has a relatively short shelf life and will need to be replaced regularly. All items must be purchased initially but reimbursement can be claimed for any personally administered drugs (see Appendix 2, Emergency equipment).

Table 4.5   Examples of sources of supply

Source	Product examples
Direct purchase from manufacturer	Travel vaccines
Purchase from wholesaler or medical mail order firm	Examination and diagnostic equipment, injectables, gloves, paper goods, dressings, IUDs and diaphragms
Purchase on account from local pharmacy	Small quantity items needed quickly
On prescription from local pharmacy	Dressings and treatments for named patients
Requisition from the primary care organisation/primary care support service	Syringes, needles, NHS stationery
Requisition from local district hospital	Pathology forms and sample bottles, cytology kits
Local health promotion department	Leaflets, posters, videos, etc. for health promotion and patient education
Contract with clinical waste service	Sharps bins, bins for unwanted medicines or vaccines, yellow bags and plastic ties

Ordering supplies and equipment

Practice policy will determine who has the responsibility for ordering supplies. Whether nurses place orders directly or via the practice manager, everyone has a responsibility for seeking value for money. Discounts may be available for bulk orders but it can be a false economy if the items do not have a long enough shelf life. Some items may appear cheaper by mail order but small orders can attract expensive delivery charges. Some examples of sources of supply are shown in Table 4.5. Copies of requisitions and receipts need to be kept for reference and accounting purposes.

TRAINING IN EMERGENCY PROCEDURES

Resuscitation

As many practice staff as possible should be able to undertake basic life support measures in emergencies. People tend to go to the surgery in times of trouble but there may not always be a doctor or other nurse in the building. Resuscitation training for nurses can usually be arranged through the local PCO, although a practice manager may arrange training in-house for all the surgery staff. Annual updating is needed to keep skills up to date.

Fire precautions

Every practice should have a procedure for dealing with a fire and an adequate supply of appropriate fire extinguishers, together with a plan of their location. Extinguishers must be serviced at least once a year and staff trained in their use at a full fire practice.

Suggestions for reflection on practice

- Review all the storage and disposal facilities in the nurses' rooms. Do they meet all the legal requirements and comply with local guidelines?
- Review:
  1. The facilities for patient care in the nurses' rooms. Are they satisfactory?
  2. The procedures for decontaminating and sterilising equipment in your practice. Are any changes needed?
- Review your own and other nurses' readiness to cope with emergency procedures. Is further training necessary? Is all the equipment needed ready for immediate use?

REFERENCES

1. Disability Discrimination Act 1995. www.disability.gov.uk (accessed 30/8/05).
2. Primary and Social Care Premises Planning and Design Guidance. www.primarycare.nhsestates.gov.uk (accessed 30/8/05).
3. Health and Safety Executive (2003) *Health and Safety Regulation . . . a short guide*. HSE Books, Suffolk.
4. Merriman, E., Corwin, P. & Ikram, R. (2002) Toys are a potential source of cross-infection in general practitioners' waiting rooms. *British Journal of General Practice*, **52**(475), 138–40.
5. Bradley, K. (2001) *The Health and Safety Act Explained*. The Point of Law Series. Stationery Office, London.
6. Health and Safety Executive (2004) *Manual Handling. Manual Handling Operations Regulations 1992 (as amended)*. HSE Books, Suffolk.
7. Health and Safety Executive (2004) *A Step by Step Guide to COSHH Assessment*. HSE Books, Suffolk.
8. British Hypertension Society (2004) *Blood Pressure Monitors*. Validated blood pressure monitor lists. www.bhsoc.org (accessed 4/9/05).
9. Department of Health (2002) *Destruction of Controlled Drugs in GP Practices*. DH Publications. www.dh.gov.uk (accessed 4/9/05).
10. News item (1992) Doctor faces charge after child drank acid. *Daily Telegraph*, 19 September 1996.
11. Department of Health (2005) Storage, distribution and disposal of vaccines. Draft Chapter 4. *Immunications against Infectious Disease* (the 'Green Book'). www.dh.gov.uk/PolicyAndGuidance/HealthAndSocialCareTopics/GreenBook/GreenBookGeneralInformation?fs/en (accessed 29/3/06).

12. Infection Control Nurses Association (2002) *Hand Decontamination Guidelines.* Fitwise, Bathgate.
13. Institute for Research in Health and Human Sciences, Thames Valley University (2003) *Prevention of Healthcare-associated Infections in Primary and Community Care.* www.epic.tva.ac.uk/epicphase2a (accessed 6/9/05).
14. Health and Safety Executive (2005) *Latex Allergies – I work in general practice.* www.hse.gov.uk/latex (accessed 6/9/05).
15. Gilbart, V., Raeside, F., Evans, B., Mortimer, J., Arnold, C., Gill, O., Clewley, J., Goldberg, D. and anonymous collaborators (1998) Unusual HIV transmission through blood contact: analysis of cases reported in the United Kingdom to December 1997. *Communicable Disease and Public Health,* **1**(2), 108–13.
16. Medicines and Healthcare Products Regulatory Agency (2000) *Single-use Medical Devices: implications and consequences of reuse.* MDA DB2000(04). www.medical-devices.gov.uk (accessed 10/9/05).
17. Medical Devices section of the Medicines and Healthcare Products Regulatory Agency (2005) *Sterilisation, Disinfection and Cleaning of Medical Equipment: guidance on decontamination from the Microbiology Advisory Committee to Department of Health, Medical Devices Agency.* www.medical-devices.gov.uk (accessed 10/9/05).
18. Medicines and Healthcare Products Regulatory Agency (2005) *Benchtop Steam Sterilisers.* www.mhra.gov.uk (accessed 11/9/05).
19. Medicines and Healthcare Products Regulatory Agency (2004) *Benchtop Steam Sterilisers – guidance on purchase, operation and maintenance.* MDA DB2002(06). www.medical-devices.gov.uk.
20. Eschmann Holdings Ltd (2005) *Best Practice in Use of Benchtop Autoclaves.* www.eschmann.co.uk/ (accessed 15/9/05).
21. Health and Safety Executive (2003) Substitution of glutaraldehyde in healthcare endoscope disinfection – WATCH findings on three possible alternatives. *Toxic Substances Bulletin,* Issue 51. www.hse.gov.uk (accessed 15/9/05).
22. Primary Ear Care Centre (2004) *Cleaning Guidelines.* www.earcarecentre.com (accessed 15/9/05).
23. Royal Pharmaceutical Society of Great Britain (2005) *Interim Practice Guidance for Community Pharmacists on 'The Hazardous Waste Regulations 2005'.* www.rpsgb.org.uk (accessed 15/9/05).

FURTHER READING

Community Infection Control Nurses Network (2003) *Infection Control Guidance for General Practice.* Fitwise, Bathgate.
Environment Agency (2005) *Hazardous Waste Legislation.* www.environment-agency.gov.uk
Health Protection Agency (2005) *Eye of the Needle: surveillance of significant occupational exposure to bloodborne viruses in healthcare workers. Seven year report.* www.hpa.org.uk
Medicines and Healthcare Products Regulatory Agency (2005) *Medical Devices Containing Mercury.* www.mhra.gov.uk
Royal College of Nursing (2005) *Good Practice in Infection Prevention and Control. Guidance for nursing staff.* Royal College of Nursing, London.

USEFUL ADDRESSES AND WEBSITES

Medicines and Healthcare Products Regulatory Agency (MHRA)
(replaced Medical Devices Agency)
Market Towers, 1 Nine Elms Lane, London SW8 5NQ
Telephone: 020 7084 2000
Website: www.mhra.gov.uk

NHS Plus – occupational health service for smaller employers
Website: www.nhsplus.nhs.uk

Chapter 5
Nursing Treatments and Procedures

The importance to the patient of hands-on nursing care should never be overlooked as the role of nurses changes and expands. Patients are entitled to care that is based on the best available evidence of effectiveness. Thoughtful preparation and skilled performance can minimise the discomfort caused by many nursing procedures and apparently routine tasks can still provide opportunities for health promotion and active listening to patients' concerns.

INJECTIONS

A variety of injections are given in general practice (specific injections are dealt with in the relevant chapters). Injections are usually prescribed by a doctor, either in a patient's records or on a prescription form. Immunisations may be given under a Patient Group Direction (see Chapter 10). Injection techniques are taught in pre-registration training and will not be described here.

Feeding seems to be the best pacifier for young babies, while a bright, musical toy will usually distract older infants. Many children, especially after the pre-school booster, welcome a stick-on badge or a certificate of bravery. Anaesthetic cream is available on prescription and can be applied to the injection site and covered by an occlusive dressing, one hour before injection, for very nervous children or those who require a large number of injections.

Records must be kept of the product name, dose and route of administration, manufacturer, batch number and expiry date. This applies to any medicine, not just injections. A nurse or doctor could be legally responsible for any harm to a patient, if unable to prove the source of the product used.[1] The site of injection should also be recorded, especially when more than one injection is given, in case of an adverse reaction to any product. The injection data may also be needed for immunisation targets or for a recall system. The nurse must observe the patient until satisfied that there are no immediate ill effects from the injection. It is not possible to specify an exact time. Some practice policies state a minimum time of 20 minutes.

Patients need information about possible side effects and the action to take if they occur. The Summary of Product Characteristics gives an in-depth account of the product and lists all the possible adverse reactions. A Patient Information

Leaflet (PIL) is provided with every drug and vaccine. Practitioners are required to supply the patient or parent of a child with the PIL. However, such leaflets can provoke anxiety and be of poor quality and hard to understand.[2] Many practices have produced their own advice sheets to be given out in addition. Many examples can be found on the internet.

Patients receiving regular injections should know when to make the next appointment. A recall system may be needed for immunisations and depot medication, together with a fail-safe system for knowing when patients are overdue for an injection.

WOUND CARE

Practice nurses are likely to encounter patients with a variety of wounds. The range of dressings can be bewildering and sales representatives produce convincing arguments for favouring their own products. A sound understanding of the principles of wound healing is necessary when selecting a dressing. A local wound care specialist will provide education and advice if needed. Some areas have wound product formularies, which can make the selection process easier.

WOUND HEALING

There are three distinct phases of healing, although some overlapping occurs between them.

1. *Inflammation* in response to the initial injury. A fibrin clot forms, to prevent further blood loss. Blood vessels in the vicinity of the wound become more permeable and leucocytes are attracted to the area to remove bacteria and debris by phagocytosis. (The normal inflammatory response, which causes slight redness around a wound, should not be mistaken for infection.)
2. *Proliferation* of cells and collagen. Fibroblasts produce collagen fibres and buds of endothelial cells and capillaries grow into the wound space to form the delicate granulation tissue. Occasionally overgranulation can occur above the level of the surrounding skin. A pressure dressing can usually arrest this. Topical triamcinolone, to be used sparingly, may be prescribed for patients who are not hypersensitive to any of the ingredients.
3. *Maturation* as the wound heals. Epithelial cells migrate across the wound until it is covered. Collagen is broken down and remoulded over subsequent months to form a firmer scar. Keloid forms when there is an overproduction of collagen. Patients with dark skin are more prone to developing keloid scars.[3]

Wounds are often classified according to their appearance or stage of healing.

- *Necrotic wounds* – when devitalised tissue forms a dry, hard, black eschar or a soft, grey slough. Surgical or chemical debridement is often necessary.

- *Infected wounds* – when bacteria overcome the body's natural defences. There may be a purulent discharge and/or cellulitis present. Systemic antibiotics may be needed. All wounds become colonised by bacteria but are not necessarily infected.
- *Clean wounds* – are those without slough or infection. They may be superficial or deep. The skin margins of incisions may be drawn together to reduce the gap to be bridged. Wider wounds heal by secondary intention.

Necrotic or infected tissue delays healing and must be treated. Sterile larvae (maggots) have been used to good effect in desloughing wounds and they are now available on prescription. Wounds have been shown to heal more quickly in the warm, moist environment created by an occlusive dressing because the epithelial cells can migrate across the wound rather than growing downwards under a scab. However, the research into moist wound healing was carried out on acute wounds and the healing process of chronic wounds may involve additional factors.[4] Infected wounds should not be covered by occlusive dressings. Moreover, the risk of infection in patients with diabetes could be so devastating that some diabetologists are totally opposed to the use of any occlusive dressings for neuropathic and ischaemic ulcers in their patients.

Dressings

The dressing range available on prescription includes the following.

- *Sterile dressing packs* provide a sterile field and contain a hand towel/paper drape, four cotton wool balls, four gauze swabs and a dressing pad. The packs are expensive and may not be needed for minor dressings. (Cotton wool is not recommended in wound cleansing because fibres can be left in the wound and impair healing.[5]) Packs of five sterile gauze swabs or 100 unsterile swabs are also available on prescription and may be more cost effective than dressing packs for minor wounds.
- *Normal saline* is available as single-use 25 ml units or from aerosol cans for irrigating wounds. Drinkable tap water can be more economical and has been shown to be safe for wound cleansing.[6] Antiseptics can damage fragile granulation tissue and are generally contraindicated.
- *Enzyme preparations* can be used to debride necrotic tissue. However, they are expensive and have not been proved to be cost-effective in some instances.[7]
- *Hydrocolloid dressings* are waterproof adhesive wafers that combine with exudate from a wound to form a gel; they are useful for desloughing wounds and promoting granulation. Hydrocolloid paste can be used in deep wounds and sinuses. These dressings may cause overgranulation if they are used for too long. The liquid that forms under the wafer can be mistaken for pus and the offensive odour of the liquid and leakage can be distressing to patients. Skin maceration can also occur if there is excessive exudate.

- *Hydrogel* is a soft gel packaged in dispenser units, which can be applied directly to a wound and covered with a film or secondary dressing. The gel helps to rehydrate wounds and create the optimum conditions for healing. It has a range of uses similar to hydrocolloids.
- *Calcium alginate dressings* are made of an extract of seaweed spun and woven into soft mats and are useful as a haemostat and for absorbing exudate. They can be used under occlusive films or other secondary dressings and they can be removed from wounds by saline irrigation. The dressings sometimes stick fast but soaking with saline will dissolve them, given time. Cavity-packing material is also produced.
- *Polyurethane foam* absorbs exudate through the non-adherent contact layer into the foam backing. It can be used under compression bandages and as a light, comfortable dressing for arterial ulcers. The foam can be cut easily and makes a good dressing after toenail surgery. It is useful for controlling overgranulation.
- *Vapour-permeable film dressings* can be used to secure a dressing or to provide a warm, moist environment for clean, superficial wounds. Some films are produced with a pad of dressing material in their centre. Film is also useful for keeping enzymatic preparations moist. Some patients are allergic to the adhesive. Skin can be damaged if the film is pulled away. The corner should be lifted and the film stretched horizontally to break the adhesive bond with the skin.
- *Low-adherent absorbent dressings* (*Melolin*) consist of a perforated film and a cotton and polyester pad with a hydrophobic backing layer. The dressing, which should be applied with the film surface in contact with the wound, is suitable for dry wounds or those with low exudate. These dressings are not suitable for highly exuding wounds because they are not sufficiently absorbent and maceration of the skin can occur.
- *Self-adhesive absorbent dressings* (*Mepore, Primapore*) are all-in-one dressings consisting of an absorbent pad situated on a piece of non-woven fabric adhesive. The dressings are available in a range of sizes and are useful for dry or lightly exuding wounds. They are not waterproof and can be difficult to remove once they get wet. Patients should be made aware of this. A shower-proof version of these dressings (*Mepore Ultra*) can be obtained.
- *Non-adherent dressings* are thin wound contact dressings designed not to stick to wounds. Nevertheless, they can adhere to a wound and damage granulation tissue so a silicone-coated product (*N-A Ultra*) was designed to prevent sticking. These contact dressings can be used for venous ulcers under compression bandages and for minor wounds. Secondary dressings are needed. Non-adherent dressings impregnated with povidone iodine (*Inadine*) are also available and can be used to prevent or treat some wound infections. Povidone iodine can sometimes be effective against MRSA.[8]
- *Soft silicone dressings* (*Mepitel*) prevent adherence to a wound and can be painless to remove.
- *Impregnated gauzes* have limited uses. Paraffin gauze might be used occasionally on skin graft sites or for minor burns. Allergic reactions to impregnated gauzes can occur.

Strapping and bandages

These may be applied to secure a dressing, to give support or provide compression to an underlying structure.

- *Adhesive tape* can be used to secure dressings or for neighbour strapping of injured fingers and toes. Many people are allergic to zinc oxide adhesive and it can be difficult to remove. One should always enquire about allergy before applying any tape.
- *Microporous tape* is light, hypoallergenic and easy to remove. Some patients can still become allergic to the adhesive. The tape is used to secure dressings but it does not stretch as the body moves. Strips of sterile reinforced microporous tape (*Steri-strips*) can be used to close minor incisions and cuts. Reimbursement of prescriptions can be claimed for these as personally administered items if they have been purchased.
- *Paper-backed tape* (*Hypafix, Mepore*) is a light, stretchable non-woven fixative.
- *Conforming bandages* are light, loosely woven bandages for securing dressings. The edges can cut into oedematous tissue if applied too tightly and those with elastic fibres can cause oedema above and below the bandage if it is overextended.
- *Tubular gauze* comes in a range of sizes and can hold dressings in place or be used under bandages to protect sensitive skin. The small sizes are useful for dressing fingers and toes. Applicators are available in a range of sizes.
- *Tubular elastic bandages*, in sizes B to G, provide support for soft tissue injuries. They are designed to be used in a double layer. Special measuring tapes can be obtained from the manufacturers for assessing the size needed.
- *Crepe bandages* can be used to secure dressings or to provide support for soft tissue injuries.
- *Paste bandages* may be used in conjunction with compression bandages to treat venous ulcers. Severe allergies to some of the constituents can develop. A skin test is recommended before applying a paste bandage. Paste bandages may also be used for treating severe eczema.[9]
- *Elastic crepe bandages* provide support but quickly lose their elasticity. Tuition and practice are needed to get the correct amount of extension when applying them.
- *Multilayer bandages* are used for compression bandaging (see venous ulcers below).
- *Compression hosiery* can be prescribed for individual patients. There are three classes of compression:
  1. Class I gives the least compression
  2. Class II gives the moderate compression needed for most patients in general practice
  3. Class III is for very firm compression.
  The stockings can have closed or open toes and be knee or thigh length. Made-to-measure hose can be prescribed for patients with unusual measurements. Black below-knee support hose is available for men.

General assessment of the patient

Wound care entails much more than applying dressings. A full assessment is needed. The factors to consider include the following.

- *Age* – elderly patients have slower rates of growth and repair, less collagen and elasticity in the skin and may have impaired circulation. The immune system can also be less effective. Care is needed to avoid damaging fragile skin with adhesives or tight bandages.
- *Mobility* – patients who are not very mobile are more likely to develop oedema or to fall. Referrals for physiotherapy or occupational therapy may be needed to help to improve mobility. Housebound patients may need to be referred to the district nurse for treatment.
- *Nutritional state* – obesity can contribute to reduced mobility and make bandaging difficult. Malnourished or cachexic patients can lack the vitamins and minerals needed for wound healing. Patients may need information about healthy eating. Those who are unable to eat a healthy diet may require food supplements or need to see a dietitian. Protein intake can be checked by liver function tests (albumin levels).
- *Medical conditions* – the general medical condition can influence the progress of any wound. Anaemia, diabetes, rheumatoid arthritis, immunosuppression and cardiopulmonary disease can all contribute to the development or continuation of tissue damage. A doctor should be consulted when necessary.
- *Psychological state* – the patient's motivation should be assessed. Patients may lack the energy or inclination to care for themselves properly or they may have self-inflicted injuries. Counselling and/or antidepressant therapy may be needed.
- *Social situation* – lonely patients have sometimes been suspected of exacerbating their wounds to maintain contact with the nurse. Referrals may be made to social services or voluntary agencies to arrange other contacts.
- *Smoking status* – smoking reduces the amount of oxygen available to the tissues and increases the damage to small blood vessels.[10]
- *Alcohol intake* – high alcohol intake can adversely affect the nutritional state and cause damage to the liver and kidneys.
- *Pain* – pain may limit mobility or affect sleep. Analgesics might be needed and the choice of dressing can be influenced if the wound is very painful.

Assessment and treatment of the wound

The wound assessment should include the type, size, stage of healing, amount of exudate and any complicating factors. The possibility of malignancy should be borne in mind in any wound that fails to heal or looks suspicious. Measurements of the wound provide an objective scale against which to judge progress. Tracing over a double plastic film is a quick and easy method, which allows the top layer to be kept free from contamination by the wound. Photographs also provide a good reference. A ruler or grid should be included in the picture to show the scale.

Choice of dressing

Considerations when choosing a dressing include:

- *Practical issues* – getting shoes on, bathing, frequency of dressing changes and patient compliance
- *Aesthetic factors* – how the dressings looks, feels or smells
- *Cost* – an important issue but should not prevent the use of the most suitable product.

Wound care is most effective if the patient is involved in planning the treatment and lifestyle changes necessary to promote healing. Advice may be sought from a tissue viability nurse if a wound poses particular difficulties.

Leg ulcers

Leg ulcers, often painful and debilitating to patients, use vast resources in manpower and dressings annually. The correct diagnosis of the ulcer type is essential before treatment is started. Tissue viability training is available in most areas and is strongly recommended before attempting to treat leg ulcers.

Venous ulcers

Approximately 80% of all leg ulcers are venous in origin. They result from inadequacy of the venous drainage of the legs. Incompetent valves in the perforator veins allow backflow and increased venous pressure in the superficial veins.
Recognition will include noting the following.

- *Skin condition* – in varicose eczema, brown discolouration is caused by the breakdown of red blood cells in the tissues.
- *Ulcer position* – commonest in the gaiter area, the pretibial and anteromedial supramalleolar areas.
- *Appearance* – often superficial with uneven edges and some granulation tissue.
- *Oedema,* due to venous insufficiency; can be exacerbated by reduced mobility.
- *Pain* – ulcers may be very painful, although some patients could be pain free.

Doppler assessment plays an essential part in the diagnosis of venous ulcers.

Aims of treatment are:

- To improve the venous return and reduce stagnation in the tissues of the affected leg

- To promote healing
- To provide clear information and encouragement to enable the patient to participate in the treatment and to maintain their legs in optimum condition after healing has occurred.

Table 5.1   Venous ulcer treatment

Treatment	Rationale
Wash the leg ulcer with warm water and dry the skin well	To remove debris without damaging the wound surface or cooling the wound
Use an emollient	To improve the skin condition
Apply a flat, non-irritant, non-adherent dressing or a hydrocolloid wafer	To prevent indentation of the surrounding skin and allow removal of the dressing without damage to healing tissues
Pad smoothly with absorbent material	To absorb exudate and protect the bony prominences
Apply graduated compression bandages	To reverse venous hypertension without compromising the arterial circulation
Advise elevation of the foot above the level of the hip when resting	To reduce oedema by using gravity
Ensure that the patient has adequate analgesia and knows when to take it, if the ulcer is painful	Pain can be debilitating and reduce mobility. Poor nutrition can result from loss of appetite due to pain
Teach suitable ankle exercises (dorsiflexing and plantarflexing the feet and circular movements of the ankles)	To aid venous return by the action of the calf muscle pump and to aid mobility
Teach the need to prevent a recurrence by good skin care, the use of compression hosiery and early treatment of injury	Patients who understand their condition can take responsibility for looking after their legs and for getting help when needed

Compression bandaging cannot be learned from a book. External compression at very high pressures will reduce blood supply to the skin and may lead to pressure damage.[11] Expert tuition and practice in multilayer bandaging are needed. Moreover, no patient should have compression bandages applied without having had a Doppler assessment.

Arterial ulcers

Arterial ulcers result from ischaemia due to arterial occlusion; often caused by atherosclerosis. Minor trauma may cause an ulcer to develop and the tissue breaks down as a result of the impaired supply of oxygen and nutrients. Smoking exacerbates the problem.

Recognition will include:

- *Position of the ulcer* – often below the ankle
- *Appearance* – often well demarcated with a pale base, necrosis and absence of healthy granulation tissue; the skin around the ulcer may be shiny and dry and the toenails thickened
- *Pain* – particularly at night and often severe
- *Foot pulses* – may be absent or diminished (experience is needed to locate foot pulses; they are not an accurate indicator). Assessment of arterial blood flow by Doppler ultrasound is more objective and early referral for arteriography should be made, if appropriate.

Aims of treatment are:

- To reduce pain
- To promote healing
- To prevent further tissue damage.

Surgery may be indicated to try and improve the blood flow for patients with ischaemia. In extreme cases amputation can become necessary.

Table 5.2 Arterial ulcer treatment

Treatment	Rationale
Ensure that the patient has adequate analgesia and knows when to take it	Ischaemic ulcers can be very painful
Identify any contributing medical conditions	Diabetes, rheumatoid arthritis, anaemia and malignancy may contribute to ischaemic ulcers
Arrange for systemic antibiotics if needed	Infection may delay healing
Apply suitable light dressings	For comfort and ease of removal and to encourage healing
Avoid compression bandages	To avoid compromising the circulation further
Encourage smoking cessation if applicable	To avoid further vascular damage and to improve the oxygen supply to the tissues

Other ulcers

Some patients have mixed ulcers caused by both arterial and venous insufficiency. Compression must be avoided where there is any risk to the arterial blood flow.

Ulcers may also be caused by diabetic neuropathy, rheumatoid vasculitis, sickle cell disease or more rare conditions such as lupus erythematosus. Each ulcer should be assessed and treated accordingly. Underlying medical causes should be addressed.

EYE TREATMENT

Patients may ask to see the practice nurse with various eye conditions. Nurses are advised to err on the side of caution and refer to the GP when in any doubt about dealing with eye conditions.

The principles of eye care are as shown in Table 5.3.

See Chapter 7 under eye problems for foreign bodies in the eye, conjunctivitis, corneal abrasions and painful eyes.

Table 5.3   Eye treatment

Action	Rationale
Avoid using antiseptic spray on the hands	It can cause irritation to the patient's eyes
Ensure there is a good light source	To be able to assess the eye properly and avoid injury during any eye treatment
Avoid shining the light directly into the eye	The patient may have photophobia
Tell the patient what action is proposed	To avoid sudden movements which could injure the eye and to obtain informed consent
Inspect the eye for signs of infection, allergy, foreign body or injury	To identify the problem and ensure the correct treatment is given
Enquire about the patient's vision; check visual acuity if necessary (see Chapter 6)	In case of any abnormality which needs investigation

EAR CARE

Ear irrigation, still called syringing by many people, is usually carried out by practice nurses for the removal of excessive earwax. Softening drops should be recommended for use up to three days beforehand. Patients with impacted wax may need to use the drops for longer. Olive oil or sodium bicarbonate is considered to be preferable to proprietary cerumolytic drops. Patients with a nut allergy should not be advised to use almond oil. Occasionally patients may require ear irrigation to remove debris or a foreign body from the auditory canal. The procedure should not be attempted for any hygroscopic foreign body, such as a dried pea, which is likely to swell in contact with water.

Any practice nurse who undertakes ear irrigation must have had adequate training and supervision to ensure that patients are not harmed. The Primary

Ear Care Centre in Rotherham runs a course in ear care accredited by Sheffield University. Ear care trainers run satellite courses and study days around the country. The practice protocol should specify the circumstances under which patients may self-refer for treatment and the contraindications to irrigation. Irrigation should be avoided:

- When there is a recent history of otitis media
- When there is acute otitis externa – an oedematous ear canal combined with pain
- With a recent history of discharging ears or current tympanic membrane perforation
- If there were untoward experiences following ear syringing in the past
- If the patient has a cleft palate, even if repaired
- If the patient has undergone any form of ear surgery (apart from grommets that have extruded at least 18 months previously and the patient has been discharged from the ENT department)[12]
- If a patient has deafness in one ear, as damage caused by irrigation of the hearing ear could be devastating: it is recommended that irrigation should not be undertaken for such patients.[13]

Metal ear syringes must not be used at all. Electric pulsed water units are safer and less likely to cause damage to the ear. The patient must understand the procedure and any possible complications in order to give informed consent.[14]

As with any nursing procedure, a full history and examination are needed before starting the treatment. Both ears should be examined with the otoscope and the necessity for irrigation decided. It is not uncommon for patients with dysfunction of the middle ear to present for ear syringing because their ears feel 'blocked'. The skin of the auditory canal will sometimes be inflamed or itchy, particularly in patients who have skin conditions such as eczema or psoriasis. Irritation or allergic reactions can also result from the use of proprietary cerumolytic drops.

Equipment needed

- Headlight or head mirror and lamp
- Waterproof cape and towel
- Otoscope with disposable speculum
- Electric pulsed water unit with new disposable jet nozzle
- Specially shaped receiver (Noots tank) or a kidney dish
- Jobson Horne probe
- Cotton wool
- Tissues
- Receivers for used tissues, cotton wool and instruments.

Procedure

The patient and nurse should both be seated and the entire procedure should be carried out under direct vision, using a headlight or head mirror and lamp.

Possibly the most important part of the consultation is educating the patient about everyday ear care. The ears should be kept as dry as possible to allow the wax to migrate normally to the external auditory meatus. Attempting to clean the ears with cotton buds, etc. should be avoided because this can cause the wax to become impacted and carries the risk of damage to the tympanic membrane as well. The old adage 'put nothing in your ear smaller than your elbow' still holds true.

Patients sometimes enquire about ear suction devices they see advertised. No research is available on their use but the specialist nurse at the Primary Ear Care Centre does not recommend using them.

Table 5.4   Ear treatment

Action	Rationale
Check whether the patient has had their ears syringed previously and identify any contraindications to the procedure	To identify any reasons for not irrigating the ear
Explain the procedure to the patient and answer any questions	To obtain informed consent and to ensure that the patient will not be unduly anxious and will remain still during the procedure
Ask the patient to sit in the examination chair with their head tilted slightly to the opposite from the affected ear (a child could sit on an adult's lap with the child's head held steady)	To allow visualisation of the auditory meatus safely
Inspect both ears with the otoscope	For comparison of the ears
Place the cape and towel in position and ask the patient to hold the receiver under the ear	To protect the patient's clothing and to catch the irrigation water
Fill the reservoir of the pulsed water unit with tap water at body temperature (39°C)	Deviations in temperature can cause dizziness by creating a caloric effect (convection currents in the semicircular canals in the middle ear)
Put on the headlight or head mirror and turn on the light and adjust as necessary	To make sure that the auditory meatus is illuminated and ensure a clear vision during the procedure
Ensure that the jet tip is firmly attached to the holder and set the pressure to the appropriate setting	To make sure it does not fly off under pressure and damage the ear

Table 5.4   (*cont'd*)

Action	Rationale
Aim the jet tip into the receiver and switch on the machine	To run any cold water or air out of the tubing to ensure that any static water is discarded and only water at the correct temperature is used. This will also allow time for the patient to become accustomed to the sound of the machine
Hold the pinna of the ear to be syringed with the non-dominant hand and pull gently upwards and backwards in an adult or directly backwards if a child	For ease of access to the auditory canal and to control any movement of the head
Twist the jet tip to point in the correct position and place the tip of the nozzle into the entrance of the external auditory meatus	At the five minutes to the hour clock position for the right ear and five minutes past the hour for the left ear
Warn the patient that the procedure is about to start and to report any pain or dizziness	So that the procedure can be stopped immediately. Irrigation may cause discomfort but should never cause pain
Switch on the machine and direct the stream of water along the roof of the meatus towards the posterior wall	To avoid direct water pressure onto the tympanic membrane
Inspect the ear with the otoscope periodically and inspect the water running into the receiver	To check on progress
No more than two reservoirs of water should be used. If wax is not removed after that, the other ear could be irrigated or the patient asked to wait for 15 minutes	Excessive irrigation could cause soreness. Further softening of impacted wax might be needed. Water has been shown to soften wax
In the case of intractable wax, the patient should be asked to use more softening drops and return at another time if necessary	The procedure should not be rushed and another consultation might be needed
Dry mop excess water from the meatus under direct vision, using best quality cotton wool and the Jobson Horne probe	Stagnation of water and any abrasion of the skin during the procedure predisposes to otitis externa and possible pseudomonas infection
Examine the meatus and tympanic membrane	In case any treatment is required or referral to the GP is necessary
Record all findings and treatments in the patient's clinical record	To comply with the standards for record keeping
Clean and disinfect all the equipment used. Dispose of single-use items in the clinical waste bin	In accordance with the control of infection policy

ASSISTING WITH MINOR SURGERY

The advantages to patients of minor surgery in general practice include reduced waiting times for treatment and a more personal service in a familiar environment. Many doctors and nurses enjoy the chance to extend their professional skills. Although some nurses have been taught to perform minor surgical procedures, it is still more usual for practice nurses to assist a GP with minor surgery. PCOs should be satisfied that practices carrying out minor surgery have such facilities as are necessary to enable them properly to provide minor surgery services.[15] The standards of care required for performing minor surgery in general practice must include the control of infection, the comfort and safety of the patient and the ability to deal with emergency situations.

The role of the nurse

Preparation of the environment

The nurse has responsibility for ensuring a high standard of cleanliness in the room used for minor surgery. The couch and lamp should be positioned to allow free access to the operation site. A comfortable room temperature is needed. Blinds should be adjusted to give privacy to patients.

Preparation of the equipment

Trolleys should be cleaned according to the local infection control policy. This might specify washing with soap and water and drying with paper towels or the use of hard-surface disinfectant wipes. If CSSD packs or disposable sterile instruments are not available, the instruments must be autoclaved and laid between sterile paper sheets; dressing packs are commonly used but special minor surgery packs can be purchased. Trolleys must not be laid up until immediately before the procedure because of the risk of contamination.

Preparation of the patient

Most people will experience some apprehension. Practice nurses can help by ensuring patients receive a clear explanation of what to expect and by encouraging the use of simple relaxation techniques. Patients commonly request to have moles and other skin lesions removed but are then surprised to learn that they will have a scar. The person performing the minor surgery is responsible for obtaining consent but the nurse can reinforce the information given. Patients should be asked to remove clothing as necessary, to make sure the operation site is accessible. Clothing not removed should be protected from any possible blood trickles; even small lesions can be surprisingly vascular. If the operation site is on the scalp, some hair may need to be trimmed but it may be possible just to tape hair out of the way. Eyebrows should not be shaved because they may not regrow.

During the operation

The nurse should comfort and observe the patient during the minor operation and assist as needed, for example, by checking the local anaesthetic, opening sterile packs, receiving specimens for histology and assisting with suturing. The nurse will usually dress the wound and select the appropriate fixative.

After the operation

The patient may need time to recover before leaving the surgery. The nurse should ensure that the patient is able to get home safely and understands how to care for the wound and when to return. Written advice sheets can be useful because verbal instructions are easily forgotten. The stress experienced by patients, undergoing what may seem to be trivial procedures, should never be underestimated.

Clearing up often falls to the nurse. Although the safe disposal of sharps is the responsibility of the person who used them, extreme caution is needed in case any have been overlooked. Items left on the bottom of trolleys can be hazardous to children, so trolleys must be cleared completely. Specimens for histology must be labelled and dispatched, with the appropriate form, to the laboratory.

Basic minor operation trolley

Each practitioner may have favourite instruments but a basic set usually comprises:

- Scalpel handle and disposable blade or disposable scalpel
- Two pairs of toothed dissecting forceps
- Two pairs of non-toothed dissecting forceps
- Curette
- Artery forceps
- Needle holder
- Scissors
- Gallipot.

Also needed are: disposable apron, chlorhexidine hand scrub, sterile surgeon's gloves, local anaesthetic, syringes and needles, skin prep solution, specimen container and formaldehyde solution, suture materials, dressings and fixative. A silver nitrate stick or cautery may also be required.

The clinician's preferences will determine the equipment for specific procedures but some of the extra instruments and equipment include the following.

Removal of sebaceous cysts

Curved scissors and mosquito forceps are needed to dissect out a cyst and keep the capsule intact. A crepe bandage should be used if a pressure dressing is needed after the minor operation, to prevent bleeding into the cyst cavity.

Incision of abscesses

Equipment required includes ethyl chloride spray (local anaesthetic) and a wound swab for microbiology. Instruments needed are sinus forceps or a probe. The dressing used will be alginate strip for light packing.

   Note: Boils, abscesses or carbuncles should raise particular suspicions about diabetes mellitus. Therefore, a blood glucose test might be needed. However, it is good practice to ensure that all patients undergoing minor surgery have had a routine check for diabetes.

Ingrowing toenails

Wedge resection or removal of an ingrowing toenail may be necessary if conservative treatment is unsuccessful. Advice and information on footcare may help to prevent a recurrence.

   Equipment required includes:

- *Plain lignocaine 1% or 2%* – as local anaesthetic for a ring block (adrenaline could cause gangrene of a digit through vasoconstriction)
- *A tourniquet to reduce bleeding* – can be made from a sterilised out-of-date unused catheter
- *Instruments* – sturdy, pointed scissors and a nail elevator
- *Dressings* need to be easily removable without causing pain, e.g. polyurethane foam, calcium alginate, soft silicone or hydrocolloid.

Skin tags

Some papillomas may be removed surgically. Small skin tags can be tied tightly with suture silk, which usually causes them to necrose and drop off after a few days.

Warts and verrucae

Warts and verrucae are caused by the human papilloma virus, which accelerates the growth of the infected skin cells and distorts them. Most people eventually acquire immunity to the virus but this can take months or years to develop. The correct diagnosis is essential before commencing treatment in the surgery. If proprietary treatments containing salicylic acid are unsuccessful, cryotherapy may work but the evidence of effectiveness is limited.[16] Some warts may require more than one treatment. Practice nurses can develop expertise in this field but must be taught to perform the treatments safely. The hazards of cryotherapy include damage to tendons, nerves and joints. The wart or verruca should be pared with a scalpel before treatment but care is needed to avoid capillary bleeding and strict control of infection procedures are necessary because the wart virus can be spread by direct contact or through contamination of the environment. Children should only receive treatment if able to cooperate. Patients must be warned to expect blistering after the treatment and be told what to do and whom to contact if advice is needed.

Insertion of intrauterine device (IUD) or intrauterine system (IUS) (see Chapter 12)

Ideally a routine IUD or IUS should be inserted around day 5 of the menstrual cycle. At this time, the cervical os will be more open, any bleeding should be light and the clinician can be sure that the patient is not pregnant. If there is any doubt about pregnancy or the patient has amenorrhoea, then a pregnancy test should be performed for confirmation of the safety of the procedure. However, an IUD can be inserted at any time, especially for emergency contraception. It is good practice to ensure that the patient has no sexually transmitted infection before inserting a coil. Screening is recommended for all women before a planned coil insertion. If time does not permit prior testing, especially for an emergency IUD fitting, then the swabs should be taken before insertion of the device and antibiotic cover given afterwards.

The following sterile equipment is required:

- Vaginal speculum
- Long artery forceps
- Sponge-holding forceps
- Volsellum or Allis tissue forceps
- Uterine sound
- Hagar's dilators
- Long round-ended scissors
- Gallipot and lotion.

In addition, sterile gloves, examination jelly, thread retriever, selection of IUDs, sanitary towel, disposal bag for clinical waste and the emergency tray will be required. Glyceryl trinitrate spray, sterile local anaesthetic gel and an introducer may sometimes be needed.

Unsterile demonstration IUDs are useful for teaching patients about the devices. A practice nurse needs to understand the insertion procedure in order to explain it to patients and to assist the practitioner when necessary.

On rare occasions, a patient may suffer cervical shock or a seizure so the emergency equipment must be accessible. A patient with epilepsy could have a reflex seizure precipitated by the insertion of an IUD.[17] The nursing care of a patient having an IUD inserted is covered in Chapter 12 (Sexual health).

Table 5.5   Insertion of IUD or IUS

Procedure	Rationale
Ensure the patient has an empty bladder	To be comfortable during the procedure
Ask her to remove tights and pants and lie on the couch	For ease of access to the vagina
Cover patient with a disposable paper sheet	To preserve dignity without any risk of cross-infection
Position the light at the foot of the couch and adjust as necessary	To illuminate the introitus
The clinician may perform a bimanual examination using examination gloves	To identify any pelvic abnormalities
A vaginal speculum is inserted and a cervical smear can be taken	To visualise the cervix If a smear is due
If the patient has an IUD in situ, the practitioner removes it with the long forceps and thread retriever if needed	A patient whose threads cannot be retrieved will be sent for ultrasound examination
A fresh, sterile speculum and sterile gloves should be used	To reduce the risk of infection
The cervix is cleaned with a swab held in the sponge-holding forceps and moistened with a cleansing solution	
The tissue forceps may then be attached (not used by all clinicians)	To hold the cervix steady
The uterine sound is inserted through the cervix	To assess the length and position of the uterine cavity
The assistant opens the outer pack of the device selected and drops the contents onto the sterile field	To keep the device sterile until needed and to make sure that it is not wasted if the procedure has to be abandoned
The clinician prepares the device and introducer and inserts it through the cervix into the uterine cavity	The device is drawn inside the introducer and will return to its normal position once the introducer is removed
Sterile anaesthetic gel or local anaesthetic may be used	To prevent pain and aid insertion
The dilators and/or GTN spray may be needed	To help to dilate the cervical canal if there is a problem with insertion
Once inserted, the introducer is withdrawn	Leaving the IUD or IUS in situ
The threads are cut with the long scissors	Leaving them long enough to be shortened later if necessary
The speculum is removed and the patient is allowed to rest until ready to dress	There may be some initial cramp-like pain

> ## Suggestions for reflection on practice
>
> - Review your most recent wound treatments in terms of healing, cost-effectiveness and patient satisfaction. What evidence supported the dressing choices?
> - Review your practice policy and procedure for ear irrigation. Are any changes to procedure needed?
> - Audit the outcomes of minor surgery. Did any patients have infections or healing problems afterwards? Are any changes to procedure needed?

REFERENCES

1. Parliament (1987) *The Consumer Protection Act 1987, Part 1– Product Liability.* HMSO, London.
2. Report of the Committee on Safety of Medicines Working Group on Patient Information (2005) *Always Read The Leaflet: getting the best information with every medicine.* Stationery Office, London.
3. British Association of Dermatologists (2004) *Patient Information Leaflet: keloids.* www.bad.org.uk (accessed 23/9/05).
4. Jones, J. (2005) Winter's concept of moist wound healing: a review of the evidence and impact on clinical practice. *Journal of Wound Care,* **14** (6), 273.
5. Cole, E. (2003) Wound management in the A&E department. *Nursing Standard,* **17** (46), 45–52.
6. Fernandez, R., Griffiths, R. & Ussia, C. (2002) Water for wound cleansing. Cochrane Database of Systematic Reviews, Issue 4. Art. No.: CD 003861.
7. National Institute for Clinical Excellence (2001) *NICE Guidance on Debriding Agents for Difficult to Heal Surgical Wounds.* www.nice.org.uk (accessed 26/9/05).
8. Royal College of Nursing (2005) *Methicillin-resistant Staphylococcus aureus (MRSA): guidance for nursing staff.* www.rcn.org.uk/mrsa (accessed 29/9/05).
9. Turnbull, R. (2003) Management of atopic eczema in children. *Journal of Clinical Nursing,* **17** (6), 34.
10. Whiteford, L. (2003) Nicotine, CO and HCN: the detrimental effect of smoking on wound healing. *British Journal of Community Nursing,* **8** (12), S22–6.
11. Cullum, N., Nelson, E., Fletcher, A.W. & Sheldon, T.A. (2001) Compression for venous leg ulcers. Cochrane Database of Systematic Reviews, Issue 2. Art. No.: CD000265.
12. Harkin, H., on behalf of the Action on ENT Steering Board (2003) *Ear Care Guidance Document.* www.entnursing.com (accessed 30/9/05).
13. British Medical Association, Royal Pharmaceutical Society of Great Britain (2005) *British National Formulary,* 50, 12.1.3. BMA & RPSGB, London.
14. Haas, F. (2003) Ear irrigation: the law and informed consent. *Practice Nursing,* **14** (7), 324–7.
15. British Medical Association (2004) *Minor Surgery: specification for a directed enhanced service.* www.bma.org.uk/ap.nsf/Content/DESsurgery (accessed 1/10/05).
16. Gibbs, S., Harvey, I., Sterling, J.C. & Stark, K. (2003) Local treatments for cutaneous warts. Cochrane Database of Systematic Reviews, Issue 3. Art. No.: CD001718.

17. Epilepsy Action (2005) *Epilepsy and Women – intrauterine device*. www.epilepsy.org.uk/info/contraception.html (accessed 3/10/05).

FURTHER READING

Brown, J.S. (2001) *Minor Surgery: a text and atlas*, 4th edn. Hodder Arnold, London.
Dealey, C. (2005) *The Care of Wounds: a guide for nurses*, 3rd edn. Blackwell Publishing, Oxford.
Dougherty, L. & Lister, S. (eds) (2004) *The Royal Marsden Hospital Manual of Clinical Nursing Procedures*, 6th edn. Blackwell Publishing, Oxford.

USEFUL ADDRESSES AND WEBSITES

Tissue Viability Society
Glanville Centre, Salisbury District Hospital, Salisbury SP2 8BJ
Website: www.tvs.org.uk

Wound Care Society
PO Box 170, Hartford, Huntingdon PE29 1PL
Telephone/fax: 01480 434401
Website: www.woundcaresociety.org

Biosurgical Research Unit (for LarvE maggots)
Bridgend, Glamorgan
Telephone: 01656 75283 Fax: 01656 752830
Website: www.larve.com/resources/

Primary Ear Care Centre
Doncaster Gate Hospital
Doncaster Gate, Rotherham S65 1DW
Telephone: 01709 304987
Website: www.earcarecentre.com/

Chapter 6

Diagnostic and Screening Tests

A practice nurse may undertake a range of investigative and screening procedures, either self-initiated or at the request of a GP. This will depend on local arrangements and guidelines and on the nurse's scope of professional practice. The standards for individual procedures should cover the following areas: nurse education, clinical guidelines, informed consent, health education, emergency procedures, records and management of specimens, and hand hygiene.

Nurse education

Some skills can be learned within the practice but for others training may be accessed through local primary care organisations and teaching establishments. Expert tuition and practice under supervision are needed for cervical screening; in-house training is not recommended. The NHS Cervical Screening Programme published national quality assurance guidelines in 1996.[1] Accredited training in cervical screening is provided through Marie Curie and family planning courses and through postgraduate study. Primary care organisations usually have a cancer lead nurse, who will advise on training available locally. Many programmes for cervical cytology are run almost entirely by practice nurses, who must therefore have a good understanding of the process.

Whatever the test or investigation, nurses owe a duty of care to their patients and must have the competence to perform the procedure satisfactorily, through the appropriate training, supervision and updating. Any equipment used must be maintained and calibrated in accordance with the manufacturer's instructions.

Clinical guidelines

Many practice nurses are given the authority to perform screening tests and to order blood tests for rubella antibodies, serum lipids, glucose, etc. Investigations have a cost implication and therefore decisions need to be made about which patient groups should be offered particular tests. Patients may self-refer for tests they have read about or discovered on the internet, so guidelines are needed to cover such eventualities. The guidelines will specify when the practice nurse should refer on to another health professional. There will also need to be reliable systems in place to react to abnormal test results.

Informed consent

Investigations must not be carried out without the patient's consent. Patients need accurate and detailed information and the opportunity to discuss possible implications of the results of the investigations to be performed. Many tests can only be performed correctly if the patient knows what to expect and can cooperate. It has been accepted practice for over ten years that tests for HIV antibodies are not performed until the patient has been fully counselled and has decided to have the test. However, it has been suggested that this same standard of care should apply equally to any investigation with serious implications because highly active antiretroviral drugs, which prolong life, have now made the diagnosis of HIV infection similar to that of other serious diseases.[2]

Health education

Patients undergoing any sort of test are likely to be concerned about some aspect of their health. Most situations, if sensitively handled, present a chance for health promotion. For example, patients frequently express half-joking hopes that clean equipment is being used for a blood test. Such expressions of concern offer a way of openly discussing worries about blood-borne virus infection. The prevention of coronary heart disease is part of the nurse's health promotion role. A patient attending for an electrocardiogram, even for medical insurance purposes, is likely to be interested in his/her health, so a discussion of the lifestyle factors likely to affect the heart could be appropriate.

Emergency procedures

Familiarity is needed with the local guidelines for dealing with needle-stick injuries, splashes or spillages of blood or bodily fluids, and for coping with a patient who collapses for any reason. Fainting is not uncommon when patients are undergoing venepuncture.

Records and management of specimens

Record keeping is a fundamental part of nursing practice.[3] Pathology forms must be completed accurately and the specimen containers labelled with the correct identification details. Details of foreign travel, fasting, medication or last menstrual period may be needed for specific tests. Failure to provide such details can affect the interpretation of the results. The practice requires a foolproof system for recording specimens sent for testing and results received.

Samples should be placed in sealed specimen bags before despatch to the laboratory. Specimens may be taken which require posting, possibly for insurance, research or other purposes, such as testing for bone marrow donors. The packaging is usually supplied for these and the instructions should be followed to the letter. There are strict regulations covering the way of packing any specimens sent by post.[4] The Royal Mail customer services will advise if there is any doubt about safe packaging.

Biohazard stickers may still be requested by laboratory staff on specimen bottles and forms of patients known to pose a high risk of infectious diseases, although in reality, all specimens should be considered as potentially hazardous and be handled accordingly.

All tests and their results must be entered in the patient's records. Patients must know how they will be notified of the results. Some investigations take longer than others, so a patient asked to telephone for results needs to know how many tests were performed and when the results are likely to be available. The electronic transfer of laboratory results is becoming routine and can save time and assist in the provision of a more reliable service. However, the use of computers will not prevent problems if the system for checking and acting on abnormal results is not robust.

Hand hygiene

Hand washing will not be mentioned in any of the procedures given below because it is taken for granted that qualified nurses are aware of this most important method of preventing cross-infection and will automatically wash their hands before and after hand contact with patients. Gloves should be worn whenever necessary.

LABORATORY TESTS

The laboratory should be consulted if there is doubt about a specimen that cannot be despatched the same day. Some tests give false results if delayed. Urine can be kept in a specimen refrigerator at +4°C overnight. This delay should be noted on the form. Swabs in transport medium can be kept in a cool place but should not be put in the fridge. Some blood samples ought not to be refrigerated. Guidance can be sought, if needed, from the laboratory on the storage of specimens awaiting collection. It is worth cultivating a good relationship with the local laboratory staff. Most pathology departments will supply a list of tests, giving the amounts of sample material needed, the type of specimen bottle and any special requirements, such as timing or diet.

Blood tests

Local pathology departments usually provide phlebotomy training, which is recommended for anyone who takes blood. Larger practices often employ a phlebotomist or a healthcare assistant whose training includes venepuncture but nurses may still need to take blood sometimes.

The following equipment is needed:

- Injection tray
- Vacuum system needles and holders
- Sample tubes and pathology forms, including sealable plastic bag
- Arm cushion with disposable protective cover
- Tourniquet
- Powder-free unsterile latex gloves (alternative gloves if nurse or patient is allergic to latex)
- Alcohol wipes and cotton wool balls or gauze swabs
- Small adhesive plasters/hypoallergenic tape/crepe bandage
- Sharps container and yellow clinical waste bag.

Vacuum systems are considered to be safer than a syringe and needle because blood is drawn directly into the specimen bottles, thus reducing the risk of contact with the patient's blood. Different sizes of double-ended needles are available and the appropriate size should be selected for each patient. Butterfly needles with adapters for vacuum systems may be needed for children or patients with 'difficult' veins. Reusable holders are no longer supplied for venepuncture because of the risks of contamination with infected blood.

Venepuncture

The procedure detailed in Table 6.1 should be followed.

Urine tests

Urine for microbiology

Midstream specimen of urine (MSU)

This test is intended to identify any organisms causing infection inside the urinary tract; hence the need to collect specimens which are uncontaminated by skin and perineal flora. The genital area should be washed and a specimen obtained after the urine flow has started. A sterile receptacle can be used if the patient cannot pass the specimen directly into the sample container. Discussing the collection of an MSU may also provide an opportunity to educate the patient about urinary tract infections and ways of preventing reinfection. Written instructions may also be needed.

Table 6.1 Venepuncture

Action	Rationale
Approach the patient confidently and explain the procedure	To reduce anxiety and to obtain the patient's cooperation and consent
Consult the patient regarding any previously identified problems and allow time to discuss these	To involve the patient in his or her treatment, to identify any factors that may influence the decision to proceed or the selection of a suitable vein
Offer an anxious patient the opportunity to lie down while blood is taken *or* Seat the patient where the arm can be supported; use a small arm pillow if needed	Recumbent patients will be less likely to faint and can be managed more easily if they do. To keep the arm extended comfortably
Verify that all identification details on the request form are correct	To ensure that the appropriate samples are taken from the correct patient
Gather required equipment and position the injection tray appropriately	Equipment needs to be easily accessible but should be kept out of the direct view of an anxious patient
Label blood tubes	With correct patient details
Ask the patient to roll up his/her sleeve or ask to remove the arm from the garment if too tight	To make sure the vein can be accessed easily (tight clothing above the elbow can contribute to haematoma formation)
Attach the double-ended needle to the holder	Vacuum sample tubes can be attached once the needle is in the vein
Apply the tourniquet above the elbow (remember, most patients have two arms so make sure the best site is selected)	To distend the vein in the antecubital fossa (there can be marked difference between the arms in the accessibility of veins)
Cleanse the skin with the alcohol wipe and wait for the alcohol to dry	To remove bacteria from the skin and avoid stinging at the puncture site
Tighten the tourniquet but make sure the radial pulse is still palpable	If the tourniquet is too tight, it can affect serum calcium, lipids and coagulation results. The tourniquet should not be on longer than 2 minutes
Insert the needle at an appropriate angle and keep it still once in situ	Depending on the depth of the vein (too steep an angle might cause the needle tip to pass right through the vein)
Attach each vacuum tube in turn, keeping the needle steady while doing so	Depending on the type of samples needed and to avoid trauma to the vein wall
Attach tubes in the order: • plain tubes • tubes with anticoagulants • other tubes with additives	To reduce the chance of contamination of clotted samples by anticoagulant or other additives

Table 6.1   *(cont'd)*

Action	Rationale
Gently invert each tube upon removal unless clotted sample needed	To mix the blood with the anticoagulant or additive without damaging the blood cells by shaking
Release the tourniquet once the blood begins to flow into the bottles	To release the pressure on the vein and reduce the risk of haematoma formation
Apply a swab over the puncture site and remove the needle and holder. Ask the patient to apply pressure for one or two minutes with the arm straight	Extravasion of the blood at the puncture site can cause bruising or a haematoma (particular care is needed with patients on warfarin or with abnormal liver function, who may bleed for longer)
Dispose of the needle and disposable holder in a sharps bin	To avoid the danger of needle-stick injury
Cover the puncture site with a small sterile adhesive plaster or bandage	To prevent infection and bleeding from the puncture site (use a bandage if patient allergic to adhesives or prolonged bleeding likely)
Ensure that the pathology form and sample tubes have all the correct details	Unlabelled specimens will not be processed, and biochemistry samples with the wrong date may also be rejected
Make sure the patient knows when and how to get the test results	

Clean-catch specimen of urine

When a midstream urine specimen cannot be obtained or is not necessary, the urine can be voided into a clean container. Special collection bags with an adhesive flange can be attached to the genital area of infants but they can be uncomfortable. The bags are expensive but small quantities can be purchased from medical supply firms. A collection pad can be placed in a child's nappy and urine can be extracted from the pad with a 5 ml syringe and transferred to a universal container. However, many laboratories will ask for a clean-catch specimen from children under three years because tests have shown less contamination than with the other two methods.[5] An advice leaflet could be given to explain how to do this.

Urine for cytology

Malignant cells in the urinary tract can sometimes be detected in urine samples. The patient should be instructed to void most of the urine and collect the sample (10–20 ml) towards the end of the stream. A positive test result may be helpful but a negative result cannot be considered definitive.[6] Urine cytology is costly because of the skilled manpower required for analysis. Guidelines are needed for the appropriate use of such tests.[7]

Nucleic acid amplification test (NAAT)

This is an acceptable test for the patient, which can give reliable results.[8] The availability of urine tests for chlamydia or gonorrhoea will depend on the facilities of the local laboratory. All sexually active men and women under 25 will be offered a test as part of a national screening programme for chlamydia, which is in the process of being rolled out across England; the other countries of the UK are likely to follow suit.[9] If a urine specimen for NAAT is requested, the patient should be asked not to pass urine for at least one hour and then to collect the first urine passed to half-fill a special sample container. Any remaining urine can be passed into the toilet. Urine samples should be refrigerated before transport to the laboratory.

Twenty-four hour urine collections

Large plastic containers and instruction sheets for collecting 24-hour specimens can be obtained from the laboratory. The containers for catecholamine analysis contain acid as a preservative and need safe storage. Dietary restrictions are needed before some tests. The patient should pass urine normally at the time of starting the collection and then save all the urine passed over the next 24 hours, finishing at the same time next day. A clotted blood sample may also be requested for serum creatinine if 24-hour urine is collected for creatinine clearance.

Cervical smear (see also Chapter 13)

There is a national call and recall system for all women aged 25–64 years of age in the UK. Practices have to reach a target of 80% or a lower target of 50% of eligible women screened in order to qualify for payments for cervical screening. The success of cervical screening depends on two factors:

• Ensuring that women attend for screening
• Obtaining adequate smears.

Practice nurses can help on both counts, by educating women about the need for screening, by facilitating access to the service and by learning to take good smears gently and sympathetically. Interpreting services may be needed when patients do not understand English and may not have had experience of cervical screening. Education in cultural awareness can have particular significance when dealing with this intimate procedure.

Liquid-based cytology (LBC) is being introduced throughout the country and obviates the need to prepare microscope slides. Samples are collected as previously using a cervical broom instead of a spatula and, depending on the system adopted locally, the head of the device is either broken off or rinsed in the preservative fluid in a sample pot. The vial must be indelibly labelled with the patient's details and sent to the laboratory, together with the usual cytology request form. In most laboratories, the process of slide preparation is automated. Samples are mixed to disperse the cells, blood and mucus are removed and the microscope slide is prepared with a thin layer of cells. Pilot tests have shown a significant reduction in the number of inadequate smears with the new method.[10] All smear takers and laboratory cytologists are being retrained. Eventually, results will be available much more quickly, which can help to lessen the anxiety of women who have the test.

Note: Smear taking cannot be learned from a book; the following is only intended as a reminder.

Equipment required

- Couch with disposable paper cover and good, adjustable, heat-filtered light
- Unsterile examination gloves
- Vaginal specula in a range of sizes (preferably single-use disposable)
- Jug of warm water or examination jelly
- Cervical broom and vials with preservative (according to the local choice of system)
- Cervical brush if needed
- Tissues
- Cytology request form.

Procedure

See Table 6.2.

Note: The smear should be taken first if a cervical swab is also required.

The patient needs to know how she will be notified of the result and to understand the significance of any abnormality.

Problems with inserting the speculum should alert the nurse to possible sexual difficulties that the patient may be encountering. Involuntary contraction of the vaginal wall muscles (vaginismus) can prevent penetration. Sensitive questions about problems with intercourse can be asked and referral made to the appropriate source of help and advice if the patient needs more help than the nurse feels competent to provide.

Swabs

Samples of infected material can be obtained from any accessible part of the body by using a sterile swab stick tipped with cotton wool or synthetic material. Commercially produced swabs are packaged with plastic tubes for transport.

Table 6.2 Procedure for taking a cervical smear

Action	Rationale
Explain the procedure and answer any questions	To obtain consent and to make sure the patient knows what to expect
Check the details with the patient and complete the cytology form	To provide the cytologist with all the relevant information for interpreting the slide and notifying the patient of the result
Note the date of the last menstrual period, hormone contraception or HRT	The microscopic appearance of cells varies during the cycle and with hormonal influences
Enquire about any discharge, abnormal bleeding or pain	Further investigations or medical examination may be needed
Write the patient's details on the sample pot	For identification and correlation with the pathology form in the laboratory
Ensure the room is warm, privacy is guaranteed and the patient has emptied her bladder	To help her relax and be comfortable during the procedure
Ask the patient to remove her undergarments and lie on the couch	
Place a suitable-sized speculum in warm water (at body temperature) if metal *or* Select a disposable plastic speculum	To warm and lubricate it
Position the patient with her knees bent and legs apart, or in left lateral position. Adjust the light	To be able to visualise the vulva and cervix
Put on examination gloves	
Observe the vulva for any lesions, bleeding, discharge or soreness	To detect any abnormalities or signs of infection or disease
Remove excess water from the speculum or use a small amount of lubricant if needed. Do not use near the tip of the blades	Water can macerate the cells and excess lubricant could affect the quality of the cell sample
Part the labia and insert the closed speculum halfway into the vagina. Turn the speculum, gently manoeuvre it and open the blades	To view the cervix without causing discomfort
Withdraw the speculum if unable to visualise the cervix. Digital vaginal examination may be necessary; a different speculum or patient position may be needed. Seek medical advice if movement of the cervix causes pain	To locate the cervix manually before a second attempt Pain on excitation of the cervix could be indicative of an infection
Note the condition of the cervix	To detect any problems, e.g. prolapse, polyps, warts, discharge or abnormal appearance
Pass the tip of the cervical broom through the speculum and with the bristles resting in the cervical os, turn the device through a full circle clockwise five times, using pencil-writing pressure	To obtain cells from the transformation zone – the junction of squamous and columnar tissue where premalignant cells are most likely to be located. The bristles are designed to collect the most material when turned clockwise

Table 6.2   (*cont'd*)

Action	Rationale
Use another cervical broom if a wide ectropion is present	A wider circle of turn may be needed to obtain an adequate sample
Take a second sample with a cervical brush if necessary. Insert the brush into the os with the lower bristles still visible. Rotate the brush through a half turn	The position of the squamocolumnar junction can lie within the cervical canal in later life, the os may be stenosed or the patient may have had previous treatment for abnormal cells. Use according to the local guidelines
Either break or cut the head off the cervical broom(s) and cervical brush (if used) and put both into the specimen vial. *or*	If *SurePath* system is being used
Push the broom vigorously in the preservative against the bottom of the vial 10 times, followed by a further vigorous rinse. Check that no visible cellular material remains and repeat the procedure if necessary. If a brush is used, press the bristles against the side of the vial 10 times and then rinse vigorously and proceed as mentioned above	If *ThinPrep* system adopted
Put the lid on the vial and tighten it to just past the marks on the lid and the vial	The vials will be centrifuged and opened automatically in the laboratory. The vial must be secure enough not to leak but the lid must not be too tight for the machine to undo it
Remove the vaginal speculum, with the blades slightly open, until almost out, noting the condition of the vaginal walls in the process.	To avoid pinching the cervix or trapping folds of skin by closing the blades too quickly
The speculum should be closed when it is removed finally	To minimise discomfort
Place the speculum in a receiver containing water *or*	To prevent secretions from drying if it is to be decontaminated in the surgery
place it in a suitable receptacle *or*	If for return to CSSD
put it into a yellow clinical waste bag.	For incineration if disposable
Invite the patient to get dressed, if a vaginal examination is not needed	Pelvic examination is not recommended for asymptomatic patients.[11] (The practice procedure should indicate the action to be taken if a patient reports abnormal symptoms)
Record any pertinent details on the cytology form	To inform the cytologist of any technical problems, bleeding or observations of the condition of the cervix
Put the form and labelled vial in the appropriate envelope	For dispatch to the laboratory

Once the patient has understood and agreed to the procedure, the swab should be gently rotated in the material for culture and transferred immediately to the container. Swabs are available for both bacterial and viral culture.

Nasal swabs

Moisten the swab with sterile saline solution because the mucosa is usually dry. Organisms will adhere more easily to a moist swab. Rotate the tip of the swab inside the anterior nares. Per nasal swabs may occasionally be needed for the diagnosis of pertussis.[12] Contact the local laboratory for details.

Throat swabs

A good light is required to visualise the throat. A tongue depressor may be needed to see the throat and prevent contamination of the sample if swabbing stimulates the gag reflex. Take the swab from the tonsil area or from any exudate.

Ear swabs

Rotate the swab tip gently at the entrance of the auditory meatus before any treatment drops are used. This will prevent infecting organisms being masked by the treatment drops.

Vaginal swabs

Gently part the labia to visualise the introitus and swab inside the vagina.

Female self-taken vulvovaginal swabs are used in chlamydia screening. Patients should be given a sterile swab and an instruction sheet on how to collect the specimen.

High vaginal swabs

Pass a speculum (as described for taking cervical smears) to visualise the cervix. Swab the discharge in the posterior fornix and withdraw the swab carefully, avoiding contact with the vaginal walls and vulva.

Endocervical swabs

An endocervical swab of any discharge may be collected for culture to test for gonorrhoea. A sample of cells, using a special type of swab, has traditionally been used to test for chlamydia by enzyme-linked immunosorbent assay (ELISA). The cervix is first cleaned with a large-headed cotton wool swab, if provided. The endocervical swab is rotated in the endocervix for 30 seconds, to obtain the specimen. The sample must immediately be placed in the transport container and be stored and transported in accordance with the manufacturer's instructions. However, nucleic acid amplification tests are replacing ELISA as a way of diagnosing infection. The NAAT may be by a urine test or a self-taken vulvovaginal swab, unless a speculum examination is needed as part of routine clinical care, when a cervical swab may be taken. NAATs are more expensive but the results are considered to be more reliable. The decision will be made locally on which type of specimens to collect.[13]

Rectal swabs

Gently pass the tip of the swab through the anus into the rectum. Rotate the swab and withdraw it.

Skin and nail samples

Skin scrapings may be collected for the diagnosis of fungal or other skin infections. A scalpel blade or special foil-wrapped U-blade is used to scrape skin scales onto dark paper or into a sterile container. Samples of hair or nail clippings may also be collected and sent to the laboratory. Mycological sample packs may be obtained from the laboratory or drug companies or be purchased from medical suppliers. A sufficient sample for testing is required for microscopy and culture.

Threadworms

Threadworms lay their eggs outside the anus at night. Either swab the perianal area or instruct the patient/parent to use a piece of clear adhesive tape next to the anus in the morning before bathing or wiping the area, in order to collect ova for microscopic examination. Seal the tape onto a ground glass slide or place it in a universal container for transfer to the laboratory.

Faeces

Patients usually collect specimens of faeces at home. Instruct the patient to empty their bladder and then to pass the stool onto toilet paper without letting it fall into the water in the lavatory pan and then to scoop a small section of the stool into the sterile container provided, using the spoon in its lid. Any remaining faeces should be flushed away.

Alternatively, the patient can use a clean receptacle, such as a potty, lined with toilet paper, pass the stool and transfer the specimen with the spoon. Any remaining faeces should be flushed away. The receptacle should be washed well with very hot water before and after use. Bleach and disinfectants could affect the test result, so should not be used before collecting the specimen. The importance of hand hygiene should be stressed. Care should be taken to avoid contaminating the outside of the specimen container. Samples for microscopy and culture must be taken directly to the laboratory.

Consult the laboratory about special instructions for collecting stool specimens for occult blood or faecal fat. Sometimes patients are asked to perform screening tests for occult blood. An instruction sheet should be given with the test cards. Three tests are requested from different stool samples, usually one a day. A smear of faeces is made in the test window of the card with a special applicator and allowed to dry. All three samples are sent to the doctor or laboratory, sometimes by post.

Practice nurses can provide information on basic hygiene and food handling to all patients with diarrhoea. Food handlers and healthcare staff with gastrointestinal infections must be clear of symptoms for at least 48 hours before returning to work.[14]

Semen

Patients may be required to produce semen samples for infertility investigations or to check the effectiveness of vasectomy operations. The sample of ejaculate should be collected in a sterile, wide specimen container and taken to the laboratory immediately or in accordance with local guidelines.

Sputum

Sputum specimens can be requested for microbiology or cytology. The patient should be given a wide sterile specimen container and asked to produce a specimen of sputum after some deep productive coughing, preferably in the morning before eating or drinking. The physiotherapist may be asked to help patients who are unable to expectorate. Nebulised normal saline can also be used to aid expectoration.

INVESTIGATIONS AND TESTS WITHIN THE PRACTICE

Blood tests

Tests performed on site allow the results to be available more quickly. However, there should be a good reason for not sending samples to a laboratory. National enhanced services provided under the latest GP Contract may be commissioned by a PCO but are not necessarily provided by every practice. Services include the management of diseases, especially in rheumatology, in which drugs need regular monitoring.

Warfarin is being given to an increasing number of patients at risk of blood clots but the risk of over- or undertreatment means that the INR needs to be kept within a set therapeutic level. Anticoagulation monitoring is another national enhanced service, using either laboratory or on-site testing and the adjustment of dosing. A computer program may be used to assist with dosing decisions. All patients having warfarin must understand why they are taking the drug and be given a yellow booklet for recording essential information, test results and dosing instructions. The booklet must be carried at all times. It also contains information about factors likely to affect INR results and what signs to report if any problems arise.

Blood glucose

Commercially produced test strips and meters give accurate results providing they are used correctly.

- Always follow the manufacturer's instructions
- Follow the instructions for quality control and keep records of control tests
- Keep the test strips dry in sealed containers
- Discard out-of-date strips
- Use a drop of blood large enough to cover the test area
- Make sure the meter is calibrated to match the strips
- Keep the meter clean and renew the battery when necessary
- Record results immediately.

The meter must be suitable for multiple patient use. An automatic device makes the fingerprick less painful by controlling the depth and speed of the puncture. A disposable sterile lancet or, preferably, a single-use retractable device must be used for each patient.

Clinical chemistry analysis

Compact microprocessor instruments are available for performing a range of blood tests on site. Point-of-care testing is described as analytical tests performed for a patient by a healthcare professional outside the conventional laboratory setting.[15] There may be advantages to such tests in remote areas without easy access to a laboratory but the advantages should be weighed against the disadvantages and there should be consultation with the pathologist before deciding to proceed. Results can be printed out for the patients' records. The advantages of point-of-care tests, such as INR, HbA1c or lipids, include the saving of time and a reduced number of visits for patients, as well as allowing for immediacy of treatment. Disadvantages include the costs of purchasing and maintaining the machines, as well as the need for robust quality control measures to ensure their accuracy at all times. Pharmacies may also offer testing as part of the development of their services under the new Pharmacy Contract.

Diabetes screening is one example of diagnostic testing, while anticoagulation monitoring is an example of the activities which can be commissioned by a primary care organisation as an enhanced service.[16]

Urine tests

A range of diptests is available for urinalysis. They have a limited shelf life once opened and some are very costly. It pays to select the most suitable product for the tests required because most have to be purchased by the practice. Some combination strips are available in smaller quantities, more suitable for use in general practice. Single-type test strips, e.g. for glucose, albumin and ketones, are prescribable for individual patients. All test strips must be kept dry, with the bottle top replaced immediately after use. The desiccant sachet must not be removed. The type of test done should be specified when recording results. Urine specimens should be emptied into a lavatory or sluice rather than a sink.

Pregnancy tests

Pregnancy tests can be bought in bulk. They detect human chorionic gonadotrophic hormone excreted in urine by pregnant women. This explains the usual requirement for testing the first specimen of the day – the early morning urine (EMU), when the urine is most concentrated. The tests give a result within minutes and are easy to use. The manufacturer's instructions should be followed. The tests are expensive and have to be purchased by the practice, so a policy is needed about using them. Patients can buy their own tests from a pharmacy and if a patient has already had a positive home test, there is usually little point in repeating it unless the patient requests a termination of pregnancy. However, not all patients can afford the expense of a home test. Patients who request tests too frequently may have other concerns about contraception and need help or advice.

The practice should also have a policy for documenting that patients have received the result of their pregnancy tests. Note the salutary tale of a patient who had a miscarriage abroad. She subsequently denied that she had been told she was pregnant and tried to blame the GP practice. The practice nurse knew that she had spoken to the patient on the telephone and had discussed the advisability of going on holiday but was unable to prove it because she had not documented the conversation.

Microscopy

The use of a microscope is mainly limited to looking for pus cells in urine when a urinary tract infection is suspected. Other uses include looking for fungal hyphae in nail or skin scrapings, *Trichomonas vaginalis* in vaginal discharge or for looking at blood smears. The degree of microscope use could depend on the accessibility of a pathology laboratory and on the skill of the operator but it might also provide the opportunity to commence treatment before laboratory results are available.

Electrocardiography

The ECG records electrical potential in the heart muscle as it beats. The various electrical pathways are altered in muscle which has been damaged or where the heart is beating irregularly. These changes give the tracing its characteristic appearance and assist in the diagnosis of cardiac problems. Some machines will even print out a report of the findings. A patient may be asked to exercise under supervision before, or as, the recording is made. This could be dangerous in the absence of full resuscitation equipment and appropriately trained staff so exercise ECGs are usually performed in hospital. Machines vary, so the maker's instructions must be followed. Nurses who have not worked in coronary care require training in the recording and interpretation of ECGs.

Equipment required

- ECG machine
- Disposable electrode patches
- Alcohol skin wipes
- Unused disposable razor
- Ballpoint pen.

Procedure

See Table 6.3.

If there is interference with the ECG tracing:

- It may be caused by other electrical equipment nearby or the metal frame of the couch
- Check that the electrodes are giving good skin contact
- Check that the wires are attached to the correct electrodes
- Check that the machine is on the correct settings, if automatic
- The machine may need servicing.

When all the tracings have been taken satisfactorily, remove the electrodes and invite the patient to get dressed.

Interpreting results

Nurses who perform electrocardiography must be able to recognise an abnormal tracing so that the appropriate actions can be taken before the patient leaves the surgery.

Table 6.3   Recording an ECG

Action	Rationale
Ensure privacy and a warm room temperature	The patient will need to undress and shivering could affect the recording
Make sure the patient knows what to expect and that it will be painless	The wires can look like something from a horror movie and cause tachycardia through unnecessary anxiety
Ask the patient to undress as needed	The chest, arms and ankles will need to be accessible
Assist him/her onto the couch and make as comfortable as possible	So he/she can lie still during the procedure
Apply the electrodes to the wrists, ankles and chest (if the skin is greasy use the alcohol wipes; very hairy skin may need to be shaved in order to achieve skin contact)	To create a good contact between the skin and the electrodes in order to detect the electrical activity as the heart muscle contracts and relaxes
Attach the correct wires to the electrodes	
Begin the recording when the patient is relaxed	Movement can cause an erratic recording
If the machine does not automatically record all the required tracings, follow the maker's instructions for recording leads I, II, III, AVR, AVL, AVF and the six V leads	To detect the electrical impulses from different directions. Twelve-lead recordings are most commonly done in general practice
Record approximately five complexes per tracing, if not done automatically	Adequate for interpretation without wasting recording paper
Record another longer tracing of II (10–12 complexes), if not done automatically	To act as a rhythm strip (lead II is usually closest to the cardiac vector – the direction and strength of electrical voltage of the heart as it contracts)
If not automatically labelled by the machine, mark each trace with the ballpoint pen	To help the reader to identify each tracing and compare it with the norm
Make sure the patient's name, date of birth and date of recording is on the ECG sheet	For filing and comparison with previous recordings

Respiratory function tests

Peak expiratory flow rate (PEFR)

Peak flow meters measure the amount of air that a patient is capable of expelling forcibly from the lungs. It is not the volume of air that is measured but the rate of expulsion. This is directly related to the elasticity of the lungs and the volume of air within the lungs and is measured in litres expelled per minute. The normal varies according to height, sex and age. Tables to give guidance on this are being revised. These guides constitute the predicted levels against which an individual patient's results can be compared. New meters were introduced in 2004 to bring them in line with European Union standard EN13826 and although patients who receive the new meters will be unaware of the change, existing patients will require help to adjust to different readings when replacement meters are prescribed. Peak flow readings can be converted online, but until all patients and clinicians are using new meters, results should be recorded as either EU or Wright. EU scale meters are clearly marked.

Use of a peak flow meter is valuable in the treatment of asthma. Indeed, many patients with asthma are encouraged to keep one at home and to use it regularly. A fall in the peak flow rate may be the first indication of the onset of severe asthma (see Chapter 7 under emergency treatment of asthma, and Chapter 16 under asthma management).

New digital peak flow meters are more compact and easier to carry. They are available on prescription and readings can be downloaded to a computer.[17] Adaptors are available for multipatient use.

The modern equivalent of the Wright's peak flow meter, the Mini-Wright's meter, is a small plastic tube with a scale along the top and a moveable indicator. This type, and similar meters, can be prescribed on FP10. New meters have a yellow scale with blue numbers, so they can be readily identified. Low-range Mini-Wright meters, with a range of 30–400 l/min, display an 'EU' symbol. They are not described as 'EN 13286 compliant' because they do not meet the criterion of measuring up to 800 l/min but EU readings should still be recorded when they are used.

Measuring peak expiratory flow rate with a Mini-Wright meter

See Table 6.4.

If the procedure has been performed correctly or the patient is not too breathless, the indicator will move along the scale and the reading can be taken. The whole manoeuvre can then be repeated twice more, if possible, and the best of the three readings recorded and compared with the predicted level for the patient's age and height. Forced expiration can make a patient feel dizzy so they should be observed carefully throughout the procedure. Patients can be taught to plot their home PEFR readings in a peak flow diary. If a digital meter is used, the manufacturer's instructions should be followed.

Spirometry

Many practices now own a spirometer for measuring lung function. The manufacturer's instructions for the use of the instrument should be followed and training in spirometry is absolutely essential (see Chapter 16 under COPD). Spirometry can be used to differentiate between obstructive and restrictive

Table 6.4   Measuring PEFR

Action	Rationale
Ask the patient to stand up or to sit straight	To allow the maximum expansion of the chest
Ask the patient to hold the meter horizontally and to keep the fingers away from the indicator, which must be set at zero	To allow the indicator to move freely along the scale
Then to take a deep slow breath, place the lips around the mouthpiece and breathe out as quickly and forcibly as possible	To expand the lungs fully and then exhale as quickly as possible into the meter. The point where the indicator stops will indicate the peak flow in litres per minute

forms of respiratory disease. A reversibility test can be performed, by recording baseline results before administering a bronchodilator and postbronchodilation spirometry 15 minutes later. Spirometry is commonly used in the diagnosis of asthma.

A spirometer can record:

- *The vital capacity* – the total amount exhaled normally after a maximum inhalation
- *The forced vital capacity (FVC)* – the amount of air forcibly exhaled after a maximum inhalation
- *The forced expiratory volume (FEV_1)* – the amount that can be forcibly breathed out in one second following a maximum inhalation. Usually, this is more than 75% of the FVC.

The results can be read from the display and compared with predicted levels. Comparisons of the actual recordings with the predicted results for each patient can demonstrate the existence and severity of respiratory disease. A calculator would usually be needed to calculate the results for a hand-held spirometer. Some spirometers make all the calculations and provide a printout together with an interpretation of the results. Some also allow the data to be downloaded to a computer. Spirometers should be calibrated by the manufacturer and serviced annually.

Spirometry may be used in health screening by demonstrating to smokers any existing lung damage and the benefits of quitting the habit. It is essential that an appointment is long enough for the procedure to be performed correctly. Practices which are not willing to commit to the use of time in this way should consider making other arrangements for the tests to be performed.

Forced expiration raises the pressure in the abdomen, chest and eye. Therefore, patients with any of the following conditions should not undertake forced expiratory tests:

- Pregnancy
- Unstable angina
- Recent surgery (especially ENT or eye surgery)
- Recent myocardial infarction or stroke
- Pneumothorax
- Haemoptysis of unknown cause.

Patients should be given written instructions about the test and the preparation needed before carrying it out.

- If possible, bronchodilator drugs should not be used for six hours before the test.
- A heavy meal should not be taken prior to the test.
- Non-restrictive clothing should be worn.
- The patient should have an empty bladder, especially if prone to stress incontinence.

Procedure

See Table 6.5.

False results will be obtained if the patient:

- Starts exhaling too slowly, when forced expiration is required
- Does not inhale and exhale fully
- Stops blowing into the spirometer too soon
- Coughs during the procedure
- Takes another breath while performing the test.

Audiometry

A national programme of screening for newborn babies has been set up, which will usually be undertaken in maternity departments and designated community clinics.[18]

Distraction hearing tests for young children undertaken by health visitors have been shown to be unreliable. Young children suspected of hearing loss may be referred to a hearing clinic. Older patients may be asked to see the practice nurse for a pure-tone audiogram. ENT consultants in some areas are not in favour of audiometry in general practice but where it is performed, the results need to be interpreted correctly. Operators must be fully trained in the use of the equipment. The procedure will usually indicate, in adults and children old enough to participate, a hearing problem that requires further investigation. A history should be noted of any ear infections or injuries, speech or learning problems, or family history of deafness. The ears should be examined and the test postponed until any conditions such as impacted wax or infection have been treated.

Table 6.5 Procedure for spirometry

Action	Rationale
Seat the patient comfortably in an upright position in a seat with arms	The procedure can cause dizziness or faintness so the patient should not be standing
Explain and demonstrate the technique	To get the patient's consent and to ensure the test is performed correctly
Prepare the spirometer. Enter any details requested	According to the manufacturer's instructions
Ask the patient to breathe in as deeply as possible, to seal the lips around the mouthpiece and exhale slowly until the lungs feel empty	To determine the relaxed vital capacity (the nurse may need to press the start button on the machine as the patient begins the inhalation)
Repeat the procedure and proceed if results are acceptable. Record as appropriate	If there is more than a 5% variation between results, the test should be rejected
Ask the patient to repeat the procedure but this time to breathe out forcibly and encourage to continue until the lungs feel empty	To determine the forced vital capacity and FEV_1 (this is a different procedure from peak flow measurement)
Ask the patient to repeat the test at least two more times (but not more than five times). Allow time to recover the breath in between	Three readings should be similar (good reproducibility) with less than 5% variation between FEV_1 results. Too many tests will exhaust the patient and could cause dizziness through reduced CO_2 levels
Record the best results for FVC and FEV_1 as well as the patient's age, height, gender and race (if not programmed in the machine). Or print the results	For comparison with the predicted levels and interpretation of the findings

A pure-tone audiogram entails recording the quietest sound the patient can hear through an earphone in a range of frequencies (usually between 500 and 8000 hertz), working down in 5–10 decibel steps from 60 or 30 dB. A quiet room is needed for the test, preferably soundproofed, with ambient noise levels of less than 35 dB.[19] Soft furnishings will dampen noise levels and appointments for audiometry could be scheduled for a quiet time of the day. Distractions must be avoided, as concentration may be lost. The machine must be checked before use and be serviced and recalibrated at least annually. A record should be kept of the service data.

Children must be old enough to understand what is required and be able to cooperate. They will get bored if the test is prolonged. If it is apparent that a patient, particularly a child, is responding inappropriately, the test should be discontinued and arrangements made for referral to the audiometry outpatients department.

A patient who has obvious hearing loss or an equivocal result should be referred. Some machines print out the results but otherwise they can be plotted by hand. It may be helpful to show patients some examples in graph form of normal and impaired hearing. Some patients might benefit from using a hearing aid. It is better to learn to use them while young enough to adapt. Practice nurses can encourage patients to persevere with their aids to prevent social isolation in later life.

Vision testing

Visual acuity is tested by reading letters of decreasing size at a measured distance from a Snellen chart. The Snellen chart should be attached to the wall and be well illuminated. A patient who normally wears spectacles for distance vision should be tested with the glasses on, with this noted on the record. Special tests, using picture or letter matching, may be used for children who are too young to read or for adults who are illiterate.

Procedure

See Table 6.6.

A person with normal sight can read the largest letter from 60 metres and the smallest letters from four metres. The result of a person reading from six metres distance who can read the sixth line (9 m) is written as 6/9. The test result of a patient with poor vision who can only see the top line is written as 6/60. Patients who cannot see any of the letters on the chart may be tested to see if they can identify hand movements or are able to perceive light.

Table 6.6 Visual acuity testing with a Snellen chart

Action	Rationale
Measure six metres from the chart and ask the patient to stand at the six-metre mark	The chart is designed to be read from this distance
Ask the patient to cover one eye gently	Each eye is tested in turn
Ask the patient to read the letters on the chart, starting from the top letter	To discover the smallest letters which can be read correctly
Record the number of the last complete line to be read accurately	The number on each line indicates the distance from which a person with normal sight can read it
Repeat the procedure with the other eye	

Suggestions for reflection on practice

Consider your role in dealing with tests and investigations.

- Could some of the work be delegated?
- Have you had all the training or updating you need?
- Could the service to patients be improved in any way?

REFERENCES

1. NHS Cervical Screening Programme: Quality Assurance and Training. www. cancerscreening.nhs.uk/cervical/(accessed 6/10/05).
2. Manevi, K. & Welsby, P.D. (2005) Editorial. HIV testing no longer needs special status. *StudentBMJ*, **13**, 133–76.
3. Nursing and Midwifery Council (2004) *Guidelines for Records and Record Keeping.* Nursing and Midwifery Council, London.
4. HSE Advisory Committee on Dangerous Pathogens (2005) *Biological Agents: managing the risks in laboratories and healthcare premises.* Appendix 2 (Table A4). www.hse.gov.uk/biosafety/biologagents.pdf (accessed 13/10/05).
5. Alam, M.T., Coulter, J.B.S., Pacheco, J., Correia, J.B., Ribeiro, M.G.B., Coelho, M.F.C. & Bunn, J.E.G. (2005) Comparison of urine contamination rates using three different methods of collection: clean-catch, cotton wool pad and urine bag. *Annals of Tropical Paediatrics: International Child Health*, **25**(1), 29–34.
6. National Library for Health Question Answering Service (2005) *How reliable is urine cytology in excluding bladder malignancy?* www.clinicalanswers.nhs.uk/ index.cfm?question =1099 (accessed 7/10/05).
7. Allen, D.J., Challacombe, B., Clovis, J.S., Chandra, A., Dasgupta, P. & Popert, R. (2005) Urine cytology: appropriate usage maximises sensitivity and reduces cost. *Cytopathology*, **16** (3), 139–42.
8. British Association for Sexual Health and HIV (2002) *Clinical Effectiveness Guidelines for the Management of Chlamydia trachomatis Genital Tract Infection.* www.bashh.org (accessed 8/10/05).
9. Department of Health (2004) *The National Chlamydia Screening Programme in England.* Stationery Office, London.
10. National Institute for Clinical Excellence (2003) *Guidance on the Use of Liquid-Based Cytology for Cervical Screening.* Technology Appraisal no 69. www.nice.org.uk (accessed 7/10/05).
11. National Library for Health, Question Answering Service (2005) *Is there any guideline available regarding whether pelvic examination should be done simultaneously when women have their routine cervical smear? How useful is this type of examination as a screening tool?* www.clinicalanswers.nhs.uk/index.cfm?question=177 (accessed 12/10/05).
12. HPA (2004) *Investigation of Specimens for Bordetella species.* National Standard Method BSOP 6 Issue 6. www.hpa-standardmethods.org.uk/pdf_bacteriology.asp (accessed 13/10/05).

13. Department of Health (2004) *National Chlamydia Screening Programme in England (NSCP): programme overview (core requirements and data collection).* www.dh.gov.uk (accessed 13/10/05).
14. Prodigy Guidance (2003) *Gastroenteritis.* www.prodigy.nhs.uk/guidance.asp?gt= Gastroenteritis (accessed 15/10/05).
15. Medical Devices Agency (2002) *Management and Use of IVD Point of Care Test Devices.* MDA DB2003(03). www.mhra.gov.uk Device bulletins (accessed 20/10/05).
16. NHS Confederation (2004) *Community Pharmacy: enhanced services.* Community Pharmacy Briefing. www.nhsemployers.org/docs/pha00201.pdf (accessed 20/10/05).
17. Asthma UK (2005) *New Digital Peak Flow Meters.* www.asthma.org.uk/news/news239.php (accessed 21/10/05).
18. Bamford, J., Uusk, K. & Davis, A. (2005) Screening for hearing loss in childhood: issues, evidence and current approach in the UK. *Journal of Medical Screening,* **12**(3), 119–24.
19. Smith, P.A. & Evans, P.I.P. (2000) Hearing assessment in general practice, schools and health clinics: guidelines for professionals who are not qualified audiologists. *British Journal of Audiology,* **34** (1): 57–62.

FURTHER READING

British Association for Sexual Health and HIV (2004) *Recommendations from the Bacterial Special Interest Group of BASHH: testing for sexually transmitted infections in primary care settings.* www.bashh.org/primarycare.htm

British Medical Association (2004) *National Enhanced Service – anti-coagulation monitoring.* www.bma.org.uk/ap.nsf/Content/NESanticoagulation

British Society for Clinical Cytology (2003) *Taking Cervical Smears,* 3rd edn. British Society for Clinical Cytology, Uxbridge.

Department of Health (2004) *Modernising Pathology Services.* www.dh.gov.uk/pathologymodernisation

General Practitioners in Asthma Group (2004) *Spirometry.* Opinion Sheet No 7. www.gpiag.org/opinions/index.php

Houlston, R.J. (2005) The new cervical smear – the implementation of liquid-based cytology. *Practice Nurse,* **30**(4), 40–3.

Medical Device Alert MDA/2004/025 – Peak Expiratory Flow Meter (PFM), all makes. www.mhra.gov.uk

Patient advice leaflet: collecting urine samples. How to collect a urine sample. www.gp-training.net/pal/gyngu/uticoll.htm

Prodigy Guidance (2004) *Fungal (dermatophyte) infection – skin and nails.* www.prodigy.nhs.uk/guidance.asp

Royal College of Nursing (2005) *Chlamydia: an educational initiative for nurses.* Royal College of Nursing, London.

USEFUL ADDRESSES AND WEBSITES

British Society for Clinical Cytology, PO Box 352, Uxbridge UB10 9TX
Website: www.clinicalcytology.co.uk

NHS Cancer Screening Programmes
Website: www.cancerscreening.nhs.uk

NHS Purchasing and Supply Agency Point of Care Testing: Pathology.
Website: www.pasa.nhs.uk/poct/

Mini-Wright peak flow meters
Website: www.peakflow.com

NHS Newborn Hearing Screening Programme
Website: www.nhsp.info/php

Education for Health (new name for National Respiratory Training Centre merged with
    Heartsave)
The Athenaeum, 10 Church Street , Warwick CV34 4AB
Telephone: 01926 493313
Website: www.educationforhealth.org.uk

Chapter 7
Emergency Situations

From time to time life-threatening crises will occur in the practice. Moreover, a practice nurse will sometimes be the only professionally qualified member of staff on the premises when an emergency call is received. She/he may be expected to assess the degree of urgency of the request and to decide on the appropriate course of action. Thorough training in emergency procedures and regular updates are needed for all the frontline staff. The fact that the skills are called upon so rarely makes it even more vital to have annual practice sessions.

Accidents, by their very nature, happen without warning but many of them could be anticipated and prevented. One of the objectives in *Saving Lives: our healthier nation* is a reduction of the death rate caused by accidents by at least a fifth and serious injury by at least a tenth by the year 2010.[1] So, apart from dealing with any emergencies that occur, medical and nursing staff also have a role in educating patients about safety.

GENERAL PRINCIPLES

While a practice nurse is unlikely to encounter situations involving multiple casualties, nevertheless he/she must always be aware that these could happen and first aid skills need to be kept up to date. The general principles in Table 7.1 always apply.

Whether giving advice over the telephone, rendering first aid at the site of an accident or dealing with an incident in the surgery, three factors have priority:

- A *Airway* – must be clear for air entry to the lungs
- B *Breathing* – must be present to oxygenate the blood
- C *Circulation* – is essential for perfusion of the brain and vital organs.[2]

This simple mnemonic can be helpful in an emergency.

Table 7.1   General principles

Action	Rationale
Check that it is safe to approach the casualty	To avoid putting self or others in danger
Maintain a calm manner and take charge confidently	To prevent panic and to resist the pressure to act in haste
Collect as much relevant information as possible	To decide on the priorities for action
Deal with life-threatening emergencies immediately	To maintain the patient's respiration and circulation
Arrange for medical help from a GP or ambulance service if necessary	(Depending on the severity of the problem)

COLLAPSE

Any sudden prostration or loss of consciousness is loosely termed collapse. The reason may be obvious when it happens in the surgery but on other occasions, an assessment of all the clues will be needed. Collapse is more likely to have a cardiac cause in adults than in children. The action to be taken will depend on the cause of the collapse and the age of the patient. Any of the following scenarios could apply. Consult the *Resuscitation Guidelines* for adults and children of all ages.[3] The Resuscitation Council UK guidelines are updated regularly in line with medical evidence. Copies of their most recent guidelines can be obtained via the internet or by post.

Collapsed but conscious patient

- Check it is safe to approach. Look for any signs of danger near the patient.
- Attempt to rouse the patient. Does he/she respond to calling or a gentle shake of the shoulders? Avoid shaking infants because of the risk of brain damage. Shaking of any patient should be avoided if a neck injury is a possibility.
- If the patent is conscious then obtain information about his/her condition, treat as appropriate and summon help if needed. Continue regular reassessments.
- Do not move the patient unless in danger.

Collapsed unconscious patient

Check as above (for collapsed but conscious patient). If there is no response, shout for help then follow the ABC.

Airway

- Check that the upper airway is clear. Leave well-fitting dentures in place but clear the mouth of any obvious obstruction. Blind finger sweeps of the mouth of a child should be avoided because they could cause swelling of the soft tissues or further impaction of a foreign body.
- Open the airway. Tilt the patient's head backwards and lift the patient's lower jaw without moving the neck. Use one finger under the chin and avoid pressing under the jaw of a child because pressure on the soft tissues can obstruct the airway.
- Take care to maintain a neutral position of the head of an infant. Use a chin lift to open the airway.

Breathing

- Check if the patient is breathing normally by looking at the chest for signs of movement, listening for breath sounds and feeling for expired air against your cheek (for no more than ten seconds). Do not confuse infrequent noisy gasps with normal breathing.
- If normal breathing is present, turn the patient into the recovery position, send or go for help and continue to reassess the breathing about once a minute.
- If the patient is not breathing or is making only occasional gasps, follow the adult or paediatric resuscitation guidelines as appropriate. Up to five attempts should be made to give five effective rescue breaths to infants and children.
- An ambulance should be called immediately for an adult and chest compressions started as soon as it established that he/she is not breathing normally.

Circulation

- It is no longer necessary to try and locate the pulse of an adult who is not responsive or breathing normally. A diagnosis of cardiac arrest should be made and chest compressions be started to help maintain the circulation.[4]
- In a paediatric patient, assess the skin colour and look for signs of life, i.e. movement or coughing. Check the carotid pulse if the patient is a child (aged from one year to puberty). The brachial pulse should be used if an infant because babies under one year do not have an obvious neck. Do not spend more than ten seconds searching for a pulse.
- If confident the child has a circulation then continue rescue breathing as necessary and reassess about once a minute.
- Move the patient into the recovery position if spontaneous breathing occurs. Continue to reassess frequently.
- If there is no pulse or sign of life in any child or the heart rate is less than 60 beats/minute, start chest compressions at a ratio of 15 compressions to two rescue breaths.

- Continue resuscitation of a child for one minute and call for an ambulance if no helper is available to do this. Carry the child to the telephone and continue resuscitation measures. In the case of a witnessed sudden collapse, when no helper is available, arrest due to a cardiac arrhythmia should be suspected and an ambulance called before starting resuscitation.

Rescue breathing

In adults, chest compressions should have priority over initial ventilations in cardiopulmonary resuscitation (CPR).

If rescue breathing is being carried out in the practice, a resuscitation mask with a one-way valve would normally be used but it is essential to have had practice in using a mask effectively. This applies equally to the use of a reservoir bag and mask. A mask will cover both the patient's mouth and the nose. If the mask has an oxygen attachment then 100% oxygen should be used. The *Basic Life Support Guidelines* are designed to deal with any eventuality and therefore the procedure will need to be adapted when using resuscitation equipment. The patient's mouth must be clear of obstruction and a clear airway position maintained.

The adult procedure is as follows.

- Pinch the patient's nose to close the nostrils.
- Open his/her mouth slightly but maintain the chin lift.
- Take a normal breath, close your mouth around the patient's mouth to obtain a good seal and breathe steadily into his/her mouth for about one second. There should be only minimal resistance.
- Turn your face sideways and watch the patient's chest fall.
- Take another breath and repeat the sequence to give two effective breaths.
- Check for obstruction and reposition the airway if rescue breaths do not make the chest rise.

The paediatric procedure is as follows.

- *Children* – as for an adult but use only as much air as is necessary to inflate the chest. Blow for one to one and a half seconds and watch for the chest to rise.
- Perform this procedure five times.
- *Infants* – as for a child but breathe into the nose and mouth of a small infant, or the mouth or nose alone of an older one. If the nose is being used, the infant's mouth may have to be held shut to prevent air escaping during the procedure.
- If there is difficulty achieving an effective breath, consider possible obstruction of the airway. Check the mouth for obstruction, reposition the airway (make sure the neck is not overextended) and make up to five attempts to achieve effective breaths. If still not successful then start chest compressions.

Chest compressions

The adult procedure is as follows.

- Kneel beside the patient, level with his/her chest, and place the heel of one hand in the centre of the patient's chest.
- Place the heel of the other hand on top of the first. Extend and lock the fingers, to keep pressure off the ribs.
- Keep the arms straight and press downwards to compress the sternum by 4–5 cm.
- Release the pressure and then repeat the process of compressions at a rate of about 100/minute.

Position the airway and give two effective breaths. Resume the compressions and rescue breaths in the ratio of 30:2 (see Figure 7.1).

The procedure for all children is as follows.

- Locate the xiphisternum at the point where the lowest ribs meet and compress the sternum at one finger's breadth above this point. Pressure applied lower than this is liable to compress the abdomen.
- Depress the sternum to about one-third of the depth of the chest. Use two fingers for an infant and one or two hands for a child, depending on his/her size. Avoid pressure over the ribs.
- Release the pressure and continue compressions at the rate of about 100/minute.

After 15 compressions, position the airway and give two effective breaths. Resume the compressions and rescue breaths in the ratio of 15:2 (see Figure 7.2).

Basic life support

The *Resuscitation Guidelines* give advice about when to go for help. In an emergency in the practice, there would usually be someone else present who would be asked to ring for an ambulance as soon as it is realised a patient is not breathing normally. Details of the patient's age, reason for collapse, if known, and the practice address must be given.

The aim of basic life support is to maintain the circulation of oxygenated blood until advanced life support measures can be taken. Do not stop the resuscitation procedure to check for a pulse (unless the patient moves). Keep going until the ambulance arrives. When more than one trained person is present, the procedure should be taken over smoothly by another person about every two minutes because resuscitation is exhausting. It is essential to maintain the quality of performance and also to minimise any interruptions to chest compressions.

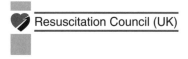
Resuscitation Council (UK)

Adult Basic Life Support

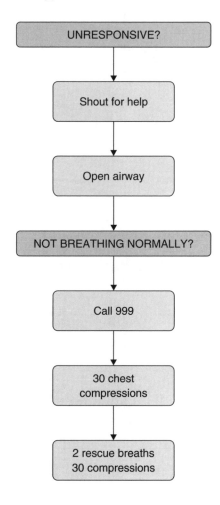

Figure 7.1

ASPHYXIA

Blockage of the airway, so that the brain is starved of oxygen, can occur in ways ranging from inhalation of a foreign body to crush injuries in an accident. Oxygen and suction could be needed. An asphyxiated patient loses consciousness quickly and the face and extremities become cyanosed. Death will follow

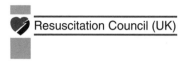

Resuscitation Council (UK)

**Paediatric Basic Life Support
(Healthcare professionals
with a duty to respond)**

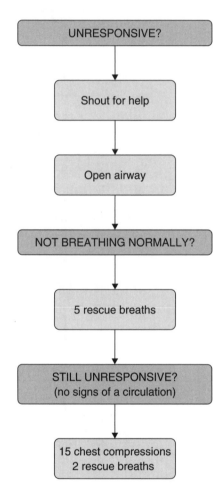

After 1 minute call resuscitation team then continue CPR

Figure 7.2

quickly unless prompt resuscitation procedures are started. The history might make the diagnosis obvious, e.g. the mother sees a child sucking something and the child then chokes and goes blue. However, in other situations such as an unconscious patient, the cause may not be known. A patient who develops respiratory distress while eating could have a foreign body obstruction but be mistakenly thought to be having a heart attack. An ambulance should be called as soon as the severity of the situation has been assessed and emergency help deemed necessary. *The Resuscitation Guidelines 2005* include the procedures for dealing with choking in adults and children.

Choking (foreign body airway obstruction)

A patient who is breathing and coughing should be encouraged to clear the obstruction him/herself. If the obstruction cannot be cleared and the patient cannot cough or speak, intervention will be needed. The aim should be to artificially increase the pressure within the chest cavity to force the expulsion of the obstruction.

Infants (up to one year of age)

- Position the baby across the lap in the prone position, with the head lower than the chest in order to make use of gravity to dislodge the obstruction and make sure it does not pass further down the airway. The head and jaw must be supported to maintain the airway in the open position.
- Tap sharply between the baby's shoulder blades up to five times with appropriate force, to try to dislodge the foreign body.
- If the obstruction is not dislodged, turn the infant into a head-down supine position and perform up to five chest thrusts, using two fingers to compress the sternum at a point one finger's breadth above the xiphisternum. Chest thrusts should be performed more sharply and slowly than those used for cardiac resuscitation. The intention in this instance is to force air out of the lungs in order to expel the foreign body.
- Check the mouth and carefully remove the foreign body if visible.
- If the infant is still conscious, continue the sequence of back blows and chest compressions if the foreign body has not been expelled. Do not attempt abdominal thrusts on an infant because of the risk of rupturing abdominal organs.
- Reposition the airway and check for breathing. If the infant is not breathing, attempt five rescue breaths.
- Start CPR if there is no response.

Children (over one year)

- Position in the prone position, with the head lower than the chest and the jaw supported in the open airway position. A small child should be placed across the lap of the rescuer.
- Give up to five back blows between the shoulder blades to try to dislodge the obstruction.

- If the obstruction has not been cleared, give up to five abdominal thrusts. Stand or kneel behind the child and encircle his/her torso. Place a clenched fist between the umbilicus and the xiphisternum, grasp the hand with the other hand and pull sharply inwards and upwards.
- Check the mouth and remove any visible foreign body carefully. If the obstruction has not been cleared, repeat the entire procedure.
- Reposition the airway and check for breathing.
- If the child is not breathing, try to give five rescue breaths and start CPR.

Adults

- If the patient is conscious, bend him/her forward with the head lower than the chest and support his/her chest with one hand.
- Give up to five sharp blows with the heel of the other hand midway between the patient's shoulder blades to try to dislodge the obstruction.
- If the obstruction is not cleared, perform up to five abdominal thrusts. Stand behind the patient, bend him/her forward and place the fist of one hand on the abdomen between the umbilicus and the xiphisternum. Grasp the fist with the other hand and pull sharply upwards and inwards under the patient's ribcage.
- If the foreign body is not ejected and the patient remains conscious, then continue alternating back blows and abdominal thrusts.
- If the patient loses consciousness, call an ambulance and start CPR even if the patient has a pulse.

A doctor must examine any adult or child who has received abdominal thrusts, in case internal injuries have been caused.

MANAGEMENT OF OTHER EMERGENCY SITUATIONS

Anaphylaxis

Anaphylactic shock is a life-threatening condition caused by an acute allergic reaction. The allergen can cause histamine and other powerful substances to be released from mast cells, which may then cause any of the following:

- Urticaria, flushed or pale skin
- Angio-oedema
- Hypotension due to peripheral vasodilation
- Tachycardia
- Dyspnoea, laryngeal stridor or bronchospasm
- Abdominal pain, vomiting or diarrhoea
- Rhinitis or conjunctivitis
- A sense of impending doom.

Table 7.2   Treatment for anaphylaxis

Action	Rationale
Begin cardiopulmonary resuscitation if needed	To maintain blood and O_2 to vital organs if condition is judged to be life-threatening
Or lie the patient flat with legs raised if this does not exacerbate respiratory distress. The patient should be comfortable	To aid venous return and counter hypotension, although a dyspnoeic patient may not be able to lie down
Administer IM epinephrine (adrenaline) in the appropriate dose (see below)	To constrict peripheral blood vessels to raise the BP and relieve bronchospasm
Repeat epinephrine after five minutes	If there is no improvement in the patient's condition
Transfer the patient to hospital	Delayed reactions may occur. Specialist follow-up is necessary

Anaphylaxis should not be confused with a panic attack or syncope. The pulse, blood pressure and peak flow rates should be recorded if possible.

The action to be taken in such an event must be established in advance, with a protocol and emergency drugs always available. Request an emergency ambulance once anaphylaxis has been diagnosed but initiate the treatment immediately. In May 2005, the Resuscitation Council UK published revised guidelines for community staff on the emergency treatment of anaphylaxis.[5] Every practice should have a copy of these guidelines and the treatment algorithms. There may also be a local anaphylaxis policy, which should be compatible.

Recommended doses of epinephrine (adrenaline) 1:1000 solution:

- Less than 6 months   50 micrograms IM (0.05 ml)
- 6 months–6 years   120 micrograms IM (0.12 ml)
- 6 years–12 years   250 micrograms IM (0.25 ml)
- Over 12 years + adults   500 micrograms IM (0.5 ml).

Epinephrine must not be administered intravenously and half the recommended dose may be safer for patients on imipramine, amitriptyline or beta blockers.

Patients at risk of anaphylactic reactions are often prescribed a disposable self-injection device containing epinephrine such as an *EpiPen* or *Anapen*. The doses in these devices may be slightly different to those given above but are considered to be acceptable. The patient or parent of a child must be aware of how and when to use it. Trainer pens are available for teaching purposes. Devices that allow for incremental dose selection should not be used for children because of the risk of overdosage.[5]

Antihistamines and corticosteroids are also used in the treatment of acute allergic reactions. They are usually administered by a doctor but the anaphylaxis protocols for nurses in some areas include the use of IM chlorphenamine.

If anaphylaxis occurs after an injection or immunisation, save the syringe and vial if possible, in case they are needed for examination. A yellow card reporting an adverse drug reaction must be sent by the GP to the Committee on Safety of Medicines.

Fainting (vasovagal syncope)

Probably the most common cause of collapse in the treatment room is a faint. Most patients get some warning of this. They become very pale and sweaty and feel nauseated; they may become confused, shaky or lose consciousness. The pulse will be slow. If a patient who feels faint lies flat or sits with the head lowered between the knees, this will often prevent the faint from occurring. (**Note**: A very pregnant woman should lie on her side because the enlarged uterus can compound the problem by slowing the venous return.) A patient who has collapsed from a simple faint will quickly recover when horizontal and this can be a useful diagnostic pointer to the cause of the collapse.

If the cause of the faint is not obvious, then the patient should be investigated for a cardiac cause, such as heart block. An ECG should be recorded to detect any conduction defect.

Myocardial infarction

Patients with severe angina or a frank myocardial infarct will sometimes arrive in surgery unaware of how ill they are. The classic symptoms are severe, crushing, central chest pain with or without radiation to the jaw and left arm. The patient may feel very unwell and look pale and sweaty. However, these gross symptoms are not always present and a patient may collapse without warning. In either case, assess the situation and call for an ambulance and a doctor, if he/she is in the surgery. If the patient is conscious, obtain as much information as possible to help make the diagnosis. Sit the patient in the most comfortable position to assist his/her breathing and if the patient carries glyceryl trinitrate or similar medication, administer a dose and encourage him/her to rest.[6] If MI is suspected give the patient one aspirin (300 mg) to chew, for its antithrombotic effect (if not severely allergic to aspirin). Check the pulse and blood pressure to monitor progress and identify a deteriorating condition. Record an ECG and insert an IV cannula, if within the nurse's competence to do so.

In the event of cardiac arrest, follow the procedure set out above (under Collapse). Prompt defibrillation during the early stage of myocardial infarction is most likely to lead to a successful outcome. All practices are recommended to have an automated external defibrillator, with the staff trained to use it. An audit should be made of the outcome of all emergencies. Cardiopulmonary resuscitation is an appropriate subject for 'critical incident debriefing' within any practice.[7]

If an emergency telephone call is received for a patient who has collapsed at home with symptoms suggestive of a myocardial infarction, then call an emergency ambulance immediately.

Transient ischaemic attack (TIA)

Most TIAs, also called mini-strokes, are caused by emboli, which lodge in small arteries of the brain. Thrombi can develop in the atria of patients with atrial fibrillation because the heart chambers are not contracting properly. Small clots break off and travel as emboli. Similarly, platelets can aggregate over atheromatous plaques in the carotid or other main arteries and result in platelet emboli. A TIA can manifest any of the symptoms of a stroke. However, the effects are not permanent. Recovery can take any time up to 24 hours as the embolus disperses but the process is likely to be frightening for the patient and carers.

A proportion of patients who have a TIA subsequently proceed to have a stroke, so the condition should be taken seriously, investigated and treated accordingly.[8] The blood pressure and pulse rate should be recorded and referral made to the GP or hospital. Prophylactic aspirin, antiplatelet drugs or warfarin may be prescribed. Atrial fibrillation and carotid artery disease are likely to require medical or surgical treatment.

Cerebrovascular accident (stroke, CVA)

Another of the targets in *Saving Lives: our healthier nation* is the reduction of the death rate from stroke in people aged under 75 by at least two-fifths by 2010. Identifying people at risk, controlling hypertension, diabetes and hypercholesterolaemia, giving prophylactic aspirin and promoting healthier lifestyles may achieve this. However, the unfortunate patients who do suffer a stroke will need appropriate care.

A cerebral thrombosis, embolus or haemorrhage can cause a cerebral catastrophe resulting in unconsciousness, hemiparesis or hemiplegia. The action to take if it occurs in the surgery is that for a collapsed patient. If it occurs at home, the relatives should be advised to make the patient as comfortable as possible wherever he/she is lying, to maintain a clear airway and to turn the patient into the recovery position if unconscious and breathing. Prompt treatment can save lives and the public are being encouraged to recognise the signs of stroke and to act quickly.[8] Facial weakness, arm weakness or speech problems are the signs likely to indicate a stroke. An emergency ambulance should be called immediately. In an ideal world, patients would be diagnosed and treatment be initiated within three hours of a stroke. The National Service Framework for Older People aims for a reduction in the incidence of stroke and to ensure prompt access to integrated stroke care services for people who have had a stroke.[9]

Table 7.3   Treatment for epileptic seizure

Action	Rationale
Give the patient as much room as possible and try to ease the fall	To prevent injury from hitting furniture or sharp corners without trying to restrain him/her
Protect the patient's head with a pillow if possible	To prevent unnecessary trauma
Do not attempt to wedge anything in the patient's mouth	More damage is likely to be caused to the patient and there is a danger of being bitten
Note the time and sequence of events	To aid the diagnosis and treatment, especially if a first seizure
Once the seizure is over, check the airway and breathing	As described above
If breathing, move the patient into the recovery position once the seizure is over	To protect the airway until consciousness is regained

Convulsions

Epileptic seizures

A generalised seizure can be frightening for both the patient and any onlookers. A practice nurse's role can involve more than simply helping a patient who has a seizure in the surgery. Some practice nurses are using their expertise to give longer term support to patients with epilepsy and their families. The Quality and Outcome Framework of the new GMS Contract includes quality indicators for the monitoring of patients with epilepsy. In the event of a tonic-clonic seizure in the surgery, the principles are straightforward (Table 7.3).

Once consciousness has been regained and the patient is talking coherently, he/she can go home with a friend or relative, after verifying some details. The nurse must check whether the patient is taking medication regularly and has an adequate supply. A medical examination is needed for any patient after a first, an unexplained or a prolonged seizure. A doctor may administer rectal diazepam to a patient having a seizure, so the emergency drugs should be available. Transfer to hospital should be arranged if repeated or uncontrolled seizures occur, or the patient does not regain consciousness after ten minutes.

Febrile convulsions

Babies and young children may develop convulsions in response to a febrile illness. A child will usually look hot, flushed and obviously feverish, with violent uncoordinated movements. He/she may be cyanosed from breath-holding and have twitching of the face and rolled-up eyes. The condition is most common between the ages of six months and six years.

Table 7.4   Treatment for febrile convulsions

Action	Rationale
Remove excess clothing and check if the parents have administered paracetamol or ibuprofen	To prevent overheating and to lower the body temperature with antipyretic treatment
Position the child on something soft	To prevent injury during convulsive movements
Explain to the parents what is happening	They are likely to be alarmed
Once the convulsions are over, check the child's airway and breathing and place in the recovery position	To keep the airway open and prevent the inhalation of any vomit
Arrange for the child to be transferred to hospital if no doctor is immediately available	To identify and treat the cause of the infection

Tepid sponging has been the traditional method for lowering the body temperature and is still recommended by first-aiders.[10] Physical methods of cooling such as fanning, cold bathing and tepid sponging are now considered to be of minimal benefit and may cause discomfort.[11] Parents can be given printed information about the condition to reassure them that the condition is caused by a feverish illness and is not a sign of epilepsy. The Prodigy Guidance on febrile convulsion contains a patient information leaflet.

Head injury

A doctor must examine a very young child and any patient who has been unconscious after a head injury. However, a practice nurse may sometimes see an active, alert child whose mother wants reassurance after the child sustained a fall or blow to the head. The assessment of a head injury should include the following.

- Establish the circumstances of the injury
- Ensure there was no loss of consciousnes, or any other injuries
- Find out if the patient remembers what happened
- Find out whether the patient has felt dizzy or nauseated, or has vomited
- Check that vision is normal
- Check for sign of cerebral compression (e.g. fixed, dilated pupil)
- Check for CSF leaking from the nose or ears.

Cerebral compression may occur at the time of injury as a result of trauma and bleeding into the brain, but can also develop some time after a head injury if a chronic subdural haematoma forms. Clear instructions about what signs to look for must be given before a patient goes home. Children should not be prevented from going to sleep as normal but the parent could be advised to try and rouse the child after an hour or so and to observe that the child is breathing normally.[12] Mild headaches, dizziness or irritability are not unusual after a head injury. The patient must go to the hospital accident and emergency department for assessment if the symptoms persist or get worse, or if severe vomiting, limb weakness, severe drowsiness, confusion, increasing irritability, convulsions or photophobia develop.

If there is any reason to suspect non-accidental injury, then the local child protection guidelines should be followed.

Hypoglycaemia

Patients with diabetes treated with insulin are always at risk of developing hypoglycaemia and should be aware of this. Part of their education about diabetes is to explain the risks of hypoglycaemia to each patient and his/her family. They should know the early signs so that action can be taken before unconsciousness supervenes.

The first sign of an impending hypoglycaemic attack is usually a feeling of faintness and hunger. This quickly passes on to confusion, aggressive behaviour and finally coma. The patient is pale, sweating and restless. Occasionally convulsions can occur, which might be mistaken for an epileptic seizure. The hypoglycaemic coma is a true emergency because the longer the patient is unconscious, the greater the risk of permanent brain damage from the low blood sugar. Thus the aim of immediate treatment is to raise the blood sugar to a normal level by the following means.

- If the patient is conscious give 10–20 g of easily digested carbohydrate, e.g. two to three teaspoons of sugar or glucose, three glucose tablets or 50 ml of non-diet *Lucozade.*
- *GlucoGel* (previously called *Hypostop Gel*) 9.2 g glucose in a 23 g oral ampoule, can be squeezed inside the patient's cheek, to be absorbed through the buccal mucosa.
- Follow up with 10–20 g of complex carbohydrate once the patient has recovered, e.g. 1–2 digestive biscuits or 150–300 ml of milk. Alternatively, the patient should be advised to have a snack or meal if it is due.
- Intramuscular glucagon can be given to an unconscious patient, followed by 30 g carbohydrate once consciousness is regained, to restore the liver glycogen. A prescription or a Patient Group Direction will be needed for administering glucagon.
- The GP may need to give intravenous dextrose if all else fails.

The patient should be reviewed after a hypoglycaemic incident, to try and identify the cause and see if adjustments are needed to the treatment, diet or lifestyle. Patients who are prone to hypoglycaemia should wear or carry something to identify them as having diabetes, e.g. a MedicAlert bracelet or medallion.

RESPIRATORY PROBLEMS

Hyperventilation

Overbreathing can be associated with anxiety or emotional distress. Rapid, deep breathing can cause faintness, trembling and carpopedal spasm as carbon dioxide is breathed out and the acid/base balance is disturbed. The symptoms can cause further anxiety and so exacerbate the problem. A firm but quiet manner should be adopted. Take the patient to a quiet room, to help him/her to calm down. Try to establish what has happened. Other causes of respiratory distress need to be ruled out. Rebreathing carbon dioxide in expired air will restore the PCO_2 to its correct level, so if necessary, the patient can be encouraged to breathe in and out of a paper bag. Once the patient has recovered, help can be offered to try and deal with the underlying problems.

Acute asthma

There are always likely to be some patients who require emergency treatment for an acute attack of asthma, despite the general improvements in asthma management. Practice nurses should have a protocol to follow in the event of an emergency when a doctor is not present. The following should be assessed.

- Age of the patient and previous history – is the patient known to have asthma?
- Details of the present episode – duration and any treatment already taken. Are there any known trigger factors?
- Degree of respiratory distress – is the patient able to talk?
- Are accessory muscles being used to breathe?
- Is the patient cyanosed?
- Peak expiratory flow rate (in comparison with the predicted level) if able to use a PEFR meter (see Chapter 6).
- Pulse and respiration rates – there may be tachycardia and rapid respiration.
- Chest sounds (if the nurse has been taught to use a stethoscope).
- Pulse oximetry (if the surgery owns a pulse oximeter).

Beta-agonist treatment can be administered by repeated activations of a metered dose inhaler through a spacer to adults without life-threatening features of acute asthma (e.g. 4–6 puffs inhaled individually and repeated at 10–20 minute intervals if necessary). This is also the preferred delivery option for

Table 7.5   Treatment for acute asthma

Action	Rationale
Call for medical help (or an ambulance if the patient's condition warrants it)	This could be a life-threatening medical emergency
Administer salbutamol via a large-volume spacer or nebulise with salbutamol (2.5 mg for children, 5 mg for adults)	For the relief of bronchospasm See *BTS/SIGN Guidelines*
Monitor the patient's pulse and appearance while using the treatment	To detect any changes or deterioration in the patient's condition
Recheck the PEFR, pulse, respiration and chest sounds after 15 minutes	To determine the effectiveness of the treatment
Give high-flow oxygen to patients over two years with severe or life-threatening acute asthma	If oxygen available in the surgery
Call for an ambulance if asthma appears life-threatening or fails to respond to bronchodilators	See *BTS/SIGN Guidelines*

children with mild to moderate asthma, the dosage depending on the severity (e.g. 2–4 puffs every 20–30 minutes, up to 10 puffs for severe asthma).[13] A spacer with a facemask should be used for children under three years. A greater amount of bronchodilator will be inhaled if a child is breathing normally and is not screaming. A nebuliser should be used for patients with severe asthma. Ideally, this should be oxygen driven but as this is unlikely to be available in general practice, a motor-driven nebuliser should be used. Inhaled ipratropium bromide is recommended to be added to salbutamol for adults and children with very severe acute asthma.

Once the bronchospasm has been relieved, the patient should see a doctor or be treated by an experienced asthma nurse. Steroids are commonly needed to deal with the inflammation of the airways. Admission to hospital may be necessary but in any event, the patient will need a follow-up appointment (see Chapter 16 under asthma management). Patients who have had near-fatal asthma or who have brittle asthma require specialist supervision. The *BTS/Sign Asthma Guidelines* specify the symptoms and behavioural or psychosocial factors that could result in death from asthma.

Single-patient use nebuliser attachments must be replaced after use.

HAEMORRHAGE

Most cuts and minor haemorrhages will soon stop if simple pressure is applied to the site of bleeding. Gloves must be worn when dealing with any bleeding because of the risk of blood-borne infections. Patients with severe bleeding should be transferred to hospital by ambulance.

Arterial bleeding

The bleeding will be profuse if an injury has severed an artery. The blood will be bright red and pumping out of the wound. If there is no foreign body embedded in the wound then direct pressure should be applied, followed by elevation of the affected limb, providing a fracture is not suspected. Large objects embedded in a wound should not be removed because of the risk of causing further bleeding.

Occasionally, pressure will have to be exerted over the artery supplying the wound area. For example, in the groin, compress the femoral artery against the symphysis pubis or in the upper arm, compress the brachial artery against the humerus. If the blood volume is reduced significantly, the patient will become shocked, with a weak rapid pulse and hypotension. Urgent transfer to hospital will be needed. Meanwhile lay the patient down and elevate his/her legs, if possible, to aid venous return. Make sure there is no tight clothing and keep the patient warm but not overheated. Do not give anything to drink because an anaesthetic may be necessary, or vomiting could obstruct the airway if consciousness is lost.

Varicose veins

Occasionally a patient with varicose veins will knock his/her leg and puncture a vein. The bleeding is impressive but being venous, the blood is darker, slower flowing and not pumping out. The wound itself may be almost invisible but still bleed copiously. The treatment is simple: lay the patient down, put a gauze pad on the wound, elevate the leg and wait for the bleeding to stop. After the patient has been lying down for half an hour with the leg elevated, a firm pad and bandage can be applied and the patient may go home if medically fit. An appointment should be made for review of the wound. The management of varicose veins and the use of support stockings can then be discussed.

Haematemesis

Haematemesis is unlikely to occur in the surgery but occasionally a nurse may be consulted about an episode of bleeding. An ambulance should be called in an emergency but whenever possible, a full history should be obtained, which includes:

- *Medication* – non-steroidal antiinflammatory drugs, steroids and warfarin can cause gastric erosion

- *Previous indigestion or peptic ulceration* – could be an ulcer or a recurrence
- *Alcohol intake* – cirrhosis of the liver, associated with alcohol abuse, commonly causes oesophageal varices
- *Unexplained weight loss* – could be caused by a carcinoma
- *Recent epistaxis* – swallowed blood from the posterior nasal space can be mistaken for haematemesis.

Most episodes of vomiting blood are significant but not desperately urgent, unless a large and obvious quantity of blood has been lost, when the patient will rapidly become shocked. This situation requires urgent hospital admission but more minor cases can be reassured and rested until a doctor can assess them. Referral may be made for upper GI endoscopy.

Melaena

Bleeding within the bowel can often be overlooked in a patient who collapses from no apparent cause. A more common presentation is unexplained iron-deficiency anaemia. NSAIDs are a common cause of gastrointestinal bleeding, especially in the elderly. Stool samples for occult blood may be requested if bleeding is suspected. The traditional black, tarry stool of severe melaena makes recognition of the problem easy for the doctor or nurse. Patients with frank melaena require further investigations in hospital. A doctor should examine all patients with unexplained bleeding. Diverticulosis is common in elderly patients. Bright blood may come from haemorrhoids but the possibility of a malignancy should always be considered, especially if the patient reports a change in bowel habits.

Constipation resulting in anal fissure is a common cause of rectal bleeding in children but non-accidental injury should be considered if a child has bleeding without an identifiable cause.

Table 7.6   Treatment of epistaxis

Action	Rationale
Seat the patient with his/her head forward over a bowl or receiver	To prevent blood from running down the back of the throat
Instruct the patient to pinch the fleshy part of the nose between his/her finger and thumb for a timed ten minutes and to breathe through the mouth	To compress the bleeding point long enough to allow clotting to take place
Use a clock or watch to measure the time	It is not possible to guess the time accurately enough

Epistaxis

Nosebleeds are very common, particularly in children. A practice nurse may have to give advice over the telephone or deal with the situation in the surgery. A calm manner will help to reassure the patient.

This action will stop a very high proportion of nosebleeds in children and some adults. A clot that has formed in the nostril should be left alone and not blown out, as this will restart the bleeding. Recurrent nosebleeds in children are often due to a dilated single capillary in the lower part of the nasal septum. Excessive dryness of the mucosa and trauma, including nose picking, can lead to bleeding. The treatment may be by antiseptic creams. Silver nitrate cautery has been shown to be painful and bilateral cautery risks perforating the nasal septum.[14]

In adults, the bleeding sometimes occurs from higher up the nose and may be precipitated by the rupture of a small arteriosclerosic capillary. Hypertension should be ruled out as a cause of a nosebleed. It is necessary to record the blood pressure and pulse. As well as identifying hypertension, this can become useful information if the bleeding becomes profuse. An INR blood test should be taken from a patient on anticoagulants. Patients with bleeding disorders who develop epistaxis need urgent medical treatment. If the simple pressure technique does not stop the bleeding, then the nose may need to be packed, either by a doctor in the surgery or in an ENT department. Occasionally a patient will need hospital admission if the bleeding will not stop.

POISONING

Young children will put anything in their mouths. An anxious parent may rush to the surgery for help when an accident occurs. If a patient is unconscious or

Table 7.7   Treatment of poisoning

Action	Rationale
Do not try to induce vomiting	Caustic substances can cause further damage to the oesophagus, and volatile substances may affect the lungs
Consult NHS Direct for advice about common poisons or suspected overdose	If there is no GP available
Consult the TOXBASE database of the National Poisons Information Service	For information about the risks and management of the poisoning incident. The practice is advised to be registered with the service
Consult the regional poisons information centre	If more specialised advice is needed
Save any vomit	In case it is needed for analysis

known to have ingested a really hazardous substance, then call for an emergency ambulance immediately. Otherwise, try to calm the situation and collect as much information as possible, including what was taken, how much and when.

This action would apply equally to adults who have been poisoned, either accidentally or through drug overdose. The abuse of alcohol, drugs and solvents should be considered as a possible cause if a patient collapses suddenly.

PAIN

Individuals have different tolerance levels for pain but a patient who attends the surgery with symptoms of pain will require a careful assessment. The nerve pathways and factors which influence the perception of pain are complex. The method of pain relief will vary with its cause and if a nurse is required to assess a patient's pain, the following points should be considered.

- *Type of pain* – constant or intermittent, throbbing, burning, stabbing.
- *Onset and duration* – how long has the patient been in pain?
- *Does anything help* – position, analgesics, antacids?
- *Intensity of pain* – on a scale of 1–10, with 1 as very mild and 10 as the worst pain imaginable.
- *Localisation* – can the patient show where the pain is?
- *Appearance* – posture, tension of facial muscles.
- *Local signs* – swelling, bruising, inflammation, deformity of joints.
- *Previous history* – e.g. of cancer, which might indicate metastases.

Mild pain may be amenable to self-medication with simple analgesics, such as paracetamol. Localised pain from a wound may be relieved once it is dressed or from an abscess once it is drained. Referral to the doctor will be necessary for patients with more severe pain. Alternative therapies may be effective in relieving chronic pain. Some practice nurses are developing expertise in reflexology, therapeutic massage or acupuncture.

TRAUMA AND MINOR INJURIES

Many of the conditions seen by a nurse in general practice will be minor injuries but they are included in this chapter because a few will have the potential to be life-threatening or to cause permanent disability. A practice nurse who treats a patient following an injury has a duty to ensure that the patient receives the most appropriate advice and treatment. A doctor should be consulted if there is any doubt about the diagnosis or management. Detailed records should be made, including diagrams of the injuries, in case a legal report is requested later. The possibility of non-accidental injury should always be borne in mind if the history is not consistent with the injury, if there has been a delay of more than 12 hours in seeking treatment or there are any other grounds for suspicion.

Whenever a patient sustains a tetanus-prone wound, the patient's antitetanus immunisation must be checked and a booster or primary course given if needed Antitetanus immunoglobulin may be needed in some instances.

Abrasions

The superficial skin loss caused by friction can be very painful because the sensory nerve endings in the skin are exposed. Thorough cleaning of the wound with water or saline is needed because residual grit can discolour the skin after healing. It may be possible to remove some particles from the wound by using fine splinter forceps. Wounds with deeply embedded dirt, especially on the face, may need to be cleaned under anaesthetic to prevent 'tattooing' of the skin.[15]

A suitable dressing will be needed to protect the wound and promote epithelialisation (see Chapter 5 under dressings).

Cuts (lacerations)

The arrest of haemorrhage is discussed above. Most simple cuts can be sutured in the treatment room. In general, all wounds which are gaping, especially on the scalp, fingers and over joint surfaces, will need suturing. However, wounds more than six hours old may have to be left to heal by secondary intention because of the risk of infection.[16] If there is any likelihood of damage to a deeper structure, such as a tendon, then the patient should be seen by a GP or referred to the A&E department. Some nurses have been taught to suture, and may be authorised to do so in the surgery. Reimbursement for purchased sutures and local anaesthetics can be claimed on prescription as personally administered items. The use of sterile adhesive strips has reduced the number of injuries that need suturing, although only one size of strips is available on NHS prescription. Tissue adhesive is also suitable for superficial small wounds. The glue is expensive but is now available on prescription. Training is needed in the technique of using skin tissue adhesive. It must not be used near the eyes and any bleeding must be stopped before application. Both the sterile strips and tissue glue obviate the need for local anaesthesia so less pain is caused, which is particularly useful in children. The disadvantages include the need to keep the wound dry and to avoid picking at it while healing occurs.

Pretibial lacerations are commonly seen in elderly patients, many of whom have very friable skin. Such wounds are rarely suitable for suturing but may be closed with adhesive strips, after careful cleaning, if the skin edges can be brought together. A dressing that will not stick to the wound should be applied. A crepe or elastic tubular bandage should be applied from toes to below knee to help reduce swelling of the leg and the patient should be advised to rest with the leg elevated.

Burns and scalds

The immediate first aid treatment for a burn or scald is to immerse the affected area into cool, preferably running, water for 20 minutes. This will considerably reduce the amount of tissue damage produced by heat but ice or very cold water should be avoided because of the risk of vasoconstriction, leading to further damage to the tissues, or of hypothermia.[17] If redness only has occurred and the area is small then probably no treatment except analgesia will be needed. An emollient cream will prevent itching as the skin heals. Sunburn is commonly seen in the treatment room as a first- or even second-degree burn. Soothing creams or after-sun lotion may be sufficient, if blistering has not occurred. A patient with severe sunburn should see a doctor.

When blistering occurs after a burn or scald, small blisters should be left intact if possible, but larger blisters may have to be drained or deroofed. A suitable dressing should be applied if it is needed. Low-adherent dressings and film dressings are suitable for burns with little exudate. Wounds with larger amounts of exudate require padding in order to avoid 'strike-through', which can increase the risk of infection.

Patients who have extensive or deep burns should be treated in hospital. Full-thickness burns will require skin grafting.

Soft tissue injuries

More frequent soft tissue injuries are likely to be seen, as patients are encouraged to take more exercise. They need to be given advice about sensible exercise for their age and general condition and to understand the reason for doing warm-up exercises. Muscle injuries are called strains and ligament injuries are known as sprains. They cause swelling, bruising and pain in the affected tissues. The history will often make the situation clear. Sometimes a fracture may also be suspected and must be treated accordingly. Patients with severe injuries should be sent to hospital. The *Prodigy Guidelines* outline the circumstances that might arouse the suspicion of domestic violence.

The initial treatment for a minor soft tissue injury includes:

- *Rest* – to avoid further damage to the tissues
- *Ice* – to constrict peripheral blood vessels to reduce bruising and oedema, e.g. a small pack of frozen peas or purpose-made cold pack applied for 10–20 minutes 3–4 times a day
- *Compression* – to reduce the swelling and provide support, e.g. crepe bandage or double tubular elastic bandage (*Tubigrip*)
- *Elevation* – to drain oedema by gravity and relieve pain
- *Analgesia* – if needed for pain. Paracetamol is the first-choice drug but ibuprofen may be used for its antiinflammatory effect if necessary[18]

- *Early mobilisation* – after two days' rest. Patients may be referred to a physio-therapist for treatment.

Fractures

Patients who have an obvious fracture will usually be transported directly to an accident and emergency department. However, minor fractures may be presented in the treatment room, often associated with other trauma such as bruises, sprains or lacerations. Particular care is needed with hand injuries because lasting deformities could result if not treated adequately. It is important to check that the tendon has not been affected in a finger injury. If there is any tenderness in the snuffbox area (the hollow between the base of the thumb and index finger) the injury must be treated as a scaphoid fracture until proved otherwise. These fractures cannot always be seen radiographically and a missed fracture could cause a long-term problem to the hand.

An injured toe or finger can be made more comfortable by strapping it to its neighbour, which acts as a splint. A piece of gauze should be used as padding between the digits and a strip of elastic adhesive tape applied above and below the joint. Tape should not be applied too tightly to avoid creating a tourniquet effect and direct contact with the skin should be avoided if the patient is allergic to the adhesive.

STINGS AND BITES

Human and animal bites can often become infected, so the patient may need antibiotics as well as treatment for the wound. The wound should be irrigated thoroughly with normal saline. Primary wound closure is not usually recommended because of the risk of infection but facial wounds or larger lacerations may need to be closed for cosmetic reasons.[19] Patients with serious wounds should be sent to hospital.

Tetanus immunity should be checked and in the case of human bites, the patient may also require immunisation against hepatitis B or antiretroviral drugs if infection with a blood-borne virus is possible. The local public health department should be contacted for advice if there is a cause for concern. Rabies prophylaxis should be considered if an animal bite occurred abroad.

Insect bites

Insect bites are usually easy to recognise as the lesions are single or in a cluster, and very irritating. Some bites cause a blister to form in the centre of the area bitten. Bites from insects such as gnats and midges only need treatment to relieve the symptoms. Recurrent bites suggest an infestation and the eradication of the source, such as fleas, is needed. Animal fleas do not usually bite humans if their animal host is available but if a pet has recently died or a patient has moved into an empty house recently, then that could suggest the cause of bites.

Uncomplicated bites can be treated with crotamiton cream or lotion to relieve itching; 1% hydrocortisone cream plus antihistamine tablets may be suggested if the irritation is intense. The risk of malaria should be considered if a patient returns from a tropical area with mosquito bites. Patients need to understand the reason for completing any malaria prophylaxis regime.

Wasp and bee stings

Insect stings usually cause pain in the lesion but require little treatment in the majority of cases. A bee may leave the sting behind and this will need to be removed as soon as possible. Grasp the sting horizontally with forceps, below the poison sac, as close to the skin as possible and lift the sting out without squeezing the sac. Topical applications of a sting relief product can provide reassurance and may ease the discomfort. Analgesics and a cold compress can also be helpful. Hydrocortisone cream 1% will help to reduce the local inflammation and antihistamine tablets may be needed if the reaction is more severe. If a patient is stung in the mouth, ice should be given to suck to reduce the swelling. Transfer to hospital should be arranged if there is any risk of oedema obstructing the airway. An anaphylactic reaction can occur in rare cases of severe allergy. Patients to whom this has happened should carry adrenaline with them everywhere throughout the summer months, and know what to do in an emergency.

Ticks

These little insects are found in long grass and woodlands. They feed off animals and can attach themselves to exposed human skin. They bury their head in the skin and grow in size as they suck blood. It is important to remove the insect without leaving the head-part still buried. Plaster remover or spirit applied to the tick should make it withdraw backwards. It can then be removed with forceps, by using sideways movements to release the head from the skin. Alternatively, cover the tick with white soft paraffin and a film dressing. The tick will withdraw from the skin because of lack of oxygen. The site should be cleaned well after the removal of the tick. Ticks can cause Lyme disease and other diseases, so the patient should be told to see the doctor and to mention the removal of the tick if a rash develops at the site of the tick-bite or he/she becomes unwell within the next fortnight.

EYE PROBLEMS

The eye may be affected by an infection, foreign body, direct force or penetrating injury. A careful examination is needed and referral for medical treatment, in all but the most straightforward cases.

Conjunctivitis

This is a common condition with a variety of causes. The signs are:

- Painful or gritty red eyes with inflammation across the conjunctiva, making the eye look pink; one or both eyes may be affected
- Discharge, which may be purulent, or just excessive tears
- The vision is unaffected.

The most common causes of conjunctivitis are infective or allergic. Very young babies can get conjunctivitis or a discharge from the eye because the tear duct system is not fully developed until the baby is about six months old. A few with blocked tear ducts eventually require surgery. Advice may be needed on how to clean discharging eyes, using swabs soaked in cooled boiled water. Each swab should be used once and then discarded.

Conjunctivitis is usually self-limiting and the need for treatment with topical antibiotics has been questioned, although the condition usually responds quickly to treatment.

Bacterial eye infections cause a purulent discharge. Chloramphenicol drops or ointment is the most commonly used antibiotic. The condition is contagious and patients should be advised about hand hygiene and the need to use separate towels and face flannels.[20] Schools will usually exclude children until the infection has been treated. If periorbital cellulitis occurs or the conjunctivitis is severe, the patient will need systemic antibiotics and to see a doctor urgently. Patients who wear contact lenses should be examined carefully to exclude trauma to the eye. The lenses should not be worn until the condition has completely resolved.

Allergic eye conditions can be caused either by hay fever or an allergy to make-up, in which case the product should not be used again. Antihistamine eye drops may be prescribed for the rapid relief of symptoms. Mast cell stabiliser drops such as sodium cromoglycate are useful for the prophylaxis of allergic eye symptoms. Oral antihistamines may also relieve allergic eye symptoms.

The important differential diagnosis for conjunctivitis is to exclude a foreign body from the surface of the eye. If a foreign body is suspected but not seen on examination then the eye should be stained with fluorescein drops to help identify a foreign body, corneal abrasion or dendritic ulcer. The history of getting a piece of dust or similar material in the eye will give an important clue to a foreign body.

Usually only one eye is affected and that will feel gritty or painful. The eye will be red and probably watering but in simple cases there will be no discharge.

Foreign bodies. Examine the eye carefully (see Chapter 5). Irrigation of the eye with saline may remove a foreign body. If it can be seen and is not embedded, then it may be possible to remove it with a moistened swab. A foreign body under the eyelid may be dislodged by drawing the upper lid over the lower lid so that the lower eyelashes sweep inside the lid. The upper lid can be everted by gently holding the stick of a cotton bud across the base of the tarsal plate of the eyelid while holding the eyelashes with the other hand and quickly drawing the eyelid outwards and upward over the cotton bud stick. No attempt should be made to remove a foreign body which is stuck or embedded. In such a situation the patient should be referred to the ophthalmic casualty department for treatment.

Corneal abrasions occur if a foreign body or a fingernail scratches the cornea. Fluorescein will stain abrasions yellow/green where epithelial cells have been removed from the cornea. A blue-light pen-torch will illuminate a fluorescein-stained abrasion more easily.

Dendritic ulcers are caused by a herpes-like virus, which can cause considerable damage to the eye if unrecognised. The symptoms are often identical to a foreign body – pain and a red eye. However, once stained, the ulcer appears as a tiny branching structure, more like the branches of a tree than the single line or mark of a corneal abrasion. Immediate referral is needed if an ulcer is seen.

Other causes of painful eyes

Of the many other causes of painful eyes which require referral, acute glaucoma is highly significant. In this condition the intraocular pressure increases, the cornea is often hazy, vision is poor and the patient is in pain. This is an emergency situation, as the eyesight can be seriously damaged. Chronic glaucoma is more common but does not usually present acutely. The onset is more insidious, possibly with headaches, but treatment is necessary to prevent loss of vision. (Patients who have a first-degree relative with glaucoma are entitled to free eye tests by an optician.)

Herpes zoster (shingles) may present as pain in the eye or forehead before the typical eruption starts. Once the vesicles begin to develop, the diagnosis is obvious; the patient should be referred for treatment urgently as soon as herpes zoster is suspected.

FOREIGN BODIES

Nose

Children are remarkably adept at putting an assortment of items up their noses. The problem may become apparent because the child has obvious difficulty breathing through the nose, or a foul nasal discharge develops. If an object is small enough to go into the postnasal cavity, it can then fall down into the posterior pharynx and be inhaled into the airway. Thus, foreign bodies in the nose should be approached cautiously and the patient be referred to a doctor if the object cannot be removed easily with nasal forceps.

Ear

A similar assortment of items may be found in the external auditory meatus. It may be possible to remove a foreign body within view with a fine forceps, but if the removal is causing pain or bleeding, then the patient must be referred to the doctor. Items such as extruded grommets may be removed by gentle irrigation of the ear but hygroscopic items, likely to swell when wet, must not be irrigated (see Chapter 5 under ear care). After removal of the object, the eardrum and auditory canal should be examined carefully to exclude any trauma.

Vagina

A woman may ask the nurse to retrieve a lost tampon. A vaginal examination should be performed and it may be possible to ease the tampon out if it can be felt easily. Often it is necessary to pass a vaginal speculum and use sponge-holding forceps to retrieve the object from the vaginal vault. Treatment will be necessary if the retained tampon has caused a bacterial vaginal infection. There may be an offensive discharge. Toxic shock syndrome is a very rare complication of tampon use. The patient will require urgent medical treatment in such an event.

EMERGENCY MIDWIFERY

A nurse could be called upon to deliver a baby in the surgery in exceptional circumstances, although there would usually be time to summon help or transfer the patient to hospital. For anyone without midwifery experience, the *First Aid Manual* has a good description and illustrations of what to do in an emergency. This book is recommended for reference in all the situations that require first aid.

> ### Suggestions for reflection on practice
>
> - Review your emergency training and the surgery's emergency equipment. How well equipped do you feel to provide first aid or emergency treatment? What further training or resources do you require?
> - Review the number of occasions on which you dealt with emergency situations over a chosen period of time. What was the outcome of your management? Could anything have been done differently?

REFERENCES

1. Department of Health Accidental Task Force (2002) *Preventing Accidental Injury – priorities for action.* Report to the Chief Medical Officer. Stationery Office, London.
2. Dean, R. (2005) Emergency first aid for nurses. *Nursing Standard,* **20** (6), 57–65.
3. Resuscitation Council (UK) (2005) *Resuscitation Guidelines 2005.* www.resus.org.uk/ siteindx.htm (accessed 4/1/06).
4. Handley, A. (2005) Adult Basic Life Support. *Resuscitation Guidelines 2005.* www.resus.org.uk/pages/bls.pdf
5. Project Team of the Resuscitation Council (UK) (2005) *The Emergency Medical Treatment of Anaphylactic Reactions for First Medical Responders and Community Nurses.* www.resus.org.uk/pages/reaction.htm (accessed 4/1/06).
6. Voluntary Aid Societies (2002) Heart attack. In: *First Aid Manual,* 8th edn. Dorling Kindersley, London.
7. Project Team of Resuscitation Council (UK) (2001) *Cardiopulmonary Resuscitation: guidance for clinical practice and training in primary care.* www.resus.org.uk/pages/ cpatpc.htm
8. Stroke Association (2005) *Stroke is a Medical Emergency.* www.stroke.org.uk/ campaigns/Latest_campaigns (accessed 23/10/05).
9. Department of Health (2001) *National Service Framework f or Older People – Standard 5.* Department of Health, London.
10. Voluntary Aid Societies (2002) Seizures in children. In: *First Aid Manual,* 8th edn. Dorling Kindersley, London.
11. Prodigy   Guidance   (2005)   *Febrile   Convulsion.*   www.prodigy.nhs.uk/ guidance.asp?gt=febrileconvulsions (accessed 25/10/05).
12. Patient UK (2002) *Head Injury Instructions.* www.patient.co.uk/showdoc/23068752 (accessed 25/10/05).
13. British Thoracic Society and Scottish Intercollegiate Guideline Network (2005) Management of acute asthma. In: *British Guidelines on the Management of Asthma.* www.brit-thoracic.org.uk/c2/uploads/asthmafull.pdf (accessed 4/1/06).
14. McGarry, G. (2005) Nosebleeds in children. In: *Clinical Evidence.* BMJ Publishing. www.clinicalevidence.com/ceweb/conditions/chd/0311/0311.jsp   (accessed 29/10/05).
15. Small, V. (2000) Management of cuts, abrasions and lacerations. *Nursing Standard,* **15** (5), 41–4.
16. Davies, P. (2005) Wound closure – getting it right for minor wounds. *Practice Nurse,* **30** (7), 60–3.
17. Prodigy   Guidance   (2004)   *Burns   and   Scalds.*   www.prodigy.nhs.uk/ guidance.asp?gt=burnsandscalds (accessed 31/10/05).
18. Prodigy   Guidance   (2005)   *Sprains   and   Strains.*   www.prodigy.nhs.uk/ guidance.asp?gt=sprainsandstrains (accessed 1/11/05).
19. Prodigy   Guidance   (2004)   *Bites – Human   and   Animal.*   www.prodigy.nhs.uk/ guidance.asp?gt=bites
20. Prodigy   Guidance   (2005)   *Conjunctivitis – Infective.*   www.prodigy.nhs.uk/ guidance.asp?gt=conjunctivitis

FURTHER READING

Prodigy Guidance: www.prodigy.nhs.uk

Purcell, D. (2003) *Minor Injuries: a clinical guide*. Elsevier Churchill Livingstone, Edinburgh.

Voluntary Aid Societies (2002) *First Aid Manual*, 8th edn. Dorling Kindersley, London.

USEFUL ADDRESSES AND WEBSITES

Resuscitation Council UK, 5th Floor, Tavistock House North, Tavistock Square, London WC1H 9HR

Telephone: 020 7388 4678 Fax: 020 7383 0773

Website: www.resus.org.uk

TOXBASE (clinical toxicology database of the National Poisons Information Centre)

Telephone: 0131 536 2298

Website: www.spib.axl.co.uk/

National Poisons Information Service

Telephone: 0870 600 6266 (calls will be transferred to the nearest regional centre)

Website: www.npis.org/NPIS/uk%20npis.htm

Chapter 8
Common Medical Conditions

Patients have several ways of getting help and advice with health problems, although the majority still tend to use their general practice.

NHS Direct is a 24-hour telephone helpline, staffed by nurses, who will give advice at any time on any health issue. They use computerised protocols to assess the problems callers present and to give advice on the action needed. In some areas NHS Direct answers out-of-hours calls to the GP and some ambulance calls are also managed in this way. NHS Direct, which covers all of England and Wales, is now a Special Health Authority.[1] NHS 24 is the Scottish equivalent service.

NHS Direct Online provides health information and advice and uses algorithms to help patients to make decisions about their health concerns. There is also a computer link whereby patients are able to record their medical details in a secure Health Space, which may eventually become part of an electronic patient record.[2]

Nurse-run NHS walk-in and minor injury centres are intended to provide easy access to advice or treatment for patients with minor illnesses or injuries in order to complement GP services. Commuters and people with limited time, who choose to pay for treatment rather than take time off work to visit their practice, can use private health centres at main railway stations. NHS walk-in centres are also planned for locations at or near to mainline stations.[3]

Nurse triage and the management of minor illnesses have become part of the role of many practice nurses. They assess the urgency of conditions when patients telephone or arrive at the surgery without an appointment and give advice and treatment themselves or refer to the GP as appropriate. In this respect there is an overlap with the role of nurse practitioners.

A practice nurse may be consulted about a variety of common conditions. Some will be self-limiting illnesses, like colds and gastric upsets, for which advice can be offered on the management of symptoms. Other problems could necessitate referral to the doctor, who has the ultimate responsibility for medical treatment. Patients who attend frequently with seemingly minor problems may be looking for a chance to discuss a deeper worry. The doctor or nurse should provide the patient with a suitable opportunity to ventilate other concerns, especially if the consultation seems inappropriate for the symptoms presented.

MEDICATION

The number of effective drugs available for purchase without a prescription changes periodically. Nurses may be asked for advice about suitable over-the-counter (OTC) medicines, so it is essential to enquire about any allergies, other medication being taken, possible pregnancy or other medical conditions before recommending proprietary products. Prescriptions may need to be issued for those who are exempt from prescription charges because cost can be a major factor for patients on low income. Information leaflets should be available in the surgery about help with NHS prescription costs. Retail pharmacists have always advised patients about a wide range of problems and treatments but the new Community Pharmacy Contract means that pharmacists are being encouraged to undertake a wider role in chronic disease monitoring and medicine management.[4] Moreover, practice nurses have been advised to consider joining forces with pharmacists in this respect.[5]

A friendly local pharmacist is a valuable source of information for doctors and nurses. Primary care organisation (PCO) pharmacists work closely with practices on a range of prescribing issues and are another resource for practice nurses.

Nurse prescribing

Nurse prescribing was first proposed in 1986 but when it finally began, only practice nurses with a district nursing or health visiting qualification were permitted to prescribe. Training and success in the examination were necessary before nurses could be recorded by the UKCC as nurse prescribers. Products could be prescribed from the *Nurse's Formulary* but they were severely restricted in number. Since that time, there has been rapid progress and all first-level registered nurses may train to prescribe in one of two ways.

1. *Independent* prescribing, by which the prescriber takes the responsibility for assessing the patient and prescribing appropriately. Doctors, dentists and some nurses and pharmacists are independent prescribers. There are two types of independent prescribing.
   - The education of all district nurses and health visitors now incorporates nurse prescribing from the limited *Nurse Prescriber's Formulary for District Nurses and Health Visitors*, which consists of dressings, appliances and some medicines.[6]
   - Extended Formulary nurse prescribers are able to prescribe for patients with specified medical conditions from a much wider range of medicines. The training is rigorous and employers must satisfy themselves that non-medical prescribers have the skills and competencies relevant to the clinical area in which they are prescribing. From Spring 2006, qualified EF nurse prescribers and pharmacist-independent prescribers will be able to prescribe any licensed medicine for any medical condition, with the exception of controlled drugs.[7]

2. *Supplementary* prescribing is a system whereby nurse and pharmacist prescribers can prescribe medicines, including some controlled drugs, provided they are included in individual patient Clinical Management Plans. Electronic CMP templates can be downloaded via the internet (see Useful addresses and websites below). However, the Nursing and Midwifery Council is adamant that the letter of the law must be followed and patients must have individual CMPs. The NMC is due to issue standards for prescribing in the near future.

All forms of nurse prescribing are recordable on the NMC register. Nurses may train as both supplementary and extended formulary nurse prescribers.

The practice nurse's responsibility regarding prescriptions

Every practice nurse has the following responsibilities in relation to prescriptions.

- To ensure that any prescription supplied by the nurse is given to the correct patient
- To be able to answer knowledgeably, or refer to the appropriate person, any enquiries by patients about their medication
- To ensure that blank prescriptions are stored securely in the nurse's room
- To be familiar with the practice repeat prescribing system
- To have appropriate reference material available
- To keep knowledge up to date.

If nurses give patients advice on self-management, they must be told to consult their GP if the condition worsens or does not resolve in the time expected. Verbal information is forgotten quickly, so important points can be reinforced with printed handouts or leaflets. The Prodigy website has a number of helpful patient information leaflets for each subject listed. The possibility of pregnancy should always be considered when advising women of childbearing age because many medicines are contraindicated in pregnancy or when breastfeeding.

It is possible to give only a brief overview of some of the medical conditions with which practice nurses may be involved. So much depends on the circumstances in individual surgeries and the knowledge and experience of the nurses concerned.

UPPER RESPIRATORY TRACT INFECTIONS

Viruses cause the majority of upper respiratory symptoms due to infection. Antibiotics should only be required if secondary bacterial infection supervenes. Advice to patients includes:

- An explanation of the nature of viral infections
- The value of analgesic/antipyretic compounds, such as paracetamol and ibuprofen, in appropriate dosage. (Aspirin is not recommended for children and adolescents under 16 years of age because of the risk of Reye's syndrome, or for anyone with a history of peptic ulceration)[8]
- Suggestions about proprietary cough linctuses and decongestants. Remember to warn patients that antihistamines in some preparations can cause drowsiness. The evidence for the effectiveness of OTC cough medicines is weak.[9] However, patients may be advised to use their favourite remedies to make themselves feel better. Pseudoephedrine is contraindicated for patients taking MAOI antidepressants and caution is needed if patients have diabetes, IHD, hypertension or hyperthyroidism
- The need for regular drinks to prevent dehydration
- Advice about the environment:
  - bedrest is not necessary unless the patient feels more comfortable there
  - central heating and crowded, smoky atmospheres can make symptoms worse
  - the only value in being away from work, if apyrexial, is to avoid passing the infection to other people
- To consult the doctor if:
  - a fever persists
  - the sputum becomes discoloured (antibiotics may be required)
  - there is pain on inspiration (could indicate pleurisy)
  - earache or facial pain occur (could indicate infection of the ears or sinuses).

Smokers may be more receptive to offers of help to quit while symptoms make them disinclined to smoke.

Catarrh

The term 'catarrh' covers a multitude of disorders related to the sensation of congestion in the nasal airways, sinuses or ears. Some patients suffer all the time (with perennial rhinitis or chronic sinusitis); others may have an acute problem related to hay fever or the common cold. The treatment will depend on the underlying cause. The patient's occupation should always be checked because there may be an acquired sensitivity to fumes, dust or chemicals at work. There could be health and safety implications.

Intermittent allergic rhinitis (hay fever)

The symptoms of hay fever – itchy, watering eyes, sneezing, blocked or running nose and sometimes wheezing chest – are caused by an allergic reaction to pollen or mould spores. Atopic individuals have an inherited tendency to develop hay fever, asthma and eczema. Patients known to suffer from seasonal rhinitis are advised to start preventive therapy a fortnight before the hay fever season begins.

The following treatments may be used (some treatments are not suitable for children).

- *Antihistamines* are used to relieve the symptoms. Cetirizine, fexofenadine and desloratadine are examples of newer antihistamines, which are claimed not to cause drowsiness. Nevertheless, they can occasionally cause this problem, so patients should be warned of the risk if driving or working with machinery. Antihistamines can also enhance the effect of alcohol.
- *Mast cell stabilisers* – sodium cromoglycate as eye drops, nasal spray or inhaler as preventive measures.
- *Steroids* – beclomethasone, budesonide and fluticasone nasal sprays. The patient may need to be shown how to use a nasal spray effectively. Oral steroids may be prescribed in extreme cases, such as before a wedding or sitting examinations. Steroid injections are not recommended for hay fever.[10]

Persistent allergic rhinitis (perennial rhinitis)

Although the symptoms and treatment are similar to hay fever, people with perennial rhinitis suffer the symptoms all the year. Instead of pollen, they may be sensitive to allergens like house dust mites or animals and sometimes will need referral for allergy testing to identify the culprit allergen. Advice can be given on possible ways of reducing the exposure to allergens. Nasal polyps should be ruled out as a cause of symptoms.

EAR CONDITIONS

A practice nurse should be able to visualise the external meatus of the ear and the tympanic membrane and be familiar with the appearance of a normal ear. Children, in particular, are susceptible to middle ear infections following a cold and any child who complains of earache should be examined. If a practice nurse examines the ears and the eardrums are not absolutely normal then the child should be referred to the doctor. Parents may be taught that antibiotics are not helpful for viral ear infections.[11] However, it is important that they understand fully the importance of compliance with any treatments prescribed.

Deafness

Blocked ears can be caused externally by excessive wax, debris from otitis externa or foreign bodies, and internally by congestion of the middle ear. Ear irrigation might be needed (see Chapter 5). Decongestants such as pseudoephedrine may be recommended for congestion of the middle ear if the patient is otherwise well (see *BNF* for contraindications). In other circumstances, the patient should be referred to a doctor.

HEADACHE

Patients with occasional headaches usually treat themselves with OTC analgesics. Most causes of headache are minor but more serious disease has to be eliminated. Patients with headaches sometimes refer themselves to the practice nurse for a blood pressure check. A medical assessment should be arranged for a patient with recurrent or severe headaches but once serious disease has been ruled out, the practice nurse can help the patient to deal with the symptoms and to devise avoidance strategies. Rebound headaches can occur as a result of large amounts of analgesics, so some patients may inadvertently be compounding the problem.

Migraine

There are several theories to explain the symptoms of migraine. The cause is still not fully understood. Episodic attacks of severe unilateral headache, nausea or vomiting, photophobia or other neurological disturbances, lasting for several hours or days, are characteristic. Attacks can be preceded by a visual or sensory disturbance (aura) and migraine is commonly classified as migraine with aura and migraine without aura. Sufferers have a family history of migraine in approximately 70% of cases. A number of trigger factors – dietary, hormonal, emotional and environmental – are implicated and sometimes an accumulation of triggers will precipitate an attack. No diagnostic test exists, so a clear history of symptoms is needed. A migraine diary can aid diagnosis and help patients to identify possible trigger factors.

There is no cure but drugs can sometimes be effective in preventing or relieving symptoms. Analgesics and NSAIDs may be used. Soluble or rectal forms may be needed when vomiting is a problem. Changes in lifestyle to avoid trigger factors, relaxation techniques and alternative therapies, like acupuncture, can be beneficial. Some nurses run migraine clinics with a holistic approach to the problem. Self-help groups also exist for sufferers.

Tension headaches

The sensation of a tight band around the head, caused by tension in the neck muscles, can be eased by relaxation, stress reduction and massage. Analgesia may also be required.

Hangover

Headache following excessive alcohol intake is not uncommon. Practice nurses can give information to sufferers on sensible drinking (see Chapter 9) and advise on the prevention of a hangover by maintaining adequate hydration.

INSOMNIA

Clinicians are often requested by patients to prescribe something 'to help me sleep'. Many patients have a high expectation of a perfect night's sleep irrespective of age, other concomitant illness or their own personal needs. A great deal more is known now about sleep and the way various drugs affect it and doctors are reluctant to prescribe drugs likely to cause addiction or habituation. Nurses may be able to help patients who are having difficulty in sleeping. A thorough assessment of the problem may present possible solutions.

- *Daytime sleep* – an elderly patient who has several short naps during the day will not sleep so well at night.
- *Pain* – people with severe pain sometimes request sleeping tablets, when adequate analgesia would be more effective.
- *Mental distress* – counselling may be offered to patients with anxiety or other distress. People with severe depression could require treatment with antidepressants.
- *Nocturia* merits investigation for urinary infection, diabetes, prostatism or the timing of diuretics.

It may also help to consider the sleeping environment; a warm bath, reading in bed, soft music and comfortable bedding all encourage the mind and body to wind down from the day's activities. Stimulants and alcohol should be avoided. Relaxation techniques can be taught. Quietness may take more innovation to achieve, especially if a partner snores. Ear plugs might provide relief or an ENT assessment of the snorer might be possible.

GASTROINTESTINAL DISORDERS

Diarrhoea and vomiting are common symptoms, particularly in children. While most of these episodes are relatively trivial and self-limiting, the risk of dehydration or the masking of more severe pathology, such as intestinal obstruction, always has to be borne in mind.

The causes of diarrhoea and vomiting are many. Age is an important consideration when trying to decide about likely cause and future management. Some of the causes of vomiting are:

- Viral, bacterial or toxic causes in all age groups
- Feeding problems in babies
- Middle ear or upper respiratory infection in children
- Pregnancy
- Ménière's disease or labyrinthitis in the middle-aged and the elderly, particularly if there have been previous episodes
- Migraine
- Gallstones
- Intestinal obstruction, particularly in babies and the elderly.

Some of the causes of diarrhoea are:

- Following vomiting, almost always infective and often viral
- On its own at any age, infection, occasionally from contaminated food (enquire about recent travel). Food poisoning and dysentery are notifiable diseases
- Other bowel disorders such as ulcerative colitis; the history will usually give the clue to these conditions
- Spurious diarrhoea caused by faecal leakage around impacted faeces.

Management of diarrhoea

- In simple uncomplicated cases where the patient is over one year of age and the history is only a matter of hours, then frequent small sips of fluid until bowel symptoms have subsided are all that is required. (Starvation is no longer recommended, so the patient may eat a normal diet if desired.)
- Explain the importance of personal hygiene measures, especially hand washing, to prevent the spread of infection.
- Advise the patient to contact the practice again if symptoms persist for more than 24 hours, if abdominal pain is persistent or severe, or blood is being passed.
- Children under a year old or any patients whose symptoms do not fit into the infective pattern should be referred to the doctor the same day.

Patients with diarrhoea who work as food handlers or in healthcare facilities should be advised to stay away from work until 48 hours after the condition has resolved.[12]

Dyspepsia

Probably more OTC remedies are bought for indigestion than for most other symptoms. Causes can include poor eating habits, pregnancy, hiatus hernia, smoking and high alcohol consumption. However, clinical diagnosis is difficult and patients with persistent symptoms will require medical investigations. The nurse may be the first person consulted, so any patient taking antacids regularly, having a lot of pain or with loss of weight needs referral.

Constipation

Patients can become anxious if their bowels do not work regularly, as witnessed by the many tons of laxatives consumed annually. Normal bowel habits vary, so a diagnosis of constipation has to be related to the norm for each individual. The advice given will depend on the age group of the patient. However, the possibility of intestinal obstruction should be considered when a patient has severe constipation. A thorough history must be taken before any advice or treatment is offered.

Babies often become constipated when their dietary intake is being changed, e.g. change from breast to bottle or milk to solids. An increase in the amount of fluid given (not just milk) may be all that is required. The health visitor will usually advise parents and refer to the GP if necessary. Young children may be slow to acquire normal toilet training habits. Health visitors will advise parents about toilet training. It is important not to focus too much attention on bowel function because a child can learn to exert power over parents by refusing to comply. Children can also be so absorbed in their daily activities that they forget to go to the toilet and so become constipated by suppressing the normal bowel reflexes. Fear of defaecation resulting from the experience of passing a painful stool or from an anal fissure can also lead to constipation.

Management of constipation in children

- Advise increased roughage in the diet (fruit puree, vegetables, high-fibre bread and cereals) and extra fluids.
- Encourage regular, unhurried toileting and reward with praise.
- Faecal softeners (e.g. docusate) and/or paediatric glycerine suppositories may be prescribed to relieve severe constipation and anaesthetic gel to be applied around the anus to relieve the pain of defaecation.

Management of constipation in adults

Constipation in adults or the elderly can be acute or chronic. Acute constipation may be the result of activity restriction by illness or injury, dehydration or drugs such as codeine. Long-term laxative use can cause chronic constipation. The bowel loses its muscle tone and reflexes, so a vicious circle is created whereby the bowel only functions when stimulated by purgatives. Poor diet and lack of exercise contribute to constipation in all age groups. Changes in bowel habits can be a sign of significant bowel disease, so constipation in a patient who has previously been regular, or alternating constipation and diarrhoea, requires medical investigation.

Acute constipation can be managed in the following ways.

- Identify the cause, if possible, and ask for a medical examination if necessary.
- Deal with the immediate problem. Advise osmotic laxatives or glycerine suppositories in mild to moderate cases.
- Advise on the prevention of a recurrence by the use of softening agents, increased fibre and fluids. (If patients have to take drugs known to cause constipation, suitable laxatives will be needed as well.)

Chronic constipation can be managed in the following ways.

- Encourage gradual re-education of the bowel with changes in diet to increase fibre and fluids.
- Change from stimulant laxatives to faecal softeners and bulking agents.
- Encourage increased mobility and sensible exercise.

Encouraging patients to change the habits of a lifetime requires patience. (Sudden increases in dietary fibre and osmotic laxatives can cause distressing flatulence, which patients should be warned to expect and be reassured will settle once the body adjusts.)

Worms

Harmless threadworms are the most common parasitic worms that inhabit the gut in Britain, especially in children. Roundworms and tapeworms are less common but can cause anorexia, weight loss and abdominal distension. Travellers may occasionally return with other helminth infections. Threadworms, true to their name, look like small white threads. They inhabit the bowel and emerge at night to lay their eggs around the anus, causing intense irritation that can disturb sleep or cause bedwetting.

Treatment should include all the family. Some anthelmintic preparations can be bought over the counter or be prescribed by a doctor or nurse prescriber. The whole family should be treated at the same time but pregnant or lactating women are advised to use hygiene methods alone to break the cycle of infection.[13] Mebendazole is only suitable for children over two years old, but in the same dose for all age groups. Piperazine can be given to children from three months of age (in a lower dose for children under six years old).

The nurse has a role in teaching parents how to avoid reinfection. Information leaflets are available from local health promotion departments and the internet. Threadworms are spread by ingestion of the eggs from hand contact. Scratching the perianal skin will transfer eggs to the hands. The following preventive measures can be advised.

- Wear close-fitting underwear at night to avoid hand contact with the skin.
- Wash hands upon rising, after using the toilet and before preparing food.
- Keep fingernails short.
- Wash the perineum daily upon rising to help to remove any eggs laid overnight.
- Make sure all family members use their own face flannels and towels.
- Launder nightclothes, bedlinen and underwear daily and avoid shaking these items to prevent eggs being released into the air.
- Vacuum carpets and damp-dust all surfaces regularly. Remember to empty the vacuum cleaner and dispose of cleaning cloths after use.

URINARY PROBLEMS

Cystitis

The complaint of cystitis may mean anything from slight burning or frequency of micturition to severe pain, nausea and febrile illness. Cystitis is very common in women and may or may not be associated with a proven urinary tract infection. Inflammation of the lower urinary tract is often associated with sexual intercourse. Changes in cell structure due to the loss of oestrogen can also make postmenopausal women prone to cystitis. Organisms that colonise the bowel will cause infection if they gain entry to the urinary tract. Anatomical differences make this much less common in men; therefore, a medical assessment is needed for any man with a urinary tract infection. The doctor must also see a pregnant woman with a urinary infection. Referral to the genitourinary clinic is advisable if a patient's cystitis is thought to be associated with a sexually transmitted disease.

Some practices use microscopy to detect urinary tract infections but more commonly, urine dip tests for nitrites and leucocytes are used. Treatment with antibiotics may be initiated immediately in some instances. Blood might also be detected on urinalysis but is not necessarily diagnostic of infection, especially if a patient is menstruating. A midstream specimen of urine should be sent to microbiology, in accordance with the practice protocol. This might include all suspected urinary tract infections or only those in specific patient groups: men, pregnant women, children and patients with haematuria or possible kidney infections. If an MSU is sent, the pathology form should specify any antibiotic prescribed so that sensitivity can be tested to that particular antibiotic.

Women who are prone to recurrent attacks of cystitis can be given information on ways to minimise problems.

- Wipe from front to back after using the toilet, to avoid bringing bowel organisms in contact with the urethra.
- Avoid using scented soaps, bath products, talc and vaginal deodorants, which can irritate the skin.

- Avoid dehydration by drinking up to two litres of fluid a day. Excess fluids can aggravate the distress of dysuria and are no longer recommended for treating a urinary infection.
- Empty the bladder regularly and completely.
- Avoid restrictive clothing and tights and wear cotton underwear in preference to nylon.
- Use a lubricant if intercourse is affected by vaginal dryness.
- If using a diaphragm, ensure it is the correct size, to avoid pressure against the urethra (recurrent UTIs could necessitate a change of contraceptive method).
- Empty the bladder after sexual intercourse.
- Consult the doctor about hormone treatment for postmenopausal urinary symptoms.

Treatments to alkalinise the urine, such as sodium citrate, potassium citrate or sodium bicarbonate, have traditionally been used and may help to relieve mild symptoms. Sachets are available from pharmacies. Cranberry juice is another favourite remedy. It is claimed that the tannins in cranberry juice prevent bacteria from attaching themselves to the walls of the urinary tract but while there is some evidence that cranberry juice and capsules can prevent recurrent infections in some women, the value of cranberries as a treatment has not been proved.[14]

Cystitis in children

The situation with children is different. Undiagnosed infection, often due to an anatomical abnormality, can lead to low-grade pyelonephritis with no symptoms, which can ultimately cause renal scarring and possibly renal failure. Therefore it is vital to examine the urine of children and refer to the doctor if there is any likelihood of a urinary tract infection. Inefficient development of the valves at the ureto-bladder junction will allow reflux of urine up the ureters on micturition. If they can be kept free of infection, most children develop the use of these valves by 8–10 years of age. A paediatric urologist may initiate prophylactic antibiotic treatment. Other causes of cystitis in children include vaginal infection or balanitis, foreign body or worms. The possibility of sexual abuse also has to be borne in mind.

VAGINAL DISCHARGE

Women have varying amounts of vaginal discharge present, either at certain times of the menstrual cycle or all the time. Infection can be caused by a variety of organisms, sometimes sexually transmitted. Offensive discharge may result from a forgotten tampon or other foreign body. It is important to establish exactly what a woman is complaining about when she says she has a vaginal discharge. A high vaginal and, possibly, an endocervical swab may be required to identify the cause of infection.

Candida albicans (thrush)

If the normal balance of commensal organisms is disturbed, an overgrowth of yeasts can result. Antibiotics, diabetes, pregnancy and, possibly, the oral contraceptive are contributory factors. The characteristic white cheesy discharge of candida infection causes severe irritation. Treatment is usually simple and consists of antifungal vaginal preparations such as clotrimazole pessaries or cream. They may be bought OTC or prescribed. Unless the patient is pregnant, oral treatment with one capsule of fluconazole or itraconazole can be used for more intractable cases or if a patient is unwilling to use topical preparations. The nurse can explain the condition to patients and advise on ways of preventing exacerbation or a recurrence.

- Avoid using scented soaps, talc, etc. which can cause irritation
- Avoid obsessive hygiene measures, which remove the normal commensal flora
- Wear stockings instead of tights because candida is more likely to develop in warm, moist conditions
- Wear loose-fitting cotton underwear and avoid tight-fitting jeans and trousers for the same reason.

Bacterial vaginosis

Anaerobic bacterial infections of the vagina can cause an offensive discharge. Sometimes patients may request a repeat of treatment for thrush, when the problem is in fact bacterial vaginosis. A high vaginal swab should be sent when necessary. Most causative organisms can be treated with systemic metronidazole or topical preparations such as clindamycin cream.

Trichomonas vaginalis

Trichomoniasis is sexually transmitted by a flagellate organism and produces a frothy yellow discharge. Metronidazole taken orally for a week will provide effective treatment, but patients must be warned to avoid alcohol totally while taking it. Patients may also require persuasion to persevere with the treatment because it can cause such an unpleasant taste in the mouth or nausea.

Chlamydia

Another protozoon, chlamydia, can cause vaginal discharge and is a major cause of pelvic inflammatory disease. Special tests are required to identify the organism (see Chapter 6). Recognition and adequate treatment with antibiotics are essential because of the serious risk to future health and fertility.

General advice

Patients may have more than one sexually transmitted infection and referral to a genitourinary clinic will sometimes be advisable. Unfortunately, the former stigma associated with these clinics may deter some patients. A practice nurse can help by explaining about the skilled diagnosis and treatment available at specialist centres and by giving practical information about clinic times and location. Appropriate advice may also be given on hygiene, safer sex, contraception and cervical screening (see Chapter 12, Sexual Health).

INFECTIOUS DISEASES

Many of the most common childhood illnesses can now be prevented by immunisation and are, therefore, seen only rarely. Patients may contact the practice nurse for information about the risk of contracting or spreading a disease or to discuss a skin rash. It will often be possible to identify the common conditions and give appropriate advice but this can be rendered extra difficult when patients want the rash to be identified by telephone.

Chickenpox (varicella zoster)

The characteristic lesion of chickenpox is a small blister-like spot with clear serous fluid in the centre. There may be many of these scattered over the trunk and face, showing various stages of development from an early red spot, through the vesicular stage, to crusting and the formation of a scab. The diagnosis will usually be obvious, especially as chickenpox tends to occur in minor outbreaks of cases. Apart from being febrile and irritable, a child is only rarely at risk from complications. Adults and adolescents tend to be more severely affected by the illness. Treatment with crotamiton cream or lotion can reduce the irritation. A sedating antihistamine, such as chlorphenamine, may help a patient to sleep. It may help the patient to have a warm bath with sodium bicarbonate added to the water to reduce the irritation.

Chickenpox infection in a non-immune woman in the first months of pregnancy can cause severe congenital abnormalities. Fetal varicella syndrome has been reported in about 1.4% of cases contracted between 12 and 28 weeks' gestation but not after that time.[15] Women are more susceptible to pneumonia if they contract chickenpox during pregnancy. Infection around the time of delivery poses a risk of overwhelming infection to the infant. This should be remembered if a pregnant woman seeks advice about chickenpox; a referral to the doctor may be necessary. If the mother has definitely had chickenpox there is no risk. Many cases in childhood are very mild. There may be no memory of the illness but a high proportion of adults do have immunity. If in doubt, an urgent blood test can be taken to check the antibody levels. A non-immune woman or neonate may be given varicella zoster immunoglobulin or antiviral drugs. Varicella vaccine is available through occupational health departments for non-immune healthcare workers who have direct patient contact.[16] Close contacts, such as siblings, of immunocompromised patients may also be immunised.

Shingles (herpes zoster)

Shingles occurs from the reactivation of varicella virus, dormant in the ganglion of a nerve, often many years after a previous episode of chickenpox, which then travels back down the nerve to affect the skin area (dermatome) served by that nerve. This is commonly around one side of the trunk but can occur on the head and seriously affect the eye. The old wives' tale about a patient dying if shingles meets in the middle arises from the rare cases of extremely debilitated people, who develop shingles affecting dermatomes on both sides of the body at the same time. Immunosuppressed patients should be aware of the risk from shingles and know the importance of seeking medical treatment immediately.

It is possible for a person who has never had chickenpox to catch the disease from someone with shingles because the same virus is responsible for both, but shingles cannot be caught from chickenpox for the reason given above.

Shingles can cause severe pain requiring regular analgesia, which occasionally leads to postherpetic neuralgia. Antiviral drugs can reduce the symptoms if taken within 72 hours of the onset of shingles and should be considered for all adult patients, especially those over 50, any patient with eye involvement, immunosuppression, atopic eczema or contact with very young infants, immunocompromised individuals or pregnant women.[17]

Measles

Measles has rarely been seen in recent years but it may become more common as a result of a reduction in the uptake of MMR vaccine. The patient may be unwell and has usually been so for several days. He or she is catarrhal with a hard, non-productive cough and a temperature of about 39°C. The eyes are often red and there is a blotchy, flat rash over the trunk, head and limbs. The rash often starts behind the ears and will slowly develop over the ensuing 24 hours. Koplik's spots look like tiny white grains of salt on the mucous membrane of the mouth and appear before the rash. They are thus a useful diagnostic pointer when measles is suspected. Laboratory diagnostic confirmation is usually required. The local consultant in communicable disease control will advise.

Mumps

Mumps is a viral infection spread by droplets that causes fever and painful swelling of the parotid glands. The incubation period can be up to three weeks. The resulting difficulty in eating and drinking can lead to dehydration in severe cases. Other organs can also be affected – the kidneys, pancreas, thyroid and testes. Orchitis can result in sterility in a small proportion of the men who develop the disease. Meningitis is another complication of mumps, which is not usually life-threatening but requires careful monitoring. Treatment for mumps is symptomatic, with bedrest while the fever is high and measures to reduce the fever and relieve pain. An adequate fluid intake is needed to avoid dehydration and constipation. The patient is infectious from about a week before the fever starts to the time the swelling subsides but close contact is usually needed for the disease to be transmitted. Outbreaks have occurred in schools and colleges and many such institutions now require proof that students have been fully immunised against mumps.

German measles (rubella)

The rash of typical rubella is much more diffuse than that of measles and is often very striking on the face. The diagnosis should not be made if the posterior occipital chain of lymph glands cannot be palpated, as many virus infections produce a transient non-specific rash very similar to rubella. The rubella rash lasts for several days whereas the imitative virus infections seldom last more than 24 hours. Usually, no treatment is required and children only need to be kept out of contact with known expectant mothers. Rubella contracted in the first trimester of pregnancy can result in the disastrous abnormalities of congenital rubella syndrome.

Paracetamol or ibuprofen may be used to treat pyrexia. Children still need to be immunised against MMR even if they are thought to have had the clinical rubella infection, because a firm diagnosis is often difficult to make. Women of childbearing age who are shown not to be immune to rubella by a blood test should be offered MMR before they conceive.

Slapped cheek syndrome (erythema infectiosum)

Also known as fifth disease, this is caused by a parvovirus, which mainly affects school-age children but can occasionally occur in adults. The infection, which is mainly spread by droplets, causes a mild flu-like illness and a red rash on the cheeks – hence the common name. Itching can be troublesome and the rash may spread to other parts of the body. Adults may get swollen painful joints. The incubation period is 1–3 weeks and the disease is not likely to be contagious once the rash has developed. The disease is usually mild but can have more serious consequences for immunocompromised individuals or occasionally, during the first half of pregnancy. In general, symptomatic treatment only is needed. Pregnant women should seek medical advice.

Hand, foot and mouth disease

This disease, not to be confused with foot and mouth disease of animals, is caused by a coxsackie virus and mainly affects children. There may be fever and a sore throat followed by the development of small blisters in the mouth, hands and feet. Blisters can also occur on the buttocks. The disease is spread partly by droplets or from contact with virus in the blisters. Faecal/oral transmission is also possible because the virus is excreted in the faeces for some time after the infection. The incubation period is short at 3–7 days. Usually, no treatment is needed but careful hygiene measures are required after toileting young children with the disease.

HUMAN PARASITES

Scabies (*Sarcoptes scabiei*)

Scabies is caused by the allergic reaction to a small arthropod, which lays its eggs in burrows just below the surface of the skin. It can only be transmitted by direct skin contact with an affected person. It causes intense irritation and the classic burrow lesions can usually be found in the web of the fingers or the wrist. Although these are common sites, it must be assumed that the whole skin except the head will be affected. Hyperkeratotic scabies (also called Norwegian or crusted scabies) mainly occurs in immunocompromised patients. It is extremely contagious and will affect the head and face as well.

Treatment choice depends on the patient's age and medical condition. All contacts should be treated at the same time to avoid reinfestation. Apply a scabicide cream or lotion (permethrin or malathion) from the head to the toes, paying particular attention to the skin folds. Treatment should be reapplied to hands after hand washing. After 12 hours the whole body can be bathed. Treat all members of the household at the same time and repeat treatment after one week. Skin irritation will continue for several days after treatment. Antipruritic treatments may be helpful.

Head lice (pediculosis capitis)

Head lice are common in all age groups but are found more often on children. They can occur in even the most scrupulously careful household and can engender concern out of all proportion to their effect. Head lice are usually first noticed as nits, the eggs, which the female louse glues to individual hairs.

Newly laid eggs will be close to the scalp and those further away and white are hatched eggs which progress outwards as the hair grows. The louse itself is very small and difficult to see. It passes from one head to another by contact. It is not necessary to keep children away from school if lice are discovered.

The patient and any family members who have definitely been proved to have live lice should be treated at the same time with malathion, permethrin or phenothrin. A second application may be needed after ten days to kill any lice that hatched after the first treatment. Pregnant and breastfeeding women must avoid using permethrin and are advised to use only the wet-combing method. Local policies exist for changing treatments in response to the developing resistance to insecticides. For this same reason, the regular preventive use of pediculosides must be discouraged. Preparations containing carbaryl are not available OTC but may be prescribed for intractable cases with suspected resistance to all other insecticides.[18] Insecticidal shampoos have been shown to be ineffective and should be discouraged. Education of the public to understand the problem and adopt simple measures, like weekly checks of children's hair with a special head lice comb for early detection, is important. 'Bug-Busting' (the regular wet-combing of hair treated with hair conditioner) requires time and commitment but can be effective if performed correctly. 'Bug Buster' kits are available on prescription or OTC.

Crab lice (pediculosis pubis)

Body lice are usually found in the pubic hair but can also be found in any other coarse hair on the body. They are more easily seen than head lice because they are larger (about the size of a pinhead). Infection occurs mainly through sexual contact. Treatment is by application of an appropriate aqueous lotion or cream (phenothrin, malathion or permethrin), left on for up to 12 hours and then washed off. All coarse hairy areas of the body, including a beard, must be treated, according to the manufacturer's instructions.

OTHER SKIN CONDITIONS

The appearance of the skin can affect the way a person is treated by society. Skin diseases are rarely life-threatening but they can devastate self-esteem. Many consultations in general practice are related to skin conditions, so there is plenty of scope for nurses with specialist skills in dermatology to help patients to improve their quality of life.

Acne vulgaris

Puberty is never the easiest time to live through but to develop acne, just when self-image becomes all-important, must rank among the crueller tricks of

Nature. An excess of sebum production results in blocked hair follicles, leading to the characteristic blackheads or whiteheads (comedones). The face and upper trunk are affected and the retained sebum provides an excellent growth medium for bacteria. Infection can result in pustules; in more severe cases, cysts can cause unsightly scarring. Patients should be advised to avoid squeezing spots if possible. There are websites which deal specifically with the problems of acne and address this issue.

Young patients with acne often need a lot of support and counselling. They should be encouraged to lead a normal social life and to avoid using thick make-up to cover blemishes that will block sebaceous glands even more. It is a myth that a diet high in carbohydrate and fats will aggravate the situation but the value of non-greasy foods and fresh fruit should be emphasised for general health reasons.

Preparations used in treating acne aim at reducing the grease in the skin and the number of blocked sebaceous ducts. Benzoyl peroxide removes the surface layer of skin to unblock the pores. Azelaic acid works in a similar fashion and also has antibacterial properties. All keratolytic products can make the skin dry and sore. A light moisturising cream may help if this occurs and treatment may also need to be stopped for a few days. Topical antibacterial products may be prescribed in some instances for inflammatory acne but antibacterial resistance can occur.

In more severe acne with persistent pustules and spots on the face and shoulders, the doctor may prescribe long-term systemic antibiotics (tetracyclines or erythromycin). Apart from their action against bacteria, they have a special action on the cells in the lower layers of the skin to make them less likely to produce pustules. Minocycline is considered to be an effective treatment for moderate acne but there are concerns about its safety and it is more expensive than other antibiotics.[19] Cyproterone acetate with ethinyloestradiol (Co-cyprindiol, Dianette) is a combined pill which reduces sebum production in the skin. It is also effective as a contraceptive but must only be prescribed as such for women who need treatment for acne as well. The prescription must indicate the fact if this 'pill' is prescribed for contraception as well; otherwise the patient will have to pay a prescription charge. It must not be prescribed for men because it works by lowering testosterone levels.

Patients with severe acne may be referred to a dermatologist for treatment with oral isotretinoin. Plastic surgery may be needed for the removal of scars.

Psoriasis

Psoriasis is a chronic skin condition with various types and degrees of severity. Arthritis is sometimes an associated condition. The patient's perception of his or her disability will often dictate the need for treatment.[20] Emollients as bath additives and soap substitutes should be used every day to hydrate the skin. In the commonest plaque form, the disease is characterised by well-demarcated, scaly, dry, red patches. Topical treatments like coal tar and dithranol, although effective, can be messy, smelly and stain clothing. Vitamin D analogues (calcipotriol, calcitriol, tacalcitol) are non-staining treatments that may be prescribed for plaque psoriasis.

Moderate sunlight may be beneficial, although sunburn can exacerbate the condition. Treatment in secondary care with psoralens and ultraviolet light (PUVA) has been shown to be effective but can increase the risk of skin cancer. There may be periods of remission but the condition frequently flares up in response to stress or other trigger factors. Techniques for stress management are likely to be helpful but have not been confirmed by research. Steroid treatments are often prescribed but their use should be monitored because inappropriate long-term use can cause thinning of the skin. The fingertip unit is a simple way of teaching patients how much cream or ointment to use to cover a given area. A patient advice sheet can be supplied.[21]

Eczema

The terms 'eczema' and 'dermatitis' are essentially the same, meaning an inflammatory condition of the skin. The skin eruption may be red and weeping in acute eczema or thickened, dry and scaly in chronic stages. The rash usually causes severe itching and can be exacerbated by infection. There are several ways of classifying eczema.

- Allergic eczema is caused by sensitisation to an allergen such as nickel, lanolin, rubber or epoxy resins.
- Atopic eczema usually starts in childhood and may accompany asthma and hay fever and allergic rhinitis. Atopic individuals develop high levels of antibodies to everyday allergens.
- Irritant eczema occurs in response to substances like detergents, chemicals or dusts. (If eczema is related to the workplace, the patient may need professional advice: information about occupational skin disease can be obtained from the Employment Medical Advisory Service.)
- Seborrhoeic eczema, clearly defined red lesions with greasy scale, commonly occurs on the scalp, face and other parts of the skin with concentrations of sebaceous glands; fungal infection is probably involved (HIV-positive patients are particularly susceptible).
- Varicose eczema is secondary to venous insufficiency and can be exacerbated by allergic reactions to topical treatments.
- Pompholyx eczema causes small vesicles on the palms and soles of the feet.

Treatment

Whatever the cause of eczema, the treatments are often similar. In acute eczema, povidone iodine or potassium permanganate soaks may be prescribed for their antiinfective action and to dry weeping areas of skin. Systemic antibiotics will be required if the eczema is infected. Steroid creams will probably be needed to control the eczema, but should be avoided until any infection is treated because steroids can suppress the local immune response. Tar-based shampoo may be prescribed for treating seborrhoeic eczema by reducing sebum production, or antifungal preparations to treat fungal infections.

Long-term therapy requires diligent skin care and avoidance of exacerbating factors when possible. The evidence for many alternative interventions is slim. Evening primrose oil, once thought to reduce inflammation, can be bought in health food shops but is no longer licensed or available on prescription. Patients who choose to take Chinese herbal medicine should be closely monitored and have regular liver function tests because the treatment can be hepatotoxic.

The nurse can help to educate patients and others about the condition and provide support and practical advice on management. This will include:

- Hydration of the skin with emollient creams such as aqueous cream and emulsifying ointment and unperfumed bath emollients. (Bathing is a good way to hydrate the skin but patients should be warned of the danger of slipping in a bath containing emollients)
- Avoiding soaps, perfumes and other irritants such as woollen clothing. (Cotton gloves can be worn inside rubber or plastic ones to protect the hands from contact)
- Applying steroid creams correctly (see above)
- Providing information about relevant support groups.

Cold sores (herpes simplex)

The common lesion caused by the herpes simplex virus is the unsightly cold sore that develops at the mucocutaneous junction of the lips. The virus is acquired, often as a child from the parent, and after the initial infection the virus lies dormant in the trigeminal nerve ganglion. Recurrent attacks can occur in response to trigger factors like stress, sunlight, illness or pregnancy. The virus is reactivated, producing a tingling sensation followed by painful blisters. The blisters weep and crack and then form scabs that heal in about seven days. The virus is contagious and can be spread to other people or to other parts of the body. Genital herpes, eye involvement and herpetic infection of eczema are some of the possible complications. Hence the need for education on ways of preventing spread of the virus by:

- Scrupulous hand hygiene
- Not kissing or engaging in oral sex when a cold sore is present
- Not sharing towels or utensils
- Not using saliva to moisten contact lenses.

Aciclovir cream, used early in the eruption, may help to minimise the effect. To be of benefit, it needs to be applied every two hours as soon as the tingling begins. Aciclovir cream can be bought over the counter. Patients with genital herpes should usually be referred to the sexual health clinic. Systemic antiviral treatment may be needed in some instances.

Boils and carbuncles

Infected hair follicles can develop into very painful swellings as a result of local inflammation and pus formation. Diabetes should always be ruled out because recurrent skin infections can be a presenting sign. Antibiotic treatment will be needed sometimes but in many instances, after hot bathing, the lesion will discharge spontaneously or be ready for incision. Carbuncles usually need incision and a light calcium alginate wick to encourage drainage, together with suitable dressings until healed.

Impetigo

Impetigo, a staphylococcal infection of the skin, can cause unsightly, weeping lesions with a yellowish crust. The face is commonly affected. Fusidic acid ointment may be used for a short time to clear small lesions but systemic antibiotics may be needed. Mupirocin should be used only for treating methicillin-resistant *Staphylococcus aureus* and is no longer recommended as a first-line treatment for impetigo. Strict personal hygiene (careful hand washing and separate towels) is needed to prevent its being spread. Children should be kept away from school or nursery until the crusting has resolved.

Fungal infections

Any part of the body may be affected by a fungal infection. Recurrent fungal infections may be indicative of diabetes mellitus and a blood glucose test should be performed in such instances. Intertrigo occurs when skin layers are in contact. Moisture and friction cause soreness and maceration of the skin. Obesity is a contributing factor and candida infection may complicate the condition. Babies can develop distressing rashes in the napkin area. Scrupulous cleansing and drying of the skin is essential. Sometimes antifungal creams containing hydrocortisone are needed for a few days to treat the inflammation of the skin. The general term 'fungal infection' covers both conditions caused by candida and those caused by dermatophytes. Most conditions can be treated with topical antifungal preparations (see *BNF*). Systemic treatment, such as terbinafine, may be needed for intractable dermatophytoses, including nail and scalp infections.

Athlete's foot (tinea pedis)

Fungal infection readily occurs in the moist skin between the toes, causing itching, maceration and painful cracks. Left untreated, this can allow entry to other organisms and result in severe infection of the legs and feet. Treatment with imidazole antifungal preparations (see *BNF*) is usually effective. Recurrence is likely if patients do not follow these basic foot care measures.

- Wash the feet at least once a day and dry carefully between the toes. (Use an antifungal treatment if athlete's foot is present)
- Wear clean socks or stockings every day
- Wear footwear which allows air to the feet
- Change footwear regularly
- See your doctor if the condition does not respond to treatment or if the toenails become affected.

Ringworm

Ringworm is an itchy dermatophyte infection that usually occurs on exposed areas of the body (tinea corporis) or on the scalp (tinea capitis). It is commonly contracted from animals but may also be spread by humans. Ringworm on the body can often be recognised by characteristic circular lesions on the skin and as circular areas of alopecia on the scalp. Skin scrapings should be taken for mycology when the diagnosis is in doubt.

Warts

Warts are caused by different types of the human papilloma virus. Warts on the hands and feet usually disappear spontaneously as the body develops immunity to the virus. Unfortunately, this can take many months and patients with unsightly warts on the hands, or pressure symptoms from verrucae, are unlikely to want to wait. Plantar warts (verrucae) are very common in children but schools will sometimes try to exclude a child from swimming or games. Although unlikely to limit the spread, verruca socks can be worn to satisfy the school rules.

If treatment is requested, topical preparations of salicylic acid can be recommended or prescribed. Many preparations also contain an occlusive substance such as collodion. The manufacturer's instructions must be followed. The treatment is applied as directed, taking care to avoid the surrounding skin. A pumice stone or emery board should be used between applications to remove dead skin. Patients need to persevere with the treatment for up to six weeks. Occlusion with duct tape may also be tried in preference to cryotherapy.[22] If there is no response, minor surgery may be considered, depending on the local policy. Chiropody may be the best treatment for plantar warts.

Genital warts

Genital warts are transmitted sexually (see Chapter 12, Sexual Health). Patients should be referred to the genitourinary medicine clinic for treatment and to be screened for other sexually transmitted diseases.

Suggestions for reflection on practice

Review your job description, professional education and experience.

- Do you feel competent to deal with the medical conditions you encounter in your practice?
- Do you have up-to-date protocols to work to?
- What further education/resources do you need?
- How does your role as a practice nurse differ from that of a doctor or nurse practitioner in dealing with patients with minor medical conditions?

REFERENCES

1. Statutory Instrument No. 569 (2004) *NHS Direct (Establishment and Constitution) Order 2004.* www.opsi.gov.uk/si/si20Sta0405.htm (accessed 5/11/05).
2. Protti, D. (2005) *Personal Health Records and Sharing Patient Information.* www.connectingforhealth.nhs.uk/worldnews/protti7 (accessed 5/11/05).
3. Department of Health (2004) New surgeries offer commuters fast-track to treatment. Press release 2004/0392. www.dh.gov.uk (accessed 7/11/05).
4. Statutory Instrument No. 641 (2005) *NHS (Pharmaceutical Services) Regulations 2005.* www.opsi.gov.uk/si/si2005/20050641.htm (accessed 7/11/05).
5. Jones, M. (2005) Profile – Mark Jones: New Zealand bound. *Practice Nursing,* **16** (11), 570.
6. Department of Health Medicines Pharmacy and Industry Group (2003) *Mechanisms for Nurse and Pharmacist Prescribing and Supply of Medicines.* www.dh.gov.uk/assetRoot/04/06/99/06/04069906.pdf (accessed 11/11/05).
7. Department of Health (2005) Nurse and pharmacist prescribing powers extended. Press release 2005/0395. www.dh.gov.uk/PublicationsAndStatistics/PressReleases/fs/en (accessed 112/11/05).
8. British Medical Association and Royal Pharmaceutical Society of Great Britain (2005) Aspirin. *British National Formulary* 49 4.7.1.
9. Schroeder, K. & Fahey, T. (2004) Over-the-counter medications for acute cough in children and adults in ambulatory settings. *Cochrane Database of Systematic Reviews,* Issue 4. Art. No. CD001831.
10. Prodigy Guidance (2005) *Allergic Rhinitis.* www.prodigy.nhs.uk/guidance.asp?gt=Allergicrhinitis (accessed 17/11/05).
11. Scottish Intercollegiate Guidelines Network (2003) *Diagnosis and Management of Childhood Otitis Media in Primary Care.* SIGN Report No 66. www.sign.ac.uk/pdf/sign66.pdf (accessed 19/11/05).

12. Prodigy Guidance (2003) *Gastroenteritis.* www.prodigy.nhs.uk/guidance.asp?gt=Gastroenteritis (accessed 22/11/05).
13. Prodigy Guidance (2004) *Threadworm.* www.prodigy.nhs.uk/guidance.asp?gt=threadworm (accessed 26/11/05).
14. Jepson, R.G., Mihaljevic, L. & Craig, J. (2004) Cranberries for preventing urinary tract infection. *Cochrane Database of Systematic Reviews,* Issue 2. Art. No. CD001321.
15. PN News (2005) New guidance on risks of chickenpox in pregnancy. *Practice Nurse,* **30** (9), 6.
16. Chief Medical Officer, Chief Nursing Officer, Chief Dental Officer and Chief Pharmaceutical Officer (2003) *Chickenpox (Varicella) Immunisation for Health Care Workers. CMO letter no 8.* Department of Health, London.
17. Prodigy Guidance (2005) *Shingles and Postherpetic Neuralgia.* www.prodigy.nhs.uk/guidance.asp?gt=Shingles (accessed 1/12/05).
18. Prodigy Guidance (2004) *Head Lice.* www.prodigy.nhs.uk/guidance.asp?gt=Headlice (accessed 2/12/05).
19. Garner, S.E., Eady, E.A., Popescu, C., Newton, J. & Li Wan Po, A. (2003) Minocycline for acne vulgaris: efficacy and safety. *Cochrane Database of Systemic Reviews,* Issue 1 Art. No. CD002086.
20. British Association for Dermatology and Primary Care Dermatology Society (2003) *Recommendations for the Initial Management of Psoriasis.* www.pcds.org.uk (accessed 5/12/05).
21. Patient UK (2004) *Fingertip Units for Topical Steroids.* www.patient.co.uk/Showdoc/27000762 (accessed 5/12/05).
22. Focht, D.R., Spicer, C. & Fairchok, M.P. (2002) The efficacy of duct tape vs cryotherapy in the treatment of verruca vulgaris (the common wart). *Archives of Pediatrics and Adolescent Medicine,* **156** (10), 971–4.

FURTHER READING

British Medical Association and Royal Pharmaceutical Society of Great Britain (2005) *British National Formulary 50.* BMA and RPSGB, London.
Coutney, M. & Griffiths, M. (eds) (2004) *Independent and Supplementary Prescribing: an essential guide.* Greenwich Medical Media, London.
Health and Safety Executive (2000) *The Employment Medical Advisory Service and You.* Health and Safety Executive, Sheffield.
Health Protection Agency (2002) *Management of Abnormal Vaginal Discharge in Women: quick reference guide for primary care.* www.hpa.org.uk (search vaginal discharge).
Johnson, G., Hill-Smith, I. & Ellis, C. (2005) *The Minor Illness Manual,* 3rd edn. Radcliffe Medical Press, Oxford.
Joseph, D. (2005) Psoriasis. *Practice Nurse,* **30**(1), 25–8.

USEFUL WEBSITES

Examples of Clinical Management Plans for supplementary prescribers
Website: www.nurse-prescriber.co.uk/education/modules/CMP_toolkit/CMP_samples.htm

Prodigy Guidance
Website: www.prodigy.nhs.uk/ClinicalGuidance/

Acne Support Group
Telephone: 0870 870 2263
Website: www.stopspots.org

Psoriasis Association
Website: www.psoriasis-association.org.uk

Chapter 9
Health Promotion

Health promotion became a natural part of the practice nurse role when the GP Contract made general practice the focus for initiatives to promote healthy lifestyles and to prevent certain diseases. Various ways of reimbursing practices for health promotional activities were introduced and later dropped. Successive governments linked health promotion to targets outlined in their strategy documents. *The Health of the Nation* (1992) and *Saving Lives: our healthier nation* (1998) were the English versions. Scotland, Wales and Northern Ireland produced similar strategies. Primary care organisations now produce plans which reflect the national and local priorities for improving health through collaboration between health and social care agencies and the public.

NATIONAL SERVICE FRAMEWORKS AND QUALITY AND OUTCOMES FRAMEWORK

A series of National Service Frameworks have been published since 1999.[1] Every practice will have a copy of the NSFs and nurses are advised to familiarise themselves with them. Since April 2004, the Quality and Outcomes Framework has provided incentives and rewards for practices to provide high-quality care, especially to patients with chronic diseases. The practice nurse's role in preventing ill health will be covered in this chapter but the reader should be aware of the wider medical and social issues.

INEQUALITIES IN HEALTH

It has long been recognised that poverty and lower social class have adverse effects on health. This was clearly demonstrated by the Black Report in 1980.[2] More recently, the Acheson Report demonstrated that inequalities still exist.[3] Unskilled working men are three times more likely to die prematurely of coronary heart disease than men in professional or managerial occupations, according to the NSF for CHD.

CULTURAL DIVERSITY

Britain is recognised as being multicultural. In terms of health promotion, this requires sensitivity to the needs of members of different cultural groups and an understanding of specific health factors. There may be a requirement for an interpreter, who is not a family member, or for literature in the appropriate language when English is not understood. Local health promotion or social service training departments usually provide sessions on cultural awareness to help nurses and doctors to examine their attitudes to members of other cultural groups and to develop strategies for meeting the needs of all their patients equitably.

EDUCATION FOR PRACTICE NURSES

Practice nurses have accepted health promotion as a fundamental part of their work but they require a thorough understanding of the process and a good grounding in using models of health promotion in order to be truly effective. Training in negotiating behaviour change and motivational interviewing is recommended as a minimum for this role. Health promotion is also covered in depth on the community specialist (general practice nursing) degree courses. Good communication skills are a prerequisite for successful health promotion. Telling people what they ought to be doing is unlikely to succeed. Motivational interviewing is a way of helping people to recognise the need to change a risky behaviour and to decide for themselves on a suitable strategy for change.

TERMINOLOGY

The term 'health promotion' is used rather freely nowadays but its exact meaning warrants some reflection. Health is a complex issue, influenced as much by environmental, political, social and genetic factors as by personal behaviour or lifestyle. Health promotion is a broad term covering all those activities that contribute to the social, physical and mental wellbeing of individuals and societies. In general practice, it mainly involves preventive care and health education although health workers may also campaign for action on the wider issues, such as cigarette smoking shown on television or alcohol advertising at the cinema.

Prevention

Preventive care aims either to prevent ill health or to minimise its effect. Three types of prevention are recognised.

- *Primary prevention* covers activities that aim to prevent disease from occurring, e.g. immunisation against infectious diseases, encouraging healthy eating and exercise.
- *Secondary prevention* aims to detect problems before symptoms develop, in order to take early remedial action, e.g. child development checks, cervical and breast screening.
- *Tertiary prevention* includes the management of existing disease or disability in order to minimise any complications and maximise the patient's quality of life, e.g. encouraging good glycaemic control in diabetes, controlling high blood pressure to prevent heart failure or a stroke.

Screening

Screening entails looking for previously unrecognised disease in particular groups of people. Screening tests have to meet various criteria in order to be of value.

- The condition being screened for should be an important health problem.
- The natural history of the condition should be well understood.
- There should be a detectable early stage.
- Treatment at an early stage should be of more benefit than at a later stage.
- The condition must be treatable.
- A suitable test should be devised for the early stage.
- The test should be acceptable.
- Intervals for repeating the test should be determined.
- Adequate health service provision should be made for the extra clinical workload resulting from screening.
- The risks, both physical and psychological, should be less than the benefits.
- The costs should be balanced against the benefits.[4]

No screening should be undertaken without informed consent. Patients could be subjected to unnecessary investigations and distress if screening tests produce false-positive results. Conversely, false-negative results may lead patients to ignore subsequent symptoms because of a false sense of security. There should be a sound evidence base for any tests performed. Private tests offered to patients might not meet such stringent criteria and caution should be advised. Patients may read about such tests in magazines or on the internet and ask for advice.

Health education

Health education seeks to provide learning opportunities about health, either by working with individuals or through the media or advertising. At the personal level, health education involves sharing knowledge about health, identifying any risks to health and helping people to develop the ability to make healthy choices.

HEALTH PROMOTION AND THE PRIMARY HEALTHCARE TEAM

Nurses who undertake health promotion must have discussed the ethical implications and have a clear philosophy of health. Many health behaviours are highly complex, yet there is a danger of attributing blame to people whose actions are perceived as contributing to their own diseases. Health promotion activities should be evidence based as far as possible. Doctors and nurses who 'practise what they preach' and act as role models for their patients may have greater credibility when offering advice to patients about healthy living.

Communication

Communication involves both the transmission and reception of information and ideas. Non-verbal communication relays messages, either consciously or unconsciously, through facial expression, gesture, general appearance and posture. All the senses pick up cues and confusion occurs when the non-verbal message conflicts with the spoken one.

A nurse should ensure that any information given is meaningful. Written material will be of little use if the patient is illiterate, cannot see well enough to read or does not understand the language in which it is written. Jargon can be useful shorthand for those in the know but it is also a way of excluding outsiders. It follows that to use jargon to patients can exclude them as well. It is better to assume nothing and always check what the patient knows and has understood. Many of the techniques of counselling can be used in health promotion.

- *Suitable ambience* – a quiet, peaceful environment, free from telephone calls and visual distractions, will help concentration on the issues.
- *Asking open questions* – closed questions such as 'Do you drink any alcohol?' will elicit yes/no type answers. Open questions (often beginning with what, why, when, where or how) allow a subject to be explored; for example 'How many days each week do you drink alcohol?' or 'What effect do you think this has on your health?'.
- *Checking on understanding* – no matter how obvious the subject may seem to the nurse, it may be totally obscure to the patient; so it pays to take stock regularly. The nurse can ask the patient to recap in his/her own words what has been discussed. Alternatively, the nurse may paraphrase what the patient has said to make sure nothing has been misunderstood.

- *Active listening* – it requires a particular skill to be able to sit and give undivided attention to another person; to maintain a calm but attentive posture, to allow eye contact without staring, to give nods of encouragement when needed, but above all, to tolerate pauses without wanting to fill them.

Motivation

Knowledge about health risks alone will not cause people to alter their behaviour. They must also feel motivated to change. This means that the rewards of change must outweigh the short-term benefits of the behaviour. Some patients are ambivalent; they want to change but are reluctant to give up the pleasures of their risky behaviour. Motivational interviewing is a technique developed by psychologists to assist ambivalent people to decide to deal with addictive behaviour.[5] The key points are:

- *Empathy* – acceptance of the patient as a person. Trying to enter into the feelings of that person
- *Developing discrepancy* – helping the patient to decide to change and to present his/her own arguments for changing
- *Avoiding confrontation* – arguments are counterproductive
- *Support for self-efficacy* – the patient is responsible for choosing and carrying out personal change.

HEALTH PROMOTION IN GENERAL PRACTICE

Opportunistic health promotion can take place during any consultation or procedure; examples are given in other chapters. The remainder of this chapter deals with planned health promotion activities.

New patient health checks

The new GMS/PMS Contracts require all new patients to be offered a registration health check, although there is no longer an item-of-service fee. Such consultations serve several purposes.

- Patients are welcomed to the surgery and given information about the services provided.
- Essential points are ascertained about a patient's health before the NHS records are transferred. (Entries can be made to the appropriate disease registers.)
- Doctors and nurses can gather details of a patient's social, medical and family history, identify potential health risks and offer appropriate help.

Questionnaires can save some time but a face-to-face interview is also needed to clarify the information and to ensure that the patient consents to personal details being recorded. It is usual to record information on a computer, most of which have a selection of templates for health promotion. Sensitivity is required in interviewing, bearing in mind that the patient is in unfamiliar surroundings and might also be feeling unwell. The questions need to be appropriate to the circumstances of individual patients. Close attention should be paid to the way questions are worded, as it would be very easy to give offence. There must be justifiable reasons for asking for information. Some of the information to be gathered is included under the following headings.

Social background

- *Title* – ask how the patient would like to be addressed. (This can also elicit whether to address a woman as Mrs, Miss or Ms, or if the patient has some other professional or honorary title.) Some patients deplore the modern trend towards addressing people by their first names.
- *Household* – ask if the patient has someone else at home. This might be a spouse or a partner, another relative or a lodger. It is wise to record the contact number and address of the person to be notified in an emergency, especially if the patient lives alone.
- *Carer* – all new patients should be asked if they are caring for someone with a long-term physical or mental disability.
- *Children* – the number and ages of any children may be relevant to the parent's health. A check can also be made on the immunisation status of children. (The health visitor should be informed about any children under five years.)
- *Employment* – check if there are any occupational hazards to consider. Increased ill health and depression can occur in the unemployed. If a woman has declared herself to be a housewife, it is insensitive to ask 'Do you work?'. It is better to enquire about any work outside the home.
- *Smoking* – record if the patient has ever smoked. The quantity per day should be recorded in any smoking history and the year of stopping, if an ex-smoker.
- *Alcohol* – if the patient is not teetotal, ask how many units a day are consumed and on how many days a week.
- *Exercise* – the frequency, duration and degree of any regular exercise undertaken should be recorded.

Past medical history

- *Illnesses* – any serious illnesses and hospital admissions should be noted.
- *Operations* – list in chronological order.
- *Allergies* – some patients confuse allergies with side effects such as nausea; any true allergies must be documented prominently.
- *Immunisations* – patients who have not completed a full course against tetanus, diphtheria or polio can be offered immunisations; routine boosters are not required (see Chapter 10).

Current health

- *Current problems* – ask particularly about indigestion, pain, any abnormal bleeding or any problems with bladder or bowel function (consider the possibility of anaemia or thyroid dysfunction).
- *Medication* – ask what, if any, prescribed, illicit or OTC medicines are taken regularly.

Women

- *Obstetric history* – ask about any pregnancies or miscarriages.
- *Menstruation* – ask questions, depending on the age of the patient, about the regularity of periods, any problems and age at menopause, HRT.
- *Rubella status* – all women who could become pregnant should be immune to rubella and should be offered rubella antibody screening if appropriate.
- *Contraception* – ask questions as appropriate. Check the method and need for further advice. If taking the pill, check for how many years. If they use an IUD or diaphragm, ask when it was last checked. If contraceptive injection or implant, check when the next one is due.
- *Cervical smear* – if appropriate, record date and result of last smear, any history of abnormal smears/treatment. (Offer a smear appointment if it is due.)
- *Breasts* – has the patient been taught breast awareness? Has she ever had mammography and if so, what was the result? (Offer advice or information if appropriate.)
- *Use of HRT* if postmenopausal.

Men

- *Testes* – has the patient been taught about testicular self-examination? The incidence of testicular cancer in young men has been increasing and public awareness of the condition has been raised by high-profile campaigns in the media.
- *Prostate* – if appropriate, ask about nocturia or any difficulty passing urine. Specific questions may detect problems which men attribute to ageing. Patients may wish to discuss testing for prostate cancer (see Chapter 14).

Men can be diffident about expressing their feelings or concerns but they may be more willing to seek help when it is needed if a rapport is established during a new patient interview.

Family history

- *Parents and siblings* – ask particularly about diabetes, CHD, hypertension, stroke, asthma, cancer, glaucoma, thyroid problems or tuberculosis, plus diagnosis and age at death (if no longer alive).

Tests

- *Height and weight* – calculate the body mass index (weight in kilograms divided by the square of height in meters) from a BMI chart or computer program. Check if the BMI is within the normal range (20–25 for men, 18.5–23.6 for women). Very muscular people may have a high BMI without having excess body fat.
- *Blood pressure* – follow the practice protocol.
- *Peak expiratory flow rate* – check this if there is a history of asthma.

Urinalysis screening for glycosuria and proteinuria is no longer considered to be reliable for diabetes or renal disease in asymptomatic individuals.[6]

Well-person checks

Patients may request a check-up at any time. Landmark birthdays, such as 40, 50 or 60 years, may trigger a sudden realisation of mortality. If a patient requests such a consultation, it is important to identify any particular health concerns and refer him/her to the doctor if necessary. Patients often have a vision of what a check-up should cover; this may be akin to the battery of tests and investigations undertaken by private health companies. Well-person health checks in general practice cover similar ground to that listed above (under new patient health checks), although the emphasis may vary, depending on the age and sex of the patient. Lifestyle factors such as smoking, alcohol consumption, diet and exercise, together with blood pressure, BMI and family history, can be used in the assessment of the risks for heart disease and to offer appropriate help. Various risk assessment tools are available, which can be used with caution in accordance with the practice protocol. Links can be found on the British Heart Foundation website.

Assessment of older people

The new GMS and PMS Contracts require all patients aged over 75 years, who request it, to be offered an annual health check.[7] Nurses are employed by some practices specifically to undertake this work. The National Service Framework for Older People contains eight standards for ensuring that older people receive a consistently high level of service and are not denied access to healthcare because of age.[8] The NSF also requires systems to be in place for ensuring that patients gain the maximum benefit from any medication and have their medication reviewed regularly. An over-75 health check can incorporate a medication review satisfactorily.[9]

The NSF calls for the integration of assessment procedures for health and social care, which entails cooperation between all the services involved and a rethinking of current assessment procedures. Practice nurses who undertake home visits must ensure that they have received appropriate education for the role. The extent of assessments depends on local policies but the following points would usually be considered.

Social assessment

- *Housing* – check whether the patient lives in his or her own home, rented accommodation or sheltered housing. Consider:
  - facilities (toilet, bathing, cooking, heating)
  - safety (any loose rugs/floorboards, trailing flexes, unguarded fires)
  - access (stairs, lift, ground floor).
- *Carers* – check whether the patient lives alone, who is next of kin, level of support from family, friends, warden or social services, age of carers, or if the carers are on the register of carers. Do the carers need more support and is there evidence of tension in the household or of any abuse of the older person? Elder abuse is recognised as a serious problem, which can take many forms. Abuse occurs in institutional settings, but more often in the home.[10]
- *Finance* – is the patient able to keep the home warm, buy nutritious food, afford holidays or employ help if needed? Are all benefits being claimed, if entitled?
- *Lifestyle* – ask about smoking, alcohol consumption, nutrition, exercise, social contacts, clubs and hobbies.

Physical assessment

- *Ability to self-care* – ask how the patient manages cooking, bathing, shopping. Check the condition of his/her skin, hair and nails and ability to take any medication correctly.
- *Mobility* – ask about how he/she walks indoors and outdoors and if able to manage stairs. Check suitability of footwear and which mobility aids are used (if needed).
- *Vision* – ask the date of last eye test, check use and condition of spectacles and ability to read.
- *Hearing* – note any hearing impairment. If the patient needs a hearing aid, check his/her ability to use and maintain it.
- *Dentition* – ask about condition of teeth or dentures and whether the patient is able to visit a dentist if needed.
- *General health* – ask about sleep, appetite, energy or any pain. Check for any signs of anaemia or thyroid dysfunction.
- *Continence* – enquire about any problems with bladder or bowel function and if continence aids/services are used or needed.
- *Tests* – check blood pressure to detect hypertension. Arrange for midstream specimen of urine if infection likely and blood tests as necessary for glucose, thyroid, kidney or liver function.

- *Medication* (if taking any medicines) – check whether the patient knows what they are for and when to take them. Ask if they were prescribed or OTC. Check they are still in date and whether any are duplicated with trade and generic names and if there is evidence of stockpiling. Make sure the patient is able to open any pill bottles or packets.

Mental assessment

- *Level of consciousness* – observe whether the patient is alert or drowsy and his/her ability to concentrate.
- *Mood* – observe whether the patient appears normal, depressed, anxious or elated.
- *Thoughts and speech* – note whether the patient's speech makes sense and any evidence of hallucinations or delusions.
- *Orientation and memory* – if appropriate, check if the patient knows the date, where he/she lives, his/her age. Ask if the patient can remember what was said five minutes ago.
- *Behaviour* – observe whether it appears appropriate to the circumstances.

A mental assessment can be more difficult than a physical assessment. Patients with early dementia can be very plausible and unless the nurse knows the family well, the problem will not always be apparent. A patient can give graphic details of his/her daily activities, which relate to years gone by and bear no relationship to the present situation.

Cautions

It would be wrong to assume that all older people are incapacitated in some way. As in every other generation, huge variations will be found. For every elderly, housebound person living in poverty, there will be another with a generous income, able to enjoy the freedom from work and family ties to travel and have fun.

Nurses should beware of promising help that cannot be delivered. False expectations can be aroused if situations are encountered for which there are few local services available. Loneliness and difficulties with bathing and foot care are probably the most common problems but many social service and chiropody departments are overstretched. Nevertheless, it would be pointless to carry out assessments of patients without acting upon any findings. A pharmacist could help with medication difficulties. Nurses must be aware of the local procedure to follow if other problems come to light. That will entail knowing:

- Which health, voluntary or social services to contact
- When to refer to the GP or to carry out further tests
- Where to find information about private agencies or suppliers of equipment for patients who can afford them and wish to use them.

DIETARY ADVICE AND MONITORING

Dieticians are responsible for providing specialised dietary advice but practice nurses are usually expected to give guidance on healthy eating and to monitor patients on some diets. Collaboration allows the expertise of dieticians and nurses to be used effectively.

Healthy eating

Food is needed to provide the protein, vitamins and minerals required for healthy tissues and to supply the energy for daily activity and a normal body weight. Malabsorption, disease and anorexia can cause malnutrition but the majority of patients seeking advice are more likely to suffer from the effects of dietary excess. The incidence of obesity continues to rise despite the increased knowledge about its detrimental effects on health. In fact, obesity has more than trebled in the last two decades.[11] Concern about childhood obesity has been particularly highlighted by the increased incidence of type 2 diabetes being found in children and adolescents.[12]

Most people would benefit from an increase in the consumption of complex carbohydrates and dietary fibre and a reduction in fat, salt and sugar. Fruit and vegetables, pasta, rice and cereals should provide the greatest proportion of the diet with smaller quantities of protein and very little fat. The current government policy is that everyone should have at least five portions of fruit and vegetables a day.[13]

Lipid-lowering diets

Patients are very aware of high cholesterol as a contributory factor for coronary artery disease. The National Service Framework for Coronary Heart Disease expects 80–90% of people to be given a statin to lower their cholesterol level after a heart attack. Patients with an inherited hyperlipidaemia can also require treatment with lipid-lowering drugs. Statins have received a great deal of publicity recently and can now be purchased over the counter. Opinions are divided about the wisdom of this development.[14,15]

The selection of asymptomatic patients for testing will depend on the practice policy, but talking to a patient who requests a cholesterol test will provide an opportunity for discussing other risk factors such as smoking, family history, raised BMI and lack of exercise. Help can be offered to consider appropriate lifestyle changes. Healthy eating and a control of dietary fat are beneficial for almost everyone. The Committee on Medical Aspects of Food and Nutrition Policy (COMA) first made recommendations in 1991. Less than 30% of the daily energy requirement should come from fat; of which not more than 10% should be saturated fat. COMA has since been replaced by the Scientific Advisory Committee on Nutrition, which will probably produce new guidance soon.

Whatever figures are chosen, they are likely to mean little to the average person, so it would be better to suggest reducing total fat intake and to replace animal fats such as full cream milk, butter and cheese with suitable low-fat alternatives by using low-fat spreads or those made with monounsaturated/ polyunsaturated fats. Olive oil, sunflower oil, corn oil and low-fat oils and salad dressings could be discussed, with suggestions for cooking methods without the use of additional fat. Aerosol cans of cooking oil can be used to grease cooking pans and electric low-fat grills are valuable for draining unwanted fats in the cooking process. Patients may need to be reminded about hidden fats in cakes, biscuits and processed foods.

The whole subject is a minefield and patients need to read food labels carefully if they are not to be misled by unrealistic claims on the packet. Prepacked meals should not contain more than 5% fat, or more than 15 g fat per serving. Low-fat spreads and yoghurts vary considerably in their fat contents. Patients who do not need to lose weight will need to increase their intake of starchy food as they reduce their fats, in order to maintain their calorie intake. Patients should also be encouraged to use wholegrain products and increase their intake of oily fish, soluble fibre (oats and pulses), fruit and vegetables.

Weight loss

The cause of obesity is simple – more calories are consumed than the body uses for energy, so the excess is stored as fat. The complexity lies in the reasons for the mismatch. Very few people enjoy being overweight but strong psychological factors and ingrained behaviour affect eating habits. There may even be genetic factors involved. Rapid weight loss can be followed by a rapid weight gain, as a result of metabolic changes. Therefore, the objective must be to help the patient to avoid drastic dieting and to substitute more suitable foods without creating an obsession with the next meal. The following steps can be helpful.

- *Obtain a full medical, social and family history*, to identify any factors that could affect the patient's weight.
- *Measure the current weight and height*, to calculate the body mass index and identify how much weight, if any, needs to be shed.
- *Assess the patient's motivation*, to find out if the patient wants to lose weight. Check if he/she perceives the increased risks to health of obesity (CHD, diabetes, osteoarthritis). Encourage the ambivalent patient to identify the personal benefits and positive reasons for change.
- *Identify the root cause of being overweight* instead of just dealing with the symptoms (i.e. by dieting).

- *Help the patient to set realistic goals.* Small steps, which can be reached in a reasonable time, will provide the encouragement to persevere. Success reinforces motivation.
- *Identify the patient's usual eating habits.* Ask the patient to keep an accurate food diary for at least a week. The diary should include the quantities as well as the types of food and drink and the circumstances when they were consumed. Alcohol consumption should also be recorded. Patients from other cultural backgrounds may eat foods with which the nurse is not familiar. The dietician can be consulted about their nutritional values. Patients from developing countries may need to be persuaded to stick to their traditional foods and to avoid the high-fat hamburgers and foods full of salt or refined sugar so popular in western diets. However, some Asian patients may also need to be persuaded to use cooking oil instead of ghee, which is mostly saturated fat, and to use less of it.
- *Negotiate changes to the diet.* Healthy eating will need to be lifelong. Drastic changes to eating habits will not be sustained if the patient does not like the substituted foods.

A nurse should be able to offer suggestions in accordance with the patient's income and religious beliefs. Sometimes compromises may be needed to help the patients to accept change. Some examples are given below.

- *Milk* – if skimmed milk is unacceptable, try semi-skimmed. Skimmed milk can be used in some cooking, where it won't be tasted. If enough milk is not drunk each day, low-fat yoghurt will provide calcium and vitamins.
- *Salads* – dieters who hate salads do not have to eat them. Alternatively, salad can be used in sandwiches, with hot food or after the main course, as they eat it in France. A teaspoonful of low-fat salad dressing can make all the difference to the taste of a salad.
- *Vegetables* – several different vegetables, even if cooked in the same pot, will be more interesting than a plate loaded with one type. Jacket potatoes make a filling meal with cottage cheese, tuna, baked beans or yogurt with onions and herbs (instead of butter).
- *Fruit* – tinned fruit in fruit juice can be found in most supermarkets. Dried fruits make a delicious snack. Fruits in season are cheaper than exotic imports, which carry high transport costs.
- *Meat* – the better cuts may be expensive but smaller quantities can be eaten. Lean meat, skinless chicken or low-fat sausages can be grilled, casseroled or baked, instead of fried. Poultry contains less fat but the skin must be removed before cooking.
- *Fibre* – if patients do not like wholemeal bread, try high-fibre white bread as an alternative. A few chopped ready-to-eat dried apricots or raisins added to breakfast cereals will add sweetness and texture. If high-fibre cereals are disliked, try mixing different cereals together to give variety and improve the taste. Porridge made with skimmed milk can make a filling breakfast.

Any of the above examples could apply equally to patients who want to eat more healthily, even without losing weight.

Once a patient has decided to lose weight the practice nurse can help by:

- *Monitoring progress* – the rapid weight loss of the first weeks will slow down. Particular encouragement is needed when a plateau is reached. Increased physical activity can be advised and keeping a food diary can help to remotivate the patient. New goals can be set as weight is lost. A good weight loss is 0.5–1 kg a week
- *Dealing with lapses* – patients need to understand that relapses are part of the cycle of change.[16] If the patient still wishes to lose weight then he/she can begin again by planning how to deal with difficult situations and have a positive attitude to change, instead of feeling like a failure
- *Encouraging maintenance of the target weight* – once the patient has reached the final goal, adjustments to the diet will need to be made to stay at the target weight. Euphoria at having achieved the goal can lead the patient to resume the old habits of eating. Throughout the period of weight loss, the benefits of permanent change must be stressed. Binge eating at this important stage of the process could be disastrous.

Discussions about diet should be accompanied by recommendations for appropriate exercise and sensible drinking.

Exercise

It is now possible in some areas to prescribe exercise in a similar way to prescribing drugs and arrangements have been made with local leisure centres for patients to take part in structured exercise. Even more innovative schemes have been reported, such as the green gyms, which link exercise to conservation work.[17] Physical activity has many benefits for health, not least in the prevention of coronary heart disease and diabetes. The level of activity must be appropriate for each individual patient. Advice booklets can be obtained from the health promotion department. Patients who are obese or who have a history of hypertension or heart disease may require specific advice from a physiotherapist.

Sensible drinking

Alcohol consumption is an important part of any health assessment. People of all ages have ready access to alcoholic drinks and millions of workdays are lost each year through drink-related absenteeism. Measurements in units of alcohol make assessment easier, providing that patients understand what constitutes a unit and give an accurate report of their consumption. One unit, equivalent to 8 g of pure alcohol, is found in:

- Half a pint of ordinary strength beer
- One single pub measure of spirits
- One small glass of wine.

Therefore, a patient who drinks an aperitif each evening and half a bottle of wine with dinner is likely to be drinking 5–6 units daily. Sensible drinking is considered to be below 28 units a week for men and 21 units for women, spread evenly over the week.[18] Patients should be made aware that drinking all the recommended units at a weekend could be more harmful than drinking regular daily amounts. They also need to know that drinking more than the recommended amount can have adverse effects on health, particularly the liver. Alcohol in pregnancy or while breastfeeding can be damaging to the fetus/baby so women must be advised not to have more than a very occasional drink in those circumstances.

Patients who answer 'yes' to two or more questions in the CAGE questionnaire are more likely to be dependent on alcohol.

- Have you ever felt you should **C**ut down on your drinking?
- Have people **A**nnoyed you by criticising your drinking?
- Have you ever felt bad or **G**uilty about your drinking?
- Have you ever had a drink in the morning to steady your nerves or get rid of a hangover (**E**ye-opener)?

The Prodigy Guidance recommends the use of a simple questionnaire called the Alcohol Use Disorders Identification Test (AUDIT), which was devised by the World Health Organisation.[19]

An elevation in one or both of two blood tests may help to confirm or monitor a patient with an alcohol problem.

- *Liver functions test* – particularly gamma-glutamyl transpeptidase (GGT).
- *Full blood count* – for mean corpuscular volume (MCV).[20]

Patients with alcohol dependence, who are willing to be helped, may require medical supervision or a support service such as Alcoholics Anonymous. Detoxification and total abstinence would be needed in such cases. Practice nurses can help patients who want to drink less to agree on a sensible limit and devise strategies for sticking to it. A drink diary can help a patient to stay within the target limit and to recognise the times and situations when the pressure to drink is greatest. Ways of cutting down which may be adopted include the following.

- Keep busy to avoid thinking about drink
- Postpone the first drink until as late as possible in the day
- Drink halves instead of pints
- Try low-alcohol drinks instead

- Dilute spirits with mixers
- Take small sips and make a drink last
- Don't get involved in buying rounds – it can involve trying to keep pace with other drinkers.
- Use a measure at home to make sure a drink is only a single, then put the bottle out of sight.

The relationship between drinking and social activities can vary. The importance of not drinking and driving can make the refusal of alcohol more socially acceptable, but in other circumstances, peer pressure can be very strong. Sadly, a lot of alcohol advertisements seem to be aimed at young people. The money spent persuading them to drink far outweighs the resources available for health education, despite some very good initiatives by schools and school nurses. It is to be regretted that actors are often seen to be reaching for a bottle in television dramas or films, whenever they need to convey that they are under some form of stress.

SMOKING CESSATION

There is an increasing awareness of the health risks from smoking and pressure on smokers to quit. Health workers are required to identify the patients who smoke, explain the dangers to health and to provide access to services to help them stop smoking.[21] It is important to understand the social and psychological pressures that lead people to take up smoking, in order to avoid being judgemental. As the overt advertising of cigarettes has been stopped, tobacco companies are finding ever more subtle ways to promote their products. Practice nurses who feel strongly about the issue could note the times actors are seen smoking on television and telephone the television company to complain.

Nicotine replacement products or the drug bupropion can be prescribed, when appropriate, together with quit-smoking counselling to help patients to overcome the addiction to nicotine.[22] Some practice nurses have undergone the training needed to become smoking cessation counsellors. Pharmacists in some areas are also taking on this role. Practice nurses should be aware of local arrangements and the support services for people who want to stop smoking. If a patient is ambivalent about quitting, the health professional has a duty to ensure that he/she has the facts about smoking and knows that help is available whenever the time is right to stop. Useful information can be downloaded from the internet. However, no one can force a patient to quit; it must be a personal decision.

The dangers of smoking to health include:

- Heart disease and hypertension
- Peripheral vascular disease
- Chronic obstructive pulmonary disease
- Cancer of the lung, throat, mouth, tongue

- Cancer of the stomach, pancreas, cervix
- Pregnant women are more likely to have smaller, unhealthy babies
- Children who live in an environment where people smoke are more likely to have respiratory problems.

Patients will sometimes develop symptoms of these conditions before they will accept help. They must be assured that it is never too late to give up smoking and that it can be a very important way of improving health. The dangers of passive smoking have received a great deal of publicity and smoking in the workplace is usually discouraged. Parents need to be aware that children learn by example and are statistically more likely to start smoking if they come from a home where people smoke. Particular emphasis is being placed on helping pregnant mothers to quit smoking.

Helping patients quit smoking

A carbon monoxide monitor and/or a spirometer can be useful tools for convincing patients of the effects of smoking. A patient who wants to quit can be helped to devise a plan.

- Work out all the reasons for stopping
- Decide a date to stop, avoiding a day likely to be stressful
- Tell people in close contact of the decision and try to persuade someone else to quit at the same time, for mutual support
- Decide how to change the routine to avoid the usual triggers for smoking
- Have nicotine replacement products ready, if needed, and contact details of support person or organisation
- The evening before the quit day, smoke the last cigarette and then throw away any remaining cigarettes.

Hints for the new non-smoker

- Avoid temptation – put ashtrays, matches and lighter out of sight
- Keep away from smokers (if possible)
- Change habits – avoid breaks when a cigarette is usually smoked
- Keep busy
- Put aside the money saved each day, for a reward later on
- Keep a supply of chewing gum, apple or carrot to nibble if necessary
- Take more exercise to avoid gaining weight.

Nicotine is highly addictive and a large number of smokers who quit smoking are likely to relapse, despite the costly input from the NHS. However, the problems caused are so serious that smoking cessation is still considered to be one of the most cost-effective of all healthcare interventions.[23]

Suggestions for reflection on practice

Consider your role in health promotion.

- How do you measure success?
- Do you need more training or resources?
- Could anything be done differently?

REFERENCES

1. Department of Health (2005) *National Service Frameworks (NSFs)*. www.dh.gov.uk Policy&Guidance (accessed 6/12/05).
2. Black, D. (Chair) (1980) *Inequalities in Health: Report of a Research Working Group*. Department of Health and Social Security, London.
3. Acheson, D. (Chair) (1998) *Independent Inquiry into Inequalities in Health*. Stationery Office, London.
4. Wilson, J.M.G. & Jungner, G. (1969) *Principles and Practice of Screening for Disease*. Public Health Paper No. 34. World Health Organisation, Geneva.
5. Miller, W. & Rollnick, S. (eds) (1991) *Motivational Interviewing: preparing people to change addictive behaviour*. Guildford Press, London.
6. UK National Screening Committee (2005) *National Screening Committee Position Papers – diabetes screening (in adults) and renal disease screening*. www.nelh.nhs.uk/screening/
7. Department of Health (2004) *Implementation of New General Medical Services and Personal Medical Services Contracts in Primary Care. Non-executive Bulletin No. 4.* www.dh.gov.uk/PublicationsAndStatistics/Bulletins/fs/en/ (accessed 9/12/05).
8. Department of Health (2001) *National Service Framework for Older People*. Department of Health, London.
9. Lowe, C., Raynor, D., Teale, C. & Lubgan, C. (2000) Can practice nurses identify medication problems using the over-75 health check? *Journal of Clinical Nursing*, 9 (5), 816.
10. House of Commons Health Committee (2004) *Elder Abuse – Second Report of Session 2003–4, Volume 1*. Stationery Office, London.
11. House of Commons Health Committee (2004) *Obesity – Third Report of Session 2003–4, Volume 1*. Stationery Office, London.
12. Aylin, P., Williams, S. & Bottle, A. (2005) Obesity and type 2 diabetes in children, 1996–7 to 2003–4. *British Medical Journal*, **331** (7526), 1167.
13. Department of Health (2003) *5 A Day General Information*. www.dh.gov.uk/PolicyAndGuidance/HealthAndSocialCareTopics/FiveADay/FiveADaygeneralinformation/fs/en (accessed 10/12/05).
14. Aronson, J.K. (2004) Editor's view – over-the-counter medicines. *British Journal of Clinical Pharmacology*, **58** (3), 231.
15. Editorial (2004) OTC statins: a bad decision for public health. *Lancet*, **363** (9422), 1659.
16. Prochaska, J. & DiClemente, C. (1989) Transtheoretical therapy: toward a more interpretive model of change. *Psychotherapy: Theory, Research and Practice*, **20**, 161–73.

17. Green Gym Home Page. Promoting Fitness, Health, Well-being and the Environ-ment. www.greengym.org.uk (accessed 10/12/05).
18. Department of Health (2005) *Alcohol and Health. How to drink sensibly.* www.dh.gov.uk/PolicyAndGuidance/HealthAndSocialCareTopics/AlcoholMisu se/AlcoholMisusegeneralinformation/fs/en (accessed 10/12/05).
19. Prodigy Guidance (2004) *Alcohol – problem drinking.* www.prodigy.nhs.uk/ guidance.asp?gt=Alcohol
20. Mead, M. (2005) Substance abuse: identifying and managing alcohol problems. *Practice Nurse*, **30** (10), 21–6.
21. HM Government (1998) *Smoking Kills: a White Paper on tobacco.* Stationery Office, London.
22. National Institute for Clinical Excellence (2002) *Guidance on the Use of Nicotine Replacement Therapy (NRT) and Bupropion for Smoking Cessation.* Technology Appraisal No. 39. www.nice.org.uk (accessed 11/12/05).
23. Ashcroft, J. (2005) Smoking . . . and how to help people to stop. *Practice Nurse*, **30** (7), 28–37.

FURTHER READING

Ewles, L. (2005) *Key Topics in Public Health: essential briefing on prevention and health promo-tion.* Elsevier, Edinburgh.
Great Britain Committee on Medical Aspects of Food Policy (1991) *Dietary Reference Values for Food Energy and Nutrients for the United Kingdom* (COMA report). HMSO, London.
HM Government (2005) *Health, Work and Well-being: caring for our future.* www.dwp.gov.uk/publications
HM Treasury and Department of Health (2002) *Tackling Health Inequalities – summary of the 2002 cross-cutting review.* Department of Health, London.
Tamkin, P., Aston, J., Cummings, J., Hooker, H., Pollard, E., Rich, J., Sheppard, E. & Tackey, N.D. (2003) *A Review of Training in Racism Awareness and Valuing Cultural Diversity.* Report for the Home Office Research, Development and Statistics Dir-ectorate. www.employment-studies.co.uk/summary/summary.php?id=1987rate

USEFUL ADDRESSES AND WEBSITES

National Electronic Library for Health (2005) Focus on screening
Website: www.nelh.nhs.uk/screening/default.asp?page=FOCUS

Quality and Outcome Framework Information
Website: www.ic.nhs.uk/services/qof

British Heart Foundation
Website: www.bhf.org.uk

Scientific Advisory Committee on Nutrition
Website: www.sacn.gov.uk

Alcohol Concern
Website: www.alcoholconcern.org.uk

Action on Smoking and Health (ASH), 102 Clifton Street, London EC2A 4HW
Telephone: 020 7739 5902
Website: www.ash.org.uk

NHS Smoking Helpline
Telephone: 0800 169 0169

Chapter 10

Child Health, Childhood and Adult Immunisation

CHILD HEALTH PROMOTION

The National Service Framework for Children, Young People and Maternity Services specifies the health promotion services to be offered to pregnant women, children and adolescents.[1] The child health surveillance programme, which applied under the GP Contract of 1990 and followed a mainly medical model of screening for defects, has been replaced by a programme of health promotion and targeting of interventions at children at risk for medical or social reasons.[2] The *Hall Report*, now in its fourth edition, has influenced changes to the organisation of services for child healthcare ever since it was first published in 1989. A child will be assessed at any age, if there is any cause for concern, so that remedial action or support can be initiated as soon as possible.

The family may have input from many members of the primary healthcare team in the first months of a child's life. A doctor usually performs the neonatal examination but trained midwives have been shown to be as good or better than paediatric senior house officers in examining the newborn.[3] A midwife carries out the heel-prick test and may administer vaccines against hepatitis B or tuberculosis if a child is at risk. The health visitor will usually establish contact with the family and assess their health needs before the delivery and take over from the midwife in the postnatal period. The 6–8 week check, performed by the GP, is to detect those disorders that do not always manifest at birth, such as some types of congenital heart disease. This examination, if performed at two months of age, coincides with a child's first immunisation course.

There are differences in the ages at which health promotion contacts are carried out and practice nurses are advised to familiarise themselves with the arrangements in their own localities. Examinations are listed in the Personal Child Health Record (PCHR). The Child Health Promotion Programme usually includes the following.

Before birth

The midwife and health visitor assess the family situation and offer help or advice as needed, especially about healthy eating and smoking. Breastfeeding is actively encouraged. Education programmes have been shown to be more effective than written material in promoting breastfeeding.[4] Arrangements are made for a smooth handover from the midwife to the health visitor at the appropriate time. Proposals outlined in the National Service Framework for Children to extend the role of the midwife for up to three months postnatally failed to recognise the importance of the health visitor's role in the early months.[5] This overlap in the professional care of mothers and babies highlights the need for partnership working.

Soon after birth

An examination in the first 36 hours is performed prior to discharge from hospital or by a GP if the mother had a home delivery or early discharge. A brief history of the health of the parents, of this pregnancy, of previous pregnancies and of brothers and sisters is taken. Any antenatal problems are identified. Any history of congenital heart disease, dislocation of the hips and hearing loss should be talked about, as parents may have anxieties about these.

Every baby has a full medical examination in the neonatal period. Posture, colour and respiratory rate can be observed while the baby is asleep. Listening to the heart for murmurs while the baby is sleeping or quiet is easier than when it has just been woken. The head circumference is measured, while also observing the fontanelles and the face. The eyes are checked for conjunctivitis or cataracts and the pupils are examined. The nose is also examined, in particular to ensure that the nares are patent (choanal atresia causes respiratory distress – the skin looks pink when resting but blue when crying or feeding). The mouth is checked by palpating and visualising the palate to exclude clefts, as well as assessing the neck for lumps and the nipples for mastitis (as a result of maternal hormones).

The abdomen is palpated, including checks for hernias and whether meconium was passed in the first 24 hours. Limbs are assessed for symmetry and the hips for signs of developmental dysplasia (previously called congenital dislocation of the hip). Head circumference, weight and length may be recorded in the PCHR. A heel-prick blood test is performed to check for congenital hypothyroidism and phenylketonuria, both of which can cause learning disabilities if not detected. Screening for cystic fibrosis and sickle cell disease is also becoming routine.[6]

Vitamin K is given in the first week after birth, either by a single IM injection or orally as drops. If given orally, a second dose is needed in that same week. A third oral dose is needed if a baby is breastfed but not if the child is mainly formula fed because formula feeds contain vitamin K.[7]

Within the first month

A neonatal hearing screen is performed. This has replaced the distraction hearing test that used to be performed by a health visitor at eight months. If hepatitis B immunisation was given at birth, a second dose is given after four weeks.

The health visitor usually makes a new birth visit once the midwife has discharged the patient. This is an opportune time to assess how the mother is coping, assessing for maternal depression and neglect or abuse. Health promotion activities will include issues such as sudden infant death syndrome, passive smoking, feeding, immunisation and safety (at home and in cars).

At 6–8 weeks

A GP who has qualified in child health and development reviews the pregnancy and family history and discusses any concerns with the parents. A full physical examination of the baby, including hips and testes, is carried out and the motor development is tested. Surgical correction of undescended testes before the age of 18 months is desirable in order to improve the chances of fertility in later life. The weight, length and head circumference are measured and the hearing and vision assessed. Normally children show a startle response to a sudden noise and can follow a moving object with the eyes to 90° on the horizontal.

At 8–12 months

Any parental concerns, especially about vision and hearing, are discussed and the motor development is assessed. At this age, a child will enjoy peek-a-boo games and the eyes are observed for squint or other possible problems with vision. Health promotion focuses around accident prevention, nutrition, dental care, safety in cars, passive smoking, developmental needs, sunburn and iron deficiency, if appropriate.

After 1 year

No further routine assessments are usually carried out until prior to school entry but the health visiting team is responsible for ensuring that health and developmental needs are being addressed. A referral is needed for specialised testing if there are any doubts about a child's vision, hearing or attainment of milestones in development.

Early recognition of learning difficulties is necessary if there is any problem with normal development. If autism is suspected, there are now several tests that can be used. The Checklist for Autism in Toddlers (CHAT) consists of a questionnaire for the parent and a series of related and confirmatory observations for the health visitor or GP.[8] Children with autistic spectrum disorders may show abnormalities of communication, social interaction and imaginative play. Children with severe developmental or growth problems can usually be detected by 21 months.

All the staff should be alert to anything that seems amiss whenever a child is seen in the surgery. A practice nurse might be as concerned about a child who seems unduly passive during a treatment as about one who wreaks absolute havoc in the nurse's room.

At 3–5 years

Any parental concerns are discussed and a physical examination carried out as necessary. The height and weight are recorded. Tests may be performed of language, gross motor and fine motor development, vision and hearing. The tests are incorporated in activities, which are presented as games to the child.

Teachers and school nurses may report any developmental problems once a child is at school.

Inherited conditions

A child who may have inherited a condition such as sickle cell disease, thalassaemia or cystic fibrosis may be referred for assessment, so that early prophylactic measures can be taken. The rapid growth in technology has made genetic screening possible and the development of gene therapy provides some hope for the future.

Sure Start

Sure Start is the government initiative to tackle child poverty and social exclusion by bringing together childcare, early education, health and other services to support families with children under five years. Until now, Sure Start has been established in the most disadvantaged areas but the government plans to have 2500 children's centres throughout the country by 2008.[9]

SAFETY

All adults have a duty to try and prevent accidents and injury to children. *Saving Lives: our healthier nation* has a target for reducing the death rate by a fifth and serious injury caused by accidents by at least a tenth by the year 2010. Health professionals can provide advice on:

- The safe storage of medicines and chemicals in the home and the use of child-proof bottle tops and cupboard-closing devices
- Potential hazards such as stairs, furniture, windows, balconies, cookers, fires, electricity, and how to make them safer
- Potentially dangerous toys and games
- The risk to health from lack of exercise

- Road safety, safety seats in cars and protection for cyclists
- How to avoid personal danger or get help if abused.

Teenage health promotion

The prevention of coronary heart disease, diabetes and lifestyle-related illness needs to begin early. Children and adolescents are particularly susceptible to pressure from their peers to experiment with smoking, alcohol, drugs or solvents. A practice nurse can sometimes initiate discussions on these health issues and be a source of information about the help and services available for worried parents and young people. Joint initiatives with school nurses and health visitors can help to ensure that a consistent message is being put across and nurses can also act as a pressure group for change.

Developing sexuality is another major concern for teenagers. Nurses with the appropriate training have an important role in promoting sexual health. The guarantee of confidentiality might encourage more teenagers to seek advice on sexual behaviour and contraception, although many of them are reluctant to visit the surgery, fearing that their parents will be informed. In some areas, nurses are successfully running services especially for young people. Details of local services should be readily available.

CHILD ABUSE

A parent could disclose information to a practice nurse, regarding the exposure of themselves or their children to physical or mental abuse. The parent may be scared and not wish to report such incidents. Every district has a formal child protection policy and staff in general practice must be aware of the procedure to follow. Primary care organisations hold regular training on child protection, which all practice nurses should attend. By knowingly keeping a child in a risk situation, there may be neglect of the nurse's duty of care. Not sharing concerns may amount to collusion. This is an extremely sensitive area, which requires tact but prompt action.

The practice nurse could be the first to suspect physical or mental abuse of a child. Suspicion may be aroused by any abnormal or frequent injuries, particularly those with special significance, such as small circular burns (cigarettes), bruises suggestive of fingertip grasps on the upper arms or from blows to the ears and lips. The relationship between the child and parent should also be noted. The cases of recognised and reported child sexual abuse have highlighted an area in which doctors and nurses have to be particularly vigilant. Any suggestion of sexual abuse, from physical findings, verbal comments or behaviour, must be taken seriously. It is important to deal with these matters confidentially and sensitively. Producing definite evidence is often extremely difficult.

A practice nurse will often be familiar with the background and problems of many local families because of the close relationship with the patients and be aware of those at risk from factors such as poverty, stress or alcoholism. However, it should be borne in mind that the incidence of abuse covers all social classes and income groups, not just the socially deprived.

THE CHILDREN ACTS (1989 AND 2004)

The first Children Act gathered all the existing legislation relating to children into a new unified law, many aspects of which concerned child protection. The 2004 Children Act complements rather than replaces the original Act. The child's welfare should be the paramount consideration at all times. This over-rides the concern for the welfare of adults or carers or concern about the future of the professional relationship. Health professionals have specific duties laid out in local policies, as well as in *Working Together*.[10] A replacement document is due to be published soon. Social services have a duty to investigate all children in their area, where there is a suspicion that a child is suffering or likely to suffer significant harm. Once a problem is identified and the decision to refer is taken, confidentiality may have to be breached in the child's best interest.

Consent to treatment

Practice nurses should be aware that any child considered mature enough to understand all the issues, regardless of age, may give or withhold his/her own consent for treatment. The Department of Health has published guidelines relating to consent for children and young people.[11]

CHILDHOOD IMMUNISATION

A practice nurse's main involvement in child health clinics may consist of giving the immunisations but parents will often ask for advice or information about other issues.

Organisation of immunisation programmes

Payments for immunisations depend on the achievement of target numbers. The GP will be eligible for a full target payment if, on the first day of a quarter, the number of courses completed in each of the groups of immunisations of all the children aged two on the surgery list on that day amounts on average to 90% of the number of courses needed to achieve full immunisation. Likewise, they will receive a lower level of payment if the average of courses completed amounts to

70% of the number needed for full immunisation. For the purpose of target payments, children should have had the following immunisations by age two:

- Diphtheria/tetanus/acellular pertussis/inactivated poliomyelitis/*Haemophilus influenzae* B
- (DTaP/IPV/Hib) – 3 doses
- Meningococcal meningitis C – 3 doses
- Measles/mumps/rubella – 1 dose.

Additional target payments are made for preschool booster doses given between three and a half and five years. These injections consist of diphtheria/tetanus/acellular pertussis/inactivated polio (DTaP/IPV or dTaP/IPV) and a second MMR dose.

Targets were introduced to improve immunisation uptake and thus reduce the spread of childhood communicable diseases. In order to do this, a monetary incentive was offered to GPs. The achievement of immunisation targets involves all the practice team and the calculation of targets takes into account immunisations carried out by others, including local health clinics. Alongside this is the collection of information relating to the percentage of children in an area who have received vaccinations. Immunisation statistics, known as Coverage of Vaccinations Evaluated Rapidly (COVER), identify pockets of susceptibility within a community and focus on services within these areas. This also enables epidemiologists to analyse whether potential outbreaks may occur as a result of a drop in coverage.

Medicolegal aspects of immunisation

Any nurse undertaking immunisation needs to be familiar with the 'Green Book', *Immunisation against Infectious Disease*. The last edition was published in 1996 and is now seriously out of date. New draft chapters are available electronically and should be printed off. The long-awaited new edition is now promised for 2006. It specifies the conditions under which nurses are covered to give immunisations. Each area will have local guidelines and the Patient Group Directions (PGDs) will enable specified nurses to administer prescription-only medications without an individual prescription from a doctor.[12] Most commonly, PGDs will apply to vaccinations in the national immunisation programme and for foreign travel. The law restricts the use of PGDs to the NHS or organisations providing care for NHS patients as part of a contract with the NHS. Nurses using PGDs in non-NHS settings should seek guidance from their professional organisation or insurer.

Immunisation criteria for nurses

Nurses must fulfil three criteria:

- To be willing to be professionally accountable
- To have received specific training and be competent in all aspects of immunisation, including contraindications to specific vaccines
- To have had adequate training in dealing with anaphylaxis.

Consent

Consent can be written, oral or non-verbal. A signature on a consent form does not prove that the consent is valid. All the necessary information must be provided about the proposed vaccine, including any contraindications or possible side effects, to inform the consent. Consent must be given voluntarily, not under any form of duress or undue influence from health professionals, family or friends. If a nanny or anyone other than the parent or legal guardian brings a child for immunisation, the nurse must ensure that their consent has been obtained. Local primary care organisations should have a policy on when a nurse needs to obtain written consent. Children under the age of 16 who are considered to be competent under the Gillick ruling may give their own consent to immunisation.[13]

Injection sites

The PGD should specify the preferred sites for immunisation, in conjunction with the manufacturer's instructions for specific vaccines. With the exception of BCG or oral typhoid and cholera, all vaccines should be given intramuscularly or by deep subcutaneous injection. Consideration should be given to the correct method of administration in people with coagulopathies.

In general, infants under one year of age should receive all vaccines in the anterolateral aspect of the thigh; over the age of one, in the anterolateral aspect of the thigh or deltoid; and for older children and adults, the deltoid is recommended. The buttock is not used because of the risk of sciatic nerve damage and it has been shown to reduce the efficacy of some vaccines, e.g. hepatitis B.[14]

Emergency situations

Anaphylaxis is a rare occurrence but it should always be anticipated. Epinephrine (adrenaline) and basic resuscitation equipment must be available. The decision on whether to give immunisations without a doctor being on the premises will depend on the practice policy, plus the individual nurse's experience and willingness to accept the responsibility. Caution seems sensible given the potential for tragedy. A plan of action for emergencies is essential, whether giving immunisations in the surgery or in patients' homes. The Resuscitation Council (UK) guidelines and algorithms can be downloaded and printed. Practice nurses must keep up to date with new guidelines and ensure that their skills are updated at least annually (see Chapter 7, page 112).

Childhood immunisation schedule (see postscript below for proposed changes to the schedule)

The primary course of immunisation is given at two, three and four months of age. This consists of two injections:

- Combined diphtheria, tetanus, acellular pertussis, inactivated polio and *Haemophilus influenzae* type B vaccine (DTaP/IPV/Hib)
- Meningitis C vaccine (MenC).

Later courses of immunisation consist of:

- Measles, mumps and rubella vaccine (MMR) at 12–18 months of age. One brand of MMR vaccine lists gelatine as an exipient; further advice should be sought from the manufacturer if this is an issue for anybody.
- A preschool reinforcing dose of DTaP/IPV or dTaP/IPV and a further MMR given to children aged between three years and five months to five years. Three years should elapse between the third dose of primary immunisations and the preschool booster but a second dose of MMR can be given three months after the first. This is recommended in some areas and can be preferable to giving two injections to a four year old.
- A school-leaving booster of a single injection of low-dose diphtheria, tetanus and inactivated polio vaccine (dT/IPV).

Meningitis C vaccine should be given up to the age of 24, if missed out previously. Hib is not given after the age of four unless there are other indications such as asplenia or haemoglobinopathies. A single dose of either vaccine should be given to a patient over one year of age, if needed.

Efficient organisation is needed, whether the call/recall system for immunisation is centrally administered or one devised by the individual practice. Opportunistic immunisation can be aided by flagging the records of patients. Flexible timing of appointments can help but home visiting may be necessary; the health visitor will undertake immunisation at home sometimes.

Birthday cards at strategic dates can provide friendly reminders about immunisation:

- Age one year for MMR
- Four years for preschool boosters
- Fifteen years for tetanus/low-dose diphtheria and polio boosters.

Patients with unknown immunisation histories

Sometimes it is impossible to discover a patient's immunisation status, especially if they have come from abroad. It should be assumed, in such instances, that the patient is unimmunised and a full immunisation schedule should be implemented. The Prodigy Guidance outlines how such vaccines should be given.[15] Vaccines containing tetanus, low-dose diphtheria and inactivated polio (Td/IPV) should be used for patients over ten years of age. If patients were given a fourth dose of DTP at 18 months, they should still have a preschool booster.

Contraindications to immunisation

Many conditions previously thought to contraindicate immunisation no longer apply. Immunisation should be postponed if the patient has an acute febrile illness. A severe local or general reaction to a previous dose would be a definite contraindication to further administration of the same vaccine until further advice has been sought. Such reactions need to be differentiated from the milder reactions that can often be expected to occur. No child should be denied the protection of immunisation without very good cause. If a patient is thought to have had an anaphylactic reaction to eggs, then immunisation may be done in hospital with vaccines, such as MMR, which are incubated in eggs.

Live virus vaccines are generally contraindicated for:

- Immunocompromised patients such as those receiving high-dose steroids and patients with malignant conditions or other diseases affecting their immune systems, such as HIV
- Pregnant women
- Patients who have received another live vaccine within the past three weeks, unless given simultaneously.

The details about specific immunisations and their contraindications are not repeated here, because the Summaries of Product Characteristics provide comprehensive information. The nurse must be sure that there are no contraindications to a specific vaccine being given. A medical opinion should be requested when necessary.

Information for parents

Written information is useful to reinforce verbal advice about possible reactions and how to deal with them. Infant paracetamol or ibuprofen is usually recommended for fever or prolonged crying. The dose varies between products (see *British National Formulary*). The products are licensed for treating infants under three months of age for postimmunisation fever. Parents should know how to get medical help if worried and be asked to report any severe reactions. Any reaction from MMR usually follows the incubation time of the actual diseases. Thus mild symptoms of measles may occur from 5–12 days, possibly with fever and a rash. Mumps incubation is slightly longer (14–21 days). There may be mild fever and parotid swelling. These reactions are non-infectious, so the children do not need to be isolated. Antipyretic medication should be advised if a fever develops after immunisation.

Special risks

Tuberculosis

Bacillus Calmette-Guerin vaccine (BCG) is a live, attenuated, freeze-dried vaccine not usually given in general practice. Routine BCG immunisation has been discontinued and is now only offered to those at particular risk.

- Infants born or living in areas with an incidence of TB of 40/100 000 or greater.
- Infants whose parents or grandparents were born in a country with an incidence of TB of 40/100 00 or greater.
- Previously unvaccinated new immigrants from countries with high prevalence of TB.

Practice nurses should be aware of the local arrangements for Mantoux testing and giving BCG to those who need it. Leaflets about tuberculosis and other immunisations can be obtained from local health promotion departments or from Department of Health Publications. Parents planning long-term travel to countries with a high incidence of tuberculosis should be advised to consider BCG immunisation for their children.

Hepatitis B

Since April 2000, women have been screened for hepatitis B status antenatally to reduce the high rate of chronic carrier state from natural passive transmission. An accelerated schedule is recommended for infants born to hepatitis B-positive mothers, with immunisation as soon as possible after birth, a second dose one month later and a third dose after another month. A booster dose is needed at one year and a further single booster when the preschool boosters are given.[16]

Hepatitis B is part of the routine schedule in some countries but if parents request the vaccine for children not at risk, then they should be asked to pay a private fee for immunisation according to the practice scale of charges.

Influenza

Children with severe respiratory disease (including asthma), chronic heart or renal disease, diabetes mellitus or immunosuppression should be offered immunisation annually against influenza. Children aged six months to three years should receive half the adult dose. Most prefilled syringes have a line marking the 0.25 ml dose. If a child aged 12 years or under is given influenza vaccine for the first time, a second dose should be given 4–6 weeks later.

Pneumococcal diseases

Pneumococcal vaccine should be offered to children at risk, including those with cochlear implants, CSF shunts or who have had a previous episode of invasive pneumococcal disease. The new chapter of the 'Green Book' on pneumococcal immunisation lists the at-risk groups and immunisation schedules. A 7-valent pneumococcal conjugate vaccine is given to children between two months and five years. A single dose of 23-valent pneumococcal polysaccharide vaccine is given after the second birthday. At least two months should elapse between the last dose of conjugate vaccine and the administration of polysaccharide pneumococcal vaccine.

Postscript

Plans for changes to the routine childhood immunisations were announced by the Department of Health in February 2006. Pneumococcal conjugate vaccine will be given to all children, not just those in risk groups. A catch-up programme will be implemented for children up to the age of two years. Two doses of meningococcal C vaccine will be given as a part of the primary immunisations, with a third dose combined with Hib at 12 months of age. The third dose of pneumococcal vaccine will be given at the same time as the first MMR.

The proposed new immunisation schedule will be as shown in Table 10.1.

The timescale for these changes has not been announced but they are likely to be introduced before the end of 2006. Information and publicity materials are likely to be made available before then and nurses will need to ensure that they have sufficient stocks of the vaccines and revised Patient Group Directions in order to implement the changes. Information can be found on the immunisation website.

Table 10.1 Proposed new immunisation schedule

Age	Vaccine(s)
2 months	DtaP/IPV/Hib + pneumococcal conjugate
3 months	DtaP/IPV/Hib + meningococcal C
4 months	DtaP/IPV/Hib + pneumococcal conjugate + meningococcal C (three injections)
12 months	Hib/Men C
13 months	MMR + pneumococcal conjugate

ADULT IMMUNISATION

The immunisation of adults may be performed for the following reasons:

- Missed or incomplete childhood immunisations (vaccines may not have been available then)

- Special risk of exposure through injury, occupation, health status or lifestyle
- Reinforcing doses are required to maintain immunity.

Tetanus immunisation

Routine immunisation against tetanus was introduced in 1961, although it was given to people in the armed forces before then. Therefore, patients born before that date who did not serve in the armed forces may never have been immunised. They require a primary course of vaccine. Tetanus vaccine is no longer available on its own; combined tetanus, low-dose diphtheria and inactivated polio are recommended (Td/IPV) in preference to tetanus and low-dose diphtheria (Td) vaccine. Three doses of 0.5 ml IM injection at monthly intervals are needed, with a booster dose five years later and a further reinforcing dose ten years after that. Any unfinished course may be completed at any time without restarting a new course. Once an individual has received five injections, boosters are only recommended if travelling to a country where antitetanus immunoglobulin may not be available in the case of a tetanus-prone wound.

Patients who are accustomed to attending for routine tetanus boosters can be shown the relevant chapter in the 'Green Book'. Unnecessary booster doses can result in adverse local reactions.

Diphtheria

Vaccine against diphtheria is now recommended in combination with vaccines against tetanus and polio. People over ten years of age should be given only low-dose diphtheria because of the risk of adverse reactions if the higher dose diphtheria vaccine is used. Tetanus and low-dose diphtheria (Td) vaccine is no longer recommended.

Poliomyelitis

Patients born before 1958 may not have been immunised against polio. Unimmunised adults should be offered the vaccine in combination with tetanus and low-dose diphtheria (Td/IPV). The primary immunisations should be given at monthly intervals.

Once five doses have been received, reinforcing doses are not required, unless at special risk from foreign travel or occupational exposure.

Rubella

It was once hoped that the immunisation of all children against measles, mumps and rubella would eventually remove the main pool of rubella infection and thus minimise the risk to a fetus of congenital rubella syndrome if a non-immune woman contracted rubella in the first trimester of pregnancy. Unfortunately, the reduction in public confidence in MMR following the unsubstantiated report of a link between the vaccine and autism and bowel disease led to a decline in the uptake of the combined vaccine. The resulting reduction in herd immunity resulted in fears of a resurgence of rubella. All women of childbearing age should be screened for rubella antibodies and immunised if necessary. Rubella vaccine was discontinued in 2003 and MMR vaccine is now advised instead. The date of the LMP should be ascertained because the vaccine should not be given if pregnancy is a possibility. Immunisation should be postponed or a pregnancy test be performed if there is any doubt. Women should also be advised not to become pregnant for at least one month after immunisation.

Mumps

The recent resurgence of mumps in schools and colleges has led to many institutions requesting proof that a young person has had two doses of MMR. Many such vaccines were given in a massive catch-up programme run by school nurses in recent times but some individuals who did not receive the immunisations are still likely to request them in general practice.

Influenza

Influenza vaccine is produced each year with the three strains of virus likely to be circulating during the winter season. Annual injections of 0.5 ml SC or IM are required. Patients at particular risk who should be targeted include:

- Patients with medical conditions likely to be exacerbated by influenza: diabetes treated with insulin or oral hypoglycaemic drugs, chronic heart, liver, renal or respiratory disease (including asthma)
- Immunosuppressed patients
- Patients resident in long-stay institutions where a rapid spread of infection would be likely to occur
- All patients aged over 65 years
- Main carers of elderly or disabled people, whose welfare may be at risk if a carer falls ill
- Frontline healthcare workers are also offered immunisation by occupational health services.[17]

Preparation for the immunisation programme should be made early. Vaccines can be bought in bulk from the manufacturer but suitable storage is needed. A profit for the practice can be made this way. Alternatively, individual patients are issued with a prescription for the vaccine, which they get from the chemist and return for the injection. Patients at risk can be identified from disease and age/sex registers. Special 'flu jab' clinics may be set up and invitations sent out. The best time to start the programme is early October. In this way the bulk of the injections will be completed before the end of the year to protect patients early in the following year when influenza epidemics are most likely.

Patients who are not in the risk categories or who do not have a valid need for immunisation should be discouraged from having flu injections in case there is insufficient vaccine available for those at true risk.

Contraindications

Contraindications to influenza vaccine include:

• Any febrile illness (postpone injection until recovered)
• Severe adverse reaction to a previous dose
• Hypersensitivity to egg (previous anaphylactic reaction)
• Pregnancy.

Adverse reactions

Adverse reactions are usually mild. Soreness can occur at the injection site. Fever, malaise or myalgia may occur a few hours after immunisation and last up to two days. Very rarely there might be an allergic reaction if the patient is hypersensitive to egg protein, because the virus is propagated in eggs to produce the vaccine. Many patients refuse the flu vaccine because they believe it gives them the flu. Discussion with the patient about the influenza vaccine, the type of vaccine, its efficacy and the benefits it provides will give patients a more informed choice. Flu vaccine is inactivated so cannot cause flu in recipients or their contacts.

Pneumococcal disease

An encapsulated strain of *Streptococcus pneumoniae* can cause pneumonia, bacteraemia or meningitis. Susceptible patients who should be offered immunisation include people with:

• Chronic lung, heart, liver or renal conditions
• Chronic respiratory disease but not asthma, unless so severe as to require continuous or repeated courses of oral steroids
• Disorders of immunity through disease or treatment
• Diabetes mellitus requiring insulin or oral hypoglycaemic drugs
• Disease of spleen or splenectomy, including homozygous sickle cell disease and coeliac disease that may lead to dysfunction of the spleen
• Cochlear implants
• Possible cerebrospinal fluid leaks, e.g. CSF shunts or head injury.

and those aged 65 years of age and older.

A single dose of 23-valent pneumococcal vaccine 0.5 ml SC or IM is required. It may be given at the same time as a flu jab, but at a different injection site.

Patients who are asplenic, hyposplenic or have chronic renal disease should be reimmunised every five years without prior antibody testing. Routine reinforcing doses are not recommended for any other patients.[18]

Hepatitis B

This highly infectious virus is spread by contact with infected blood or bodily fluids, for example through contaminated sharps or needles, sexual intercourse, mother to child at birth or a bite from an infected person.

Immunisation is recommended for people at particular risk.

- Drug abusers and their sexual partners and children
- Patients at increased risk due to sexual activities, including commercial sex workers and men who have sex with men
- Close family contacts of patients with hepatitis B or healthy carriers of the virus
- Families adopting children from countries with a high or intermediate prevalence of the disease
- Foster carers
- Individuals receiving regular blood transfusions or blood products
- Patients with chronic liver disease or renal failure. Seroconversion rates are lower in patients with renal failure. Adults should be given the higher (40 mcg) dose vaccine
- Inmates of custodial institutions
- People travelling to or planning to reside in areas of high or intermediate prevalence of hepatitis B
- Occupational risk, especially healthcare workers and laboratory staff.[19]

The recombinant hepatitis B vaccine is prepared from yeast cells. Three intramuscular doses of 1 ml are required for adults at zero, one and six months. An accelerated schedule may be used and immunoglobulin may also be needed in some circumstances (see 'Green Book'). Injection should be into the deltoid muscle instead of the buttock. Patients with bleeding disorders, in whom an intramuscular injection could cause bleeding into the muscle, may be given subcutaneous injection at the discretion of the GP.

Antibody levels should be checked about 1–4 months after the completion of the primary course in patients at occupational risk only. Further doses are sometimes required to achieve initial immunity levels of 100 iu/ml. One reinforcing dose five years after the primary course is recommended for all patients at continued risk. Serology testing is not required.

Adverse reactions include redness and soreness at the injection site. More rarely there is fever, rash, flu-like symptoms, arthralgia and/or abnormal liver function tests.

Hepatitis A

Protection against hepatitis A is usually required for travellers to endemic areas. However, preexposure immunisation should also be considered for the following groups at particular risk.

- Patients with chronic liver disease
- Patients with haemophilia
- Men who have sex with men
- Injecting drug users
- Those at occupational risk – some laboratory workers, staff in large residential institutions, sewerage workers or those who work with primates.

Two injections are required for lasting immunity, given intramuscularly into the deltoid muscle (or subcutaneously if haemophiliac, etc.), the second dose administered 6–12 months after the first. Reinforcing doses should be given after 20 years to patients at ongoing risk.[20] Human normal immunoglobulin (HBIG) is no longer used for travellers but may still be used in certain outbreak situations. Combined hepatitis A and B vaccine may be used for patients who need immunisation against both diseases.

Chickenpox (varicella)

Healthcare workers involved in direct patient care who are not immune to chickenpox are being offered immunisation through NHS occupational health services.[21] Practice nurses are therefore unlikely to have to administer this vaccine but should be aware of the recommendations and may even need immunisation themselves.

CONCLUSION

The input by health professionals is usually greatest in the early years of an individual's life. Events such as the Victoria Climbié case highlight the importance for professionals of working within a multidisciplinary team with good communication.[22] It is important for health professionals to understand their roles and responsibilities when working with children and to be trained adequately. People say 'this must never happen again' every time there is a tragic case of cruelty to a child but sadly, such cases continue to happen.

Many parents will not have seen first hand the effects of the diseases that have now largely been prevented owing to the success of the national vaccination programme. The introduction of meningitis C in recent times has shown the effectiveness of the immunisation programme and it is when the incidence of disease is low that vaccine safety becomes an issue. Due to public anxiety about the safety and efficacy of pertussis vaccine, the uptake rate fell to 30% in 1975. At that time, health professionals were not confident with the evidence presented and felt that by offering a choice (DTP or DT), they could allow parents to choose the safest option for their child. Unfortunately this resulted in several major epidemics with over 100 000 notified cases of pertussis. The recent fall in MMR uptake can be directly attributed to public anxiety about the safety of the combined vaccine and a lack of confidence in 'expert' advice.

Achieving a high uptake of immunisation makes a worthwhile contribution to the health of the population. Practice nurses provide a vaccination service but time also needs to be made available, when planning appointments, to help educate the public about the transmission of infectious diseases and what immunisation means. It is important that health professionals are kept up to date with information about vaccines and vaccine policy.

Suggestions for reflection on practice

What are the arrangements in your locality and practice for:

- Midwifery and health visiting services?
- Child protection?
- Immunisation call and recall?
- Using Patient Group Directions?
- Obtaining informed consent?
- Providing written material about immunisations?
- Dealing with allergic reactions?

What further training/updating or resources do you need?

REFERENCES

1. Department for Education and Skills and Department of Health (2004) *National Service Framework for Children, Young People and Maternity Services: Key Issues for Primary Care.* www.dh.gov.uk/assetRoot/04/10/40/33/04104033.pdf (accessed 12/12/05).
2. Hall, D.M.B. & Elliman, D. (eds) (2003) *Health for All Children*, 4th edn. Oxford University Press, Oxford.
3. Townsend, J., Wolke, D., Hayes, J., Dave, S., Rogers, C., Bloomfield, L., Quist-Therson, E., Tomlin, M. & Messer, D. (2004) Routine examination of the newborn: the EMREN study. Evaluation of an extension of the midwife role including a randomised controlled trial of appropriately trained midwives and paediatric senior house officers. *Health Technology Assessment*, **8** (14).
4. Centre for Reviews and Dissemination (2003) *Effectiveness of Primary Care-Based Interventions to Promote Breastfeeding*. Health Technology Assessment 20031101. www.york.ac.uk/inst/crd (accessed 12/112/05).

5. Community Practitioners' and Health Visitors Association (undated) *CPHVA Response to the National Service Framework for Children, Young People and Maternity Services.* www.amicus-cphva.org (accessed 18/12/05).
6. UK Newborn Screening Programme (2005) *What is the Heel Prick Test and How is it Done?* www.ich.ucl.ac.uk/newborn/screening/what.htm (accessed 12/12/05).
7. British Medical Association and Royal Pharmaceutical Society of Great Britain (2005) Vitamin K. *British National Formulary 49*, 9.6.5. BMA and RPSGB, London.
8. Baren-Cohen, S., Wheelwright, S., Cox, A., Baird, G., Charman, T., Swettenham, J., Drew, A. & Dehring, P. (2000) The early identification of autism: the Checklist for Autism in Toddlers (CHAT). *Journal of the Royal Society of Medicine, 93*, 521–525.
9. HM Government (2005) *A Sure Start Children's Centre for Every Community: Phase 2 planning guidelines.* www.surestart.gov.uk/publications/?Documents=50 (accessed 16/12/05).
10. Department of Health (1999) *Working Together to Safeguard Children.* HMSO, London.
11. Department of Health (2001) *Consent – what you have a right to expect: a guide for children and young people.* Department of Health, London.
12. Department of Health (2000) *Patient Group Directions (England only).* Health Service Circular HSC2000.026. Department of Health, London.
13. Department of Health (2001) *Reference Guide to Consent for Examination or Treatment.* Department of Health, London.
14. Vaccine Administration Taskforce (2001) *UK Guidance on Best Practice in Vaccine Administration.* Shirehall Communications, London.
15. Prodigy Guidance (2005) *Immunizations – childhood vaccination programme.* www.prodigy.nhs.uk/guidance.asp?gt=Immunizations (accessed 15/12/05).
16. Department of Health (2005) *Immunisation against Infectious Disease*, Draft Chapter 19, Hepatitis B. www.dh.gov.uk (accessed 19/12/05).
17. Chief Medical Officer (2005) *The Influenza Immunisation Programme* (letter). PL/CMO/2005/2.
18. Department of Health (2005) *Immunisation against Infectious Disease*, Draft Chapter 26, Pneumococcal. www.dh.gov.uk (accessed 23/12/05).
19. Department of Health (2005) *Immunisation against Infectious Disease*, Draft Chapter 19, Hepatitis B. www.dh.gov.uk (accessed 24/12/05).
20. Department of Health (2005) *Immunisation against Infectious Disease*, Draft Chapter 18 Hepatitis A. www.dh.gov.uk (accessed 24/12/05).
21. Chief Medical Officer, Chief Nursing Officer, Chief Dental Officer and Chief Pharmacy Officer (2003) Chicken Pox (Varicella) *Immunisation for Health Care Workers* (letter). PL/CMO/2003/8.
22. Lord Laming (2003) *The Victoria Climbié Report.* CM5730. Stationery Office, London.

FURTHER READING

Department of Health (1996) *Immunisation against Infectious Disease.* HMSO, London. Revised draft chapters available electronically: www.dh.gov.uk search for 'Green Book'.
Hall, D.B. & Elliman, D. (eds) (2003) *Health for All Children*, 4th edn. Oxford University Press, Oxford.

HM Government (2005) *Every Child Matters: change for children.* DfES, London. www.everychildmatters.gov.uk

HM Government (1989) *Children Act 1989.* Stationery Office, London.

HM Government (2004) *Children Act 2004.* Stationery Office, London.

USEFUL ADDRESSES AND WEBSITES

Health for All Children
www.healthforallchildren.co.uk

Sure Start
www.surestart.gov.uk

UK Newborn Screening Centre
www.newbornscreening-bloodspot.org.uk

Neonatal screening
www.omni.ac.uk/browse/mesh/D015997.html

NHS immunisation information
www.immunisation.nhs.uk

Department of Health Publications
Telephone: 08701 555 455
E-mail: dh@prolog.uk.com

Health Protection Agency
www.phls.co.uk

NHS Patient Group Directions
www.portal.nelm.nhs.uk/PGD/default.aspx

Resuscitation Council (UK)
www.resus.org.uk

Chapter 11
Travel Health

With travellers becoming increasingly adventurous and virtually no country inaccessible, pre-travel consultations should concentrate mainly on giving advice and stressing the importance of following reliable guidelines on subjects such as food hygiene and bite prevention. Sensible behaviour is the key to good health; vaccination and preventive medicine are simply added safeguards.

Between 1000 and 2000 UK nationals die abroad each year.[1] Many deaths are from natural causes, particularly cardiovascular events, but accidents are the cause of a significant number of deaths, especially in younger people.

Preexisting conditions that could present problems should be identified before travel. With the frequency of travel to exotic destinations rising in the older age group, it is wise for the adviser to take a careful history and to tailor advice and preventive measures to individual patients. Many practice nurses have assumed the responsibility for travel health which, because of its complexity, calls for high standards of care. The nurse should have had adequate education and have up-to-date knowledge about travel health, access to suitable reference materials and work to appropriate guidelines. Guidance has been published by the Royal College of Nursing on the provision of general and specialist travel health services.[2]

NURSE EDUCATION

Practice nurses who provide a general travel health service are advised, as a minimum, to obtain a foundation-level qualification. Updating is also necessary at least annually, through study days, by attendance at travel conferences or by private study.

Accredited training is available in several ways.

- Short courses in travel health are run at many institutions, several of which also offer the chance to progress to Diploma and MSc levels. Examples include Sheffield Hallam University, Health Protection Scotland, the London School of Hygiene and Tropical Medicine and the Royal Free Hospital, London.

- Distance learning can be undertaken with the Magister Learning Unit in Travel Health.

Sources of information

The following are recommended.

- An up-to-date atlas to identify the areas being visited.
- *Immunisation against Infectious Diseases* (the 'Green Book') and *Health Information for Overseas Travel* (the 'Yellow Book'). These have always been standard reference texts but are no longer up to date. New draft chapters of the 'Green Book' are available electronically and revised chapters of the 'Yellow Book' will be available soon on the National Travel Health Network and Centre (NaTHNaC) website.
- *International Travel and Health*. This is a more up-to-date publication by WHO which has regular updates on the internet.
- A computerised system via a modem link to provide current information and advice to help with risk assessment for individual travellers. The practice policy should specify the agreed source of information to be used. TRAVAX, run by Health Protection Scotland, is free to NHS users in Scotland but a fee is charged for the service in other parts of the UK. Many primary care organisations pay a lump sum to obtain access for all their practices. NaTHNaC has an advice line for health professionals as well as a website and so does the Medical Advisory Service for Travellers (MASTA). Telephone and on-line information services run by vaccine companies Sanofi Pasteur MSD and Glaxo SmithKline give advice about health risks and recommended vaccines. Health professionals need to register to use the on-line services.
- There are many textbooks providing information on all aspects of travel health but textbooks become out of date quickly and must be replaced. The TravelHealth website has a list of recommended books.
- Health advice for travellers is available from the Department of Health website.

It is helpful if patients fill in a pre-travel questionnaire outlining their travel plans and immunisation status, so that advice can be tailored to their individual needs. These forms could be created on the practice computer or be obtained from the PCO or via the internet. The TravelHealth website provides a form for patients to complete. Appointment times should be long enough to deal fully with travel risk assessments, patient education and immunisations. Further appointments should be given if necessary and the patient can be asked to carry out his/her own fact finding. Referral to a specialised clinic may be needed for complicated itineraries. Patients can obtain personalised health briefs from MASTA or the IV Telecom hotline for a small cost if they provide details of their travel plans.

ADVICE FOR TRAVELLERS

Food and water

Diarrhoea is the most common problem for travellers. Detailed advice on hygiene and food and water safety may prevent a journey from becoming a disaster. Careful hand washing after using the toilet and before eating can significantly reduce the risk of developing diarrhoea.[3] Wet wipes are very useful for maintaining hand hygiene. Some experts have challenged the value of preventive advice but the points in Table 11.1 are usually recommended for situations where hygiene standards are suspect.

Table 11.1 Advice for travellers

Advice	Rationale
Eat freshly prepared and well-cooked hot food	Before bacterial growth can occur in cooked food and after any bacteria have been destroyed by heat
Make sure cutlery and crockery are clean	
Avoid salads and choose raw fruits and vegetables that can be peeled	Human excreta may be used as fertiliser or unsafe water may be used to wash the food
Avoid shellfish	Their feeding method concentrates microorganisms from their environment within their bodies
Boil or avoid unpasteurised milk	Risk of tuberculosis or brucellosis
Avoid ice creams, especially those in multi-portion containers	Ingredients could be hazardous, especially if ice cream has melted and been refrozen
Avoid raw meat and fish	Worm infestation risk
Boil or sterilise unsafe water or use bottled water for drinking	Water could be contaminated with human or animal excreta
Check the seal is unbroken on any bottled water purchased	To ensure that the bottle has not been refilled with tap water
Use carbonated water if possible	It is more difficult to counterfeit
Avoid ice cubes in drinks and use safe water for cleaning teeth	Even small amounts of unsafe water could be hazardous
Check that recreational water is safe	Swimming pools may be contaminated if not well maintained; there is a risk of bilharzia in some fresh-water areas; seawater may have sewage contamination

Diarrhoea advice

Most cases of diarrhoea will resolve within 2–3 days. Whatever the cause, dehydration is the major complication, so fluid replacement is essential. Mildly affected healthy adults may only need plenty of non-alcoholic drinks, including fruit juices and soups, but in all other cases, rehydration fluid should be used – either a solution made from a commercially produced sachet or four heaped teaspoonfuls of sugar or honey and one level teaspoonful of salt in one litre of safe drinking water. One glass should be drunk after each motion. Small, regular amounts should be continued even if vomiting occurs. Starvation is not recommended. Breastfeeding for infants should also be continued.[4] Medical help should be obtained for very young children, elderly or frail people, those with other medical conditions like diabetes, if diarrhoea contains blood or the patient becomes more ill.

Antidiarrhoea medication may be needed by adults, e.g. on long bus journeys or on business trips. Antidiarrhoea drugs are not recommended for children or for patients with bloody diarrhoea. A short course of antibiotics can reduce the severity and duration of travellers' diarrhoea.[5] The decision on which patients should carry self-treatment will depend on the practice policy. Private prescriptions should be issued for any medication prescribed for this purpose. Diarrhoea can make the contraceptive pill ineffective so patients should be advised to carry alternative methods of contraception. Diarrhoea can also affect the absorption of other medication such as antimalarials.

Malaria

Female anopheles mosquitoes transmit the parasites that cause malaria in their saliva. Protection against bites is often more important than drug prophylaxis because drug resistance is becoming such a serious problem. Of the four species of malaria parasites, *Plasmodium falciparum* is the most serious. There are approximately seven deaths from malaria of the 2000 cases imported into the UK each year.[6] The Malaria Reference Laboratory supplies up-to-date information on antimalarial drugs. Travellers at risk on long trips to remote places should also have drugs and information for treating malaria, in case infection does occur. People who previously have lived in a malarious area must be warned of their particular risk when returning, as they may have lost any immunity they had acquired but fail to take adequate precautions against mosquito bites. Advice on malaria should cover the following points.

- Personal protection: since mosquitoes feed mainly after dusk and at dawn, keep arms, legs and feet covered after sunset and avoid perfume and dark clothing, which attract mosquitoes.
- Use insect repellents containing diethyltoluamide (DEET) or natural repellents such as lemon eucaplyptus oil, to deter biting. Adults can use preparations

with a DEET content of up to 50% but a much lower strength of 10% or less should be used for infants and young children because they have a greater risk of absorption through the skin. An alternative repellent might be wiser for children. Repellents may be applied directly to the skin or clothes can be impregnated with DEET or permethrin for a more lasting effect; impregnated wrist and ankle bands may also be helpful. DEET should not be ingested, so should not be put on the hands of children, who are likely to suck their hands. Follow the maker's instructions for using any repellent product.

- Protection at night: if using air conditioning, make sure that windows and doors are closed properly and use a knock-down insecticide spray if necessary.
- If mosquitoes are able to enter at night, use a mosquito net. Make sure it has no holes or tears and tuck it properly under the mattress, preferably before dusk. Ensure that the net is large enough to allow plenty of space between the sleeper and the net because if their body is in contact with the net the mosquitoes can still attack through it. Nets impregnated with permethrin will kill or repel mosquitoes, so are more effective. Nets should be reimpregnated every six months or if they are washed.
- Pyrethroid mosquito coils may also be of use.
- Malaria can develop whilst travelling and, in some instances, up to a year after it. If travellers experience flu-like symptoms and fever, especially if associated with rigors, they should seek medical help as soon as possible. If they have already returned home, they should inform the doctor that they have been to a malarious area.
- Early treatment of malaria can prevent a fatal outcome.

Information about malaria is available on the Prodigy website.[7] The potential risk of malaria needs to be established and the appropriate prophylaxis advised. The websites mentioned above all advise on antimalarials. All team members should use the same information source in order to ensure consistency of advice. Chloroquine and proguanil can be purchased in a pharmacy. A private prescription is required for mefloquine, doxycycline and Malarone. Only chloroquine is available in liquid form for children. Tablets for children can be crushed and administered with honey or jam.

No antimalarial tablets are 100% effective. The best way to avoid malaria is to avoid mosquito bites. The main effect of antimalarials is to impede the life cycle of the parasite after the liver stage. Hence the need to continue taking most tablets for at least four weeks after leaving the risk area. Malarone is the exception because it prevents reproduction of the parasite both in the liver and in the blood; therefore it only needs to be taken for one week afterwards. Patients must be advised to seek medical advice and to mention having visited a malaria-endemic area, if symptoms occur at any time up to three months and possibly up to one year afterwards. All the tablets can cause nausea and gastric disturbance and should be taken with food and swallowed with plenty of water. The inconvenience of side effects can be minimised by evening dosing and a milky drink.

Unless otherwise stated, tablets should be started one week before arrival, to ensure an adequate level of drug in the bloodstream, taken continuously throughout the stay and for four weeks after leaving the malarious area. Tablets should be taken as prescribed. Missing doses can be as bad as taking no tablets at all. Patients should be warned about possible side effects (see *BNF*).

Malaria prophylaxis

All antimalarial drugs can have unwanted side effects. Patients should be advised to read the patient information leaflet supplied with the tablets and know what problems could occur.

Sun exposure

Patients should be warned about the risks of exposure to too much sun. Long-term exposure can cause skin cancer, especially as the ozone layer, which filters out dangerous ultraviolet radiation, is being destroyed. Sunburn may ruin a holiday and could be fatal in extreme cases. Falling asleep in the sun is a big danger and is often caused by excessive alcohol intake. Generally speaking, the fairer the skin, the greater the risk of burning. Children need special vigilance and protection from the sun.

Sensible precautions for sunbathers should include gradual acclimatisation (beginning with only 10–15 minutes a day in the morning or mid-afternoon) and the regular application of sunscreens with a minimum of SPF 15. Reapplication will be needed after swimming or showering. Water, sand and snow will all increase the reflection of ultraviolet, so extra care is needed to protect skin on beaches and ski slopes or when taking part in water sports. A moisturising cream should be applied after exposure to the sun and regular drinks are needed to replace fluid loss. Alcohol causes dehydration and so should be limited. If urine is dark and concentrated then more fluids are needed. Salt lost in sweat will also need replacing, either in the diet or by adding half a level teaspoonful of salt per litre of liquid for drinking. Severe sunburn will need medical treatment.

Heat illness

Heat exhaustion is common, especially in elderly patients. The causes may include dehydration, salt deficiency or impairment of the ability to sweat. Prolonged heat stress may result in the more serious condition of heatstroke.

Heatstroke can happen without direct exposure to the sun. Impairment of the heat-regulating system causes a dangerous rise in body temperature as sweating

Table 11.2 Malaria prophylaxis

Drug	Contraindications/cautions	Advice
Proguanil (***Paludrine***) Daily dose Often recommended to be used in conjunction with chloroquine	Caution in renal impairment May potentiate the effect of warfarin Folate supplements needed in pregnancy	Seek specialist advice Blood test pre- and post-travel to stabilise warfarin dose 5 mg, daily recommended dose of folic acid
Chloroquine (***Avloclor, Nivaquine***) Weekly dose Start 1 week before entering malarious area	Contraindicated with epilepsy May aggravate psoriasis Caution with liver and renal impairment	Consider doxycycline as an alternative Seek specialist advice
Mefloquine (***Lariam***) Daily dose Commence tablets 2.5–3 weeks before departure to allow time to change to another drug if side effects occur	Contraindicated if: – history of mental illness – convulsions or epilepsy – pregnant, breastfeeding or planning a pregnancy within three months of trip – severe liver, heart or kidney disease Vivid dreams and dizziness can occur	Use alternative antimalarial Ensure adequate supplies of contraceptives Get medical advice Caution if driving
Doxycycline Daily dose	Contraindicated in: – pregnancy and lactation – children Caution with liver disease Can cause sun sensitivity Can cause oesophagitis	Use alternative drug or seek specialist advice Cover up and use high factor suncream Take after food with plenty of water, while standing or sitting straight
Atovaquone with proguanil (***Malarone, Malarone Paediatric***) Daily dose Commence 1–2 days before arrival and continue until seven days after leaving the malaria-endemic area	Licensed for trips up to 28 days, i.e. up to 37 tablets	The tablets are expensive Patients should be aware of the cost before the private prescription is written

diminishes. Death can occur within a few hours if not treated. Immediate cooling by evaporation is needed, using wet sheets or towels on the skin and fanning. Rehydration with cool drinks is also essential and emergency medical treatment should be obtained. Patients should be warned of the contributing factors to heatstroke, especially for anyone with a skin condition that impairs sweating. These include:

- Continuous heat stress
- Lack of fitness, obesity
- Alcohol excess
- Strenuous exercise
- Too much or unsuitable clothing
- Some drugs, including cold remedies and diuretics.[8]

Blood-borne viruses and sexually transmitted diseases

The holiday atmosphere and alcohol may combine to remove inhibitions but can also result in unwanted souvenirs. Casual sexual encounters lead to the spread of sexually transmitted diseases (including blood-borne viruses). The prostitutes in many countries could be infected and patients should be warned of the serious risks. If used correctly, condoms provide a degree of protection but they should be stored in a cool place away from direct sunlight and particular care is needed to prevent their being damaged in transit. The quality of condoms available in countries outside the UK may not be as high, so travellers, both male and female, should be encouraged to take a supply with them.

Tattooing, acupuncture and body piercing should be avoided. Emergency medical or dental treatment may expose travellers to risk in countries where the reuse of equipment is likely. Sterile emergency packs containing syringes, needles, sutures and blood transfusion needles can be purchased for a reasonable price but blood transfusion and dental work should be avoided if at all possible in high-risk countries. Travellers should be advised to have sufficient health insurance to be repatriated in an emergency.

Accidents and injury

Some patients worry about catching exotic diseases and request a plethora of immunisations, whereas in reality, they are probably far more at risk of accidental injury or even death. Some of the hazards travellers need to consider seriously include: drowning, alcohol excess leading to risk taking, or dangerous transport and driving conditions. Travellers should also consider the risks of violence or kidnapping, particularly in countries with civil unrest. Nurses must advise patients to do their homework and be aware of any potential problems. The choice of where to travel lies with the patient. Every attempt should be made to obey the laws of the country being visited.

High altitude

The reduced atmospheric pressure at high altitudes means that less oxygen is available to the tissues. The body adapts by deeper respirations and a faster heart rate, but time for acclimatisation is necessary and fatalities do occur. Patients planning journeys to high altitudes (over 2400 m) should seek medical advice, especially if they have respiratory or cardiac conditions or sickle cell anaemia. Patients who fly directly to areas at high altitude, as in the Andes and Himalayas, may be unaware of the risk and therefore not allow sufficient time to acclimatise. Some authorities recommend prophylactic acetazolamide 250 mg and patients may request a prescription but drugs for prophylactic use abroad must be issued on private prescription. Patients should be made aware of the need to descend to a lower level if they are seriously affected by altitude sickness.

Air travel

Flying at high altitude, despite cabin pressurisation, may also cause problems of hypoxia for some people, particularly those who smoke heavily. The ears are likely to be affected by changes in air pressure and severe discomfort may be caused if congestion blocks the Eustachian tubes. Patients with medical problems should ask a doctor to check their fitness to fly.

The venous return can be slowed when sitting for long periods and can cause a deep vein thrombosis (DVT). The effects of air travel on health were the subject of an enquiry by a Select Committee of the House of Lords in the year 2000. Among the recommendations on seating, ventilation and air quality was advice that health professionals stop using the term 'economy class syndrome' because first-class and business passengers or people using other forms of long-distance transport could be equally vulnerable. Travellers' thrombosis is now the generally accepted term.[9] Publicity around the risk of DVT has led to several preventive recommendations. These include:

- Wearing comfortable clothing that will not restrict the legs or abdomen
- Regular ankle exercises, standing up and deep breathing to aid the venous return
- Drinking plenty of water but reducing alcohol intake to avoid dehydration, which can make the blood more likely to coagulate
- Compression hosiery for long-haul flights and for patients with specific risk factors for DVT.

Travellers at increased risk of DVT should see their GP before travel. Low molecular weight heparin may be prescribed. Those at risk include patients who:

- Have a history of DVT or pulmonary embolism
- Have had a recent myocardial infarction
- Are taking oestrogen in the contraceptive pill or HRT
- Have a malignancy
- Have had any recent major surgery

- Are pregnant
- Have a haematological disorder such as thrombocytosis.

Research is ongoing into the causes and prevention of travellers' thrombosis. The use of low-dose aspirin is still popular but aspirin can cause gastric irritation and it has been suggested that 17 000 travellers would have to be treated with aspirin to prevent one case of DVT.[10]

Travel in pregnancy

Always ask 'Is your journey really necessary?' Pregnant women should be advised not to travel to remote areas but if such travel is essential, then during the second trimester is considered to be the most suitable time. The risk of early miscarriage or of preterm birth is lower than at other times. Air travel in normal pregnancy is generally considered safe up to 35 weeks, but women should check with their particular airline. They should also remember that they may not be allowed to travel back after a long stay if the pregnancy is too advanced. There is a greater risk of thromboembolic disease in pregnancy. A doctor's letter may be required and adequate health insurance, which covers pregnancy, is essential.

Immunisation should be avoided in pregnancy, except when the risk from the disease outweighs the risk from the vaccine. All risks should be discussed with the woman and any immunisation must be prescribed by a GP. Pregnant women are more likely to be seriously affected by malaria, which can induce maternal death, miscarriage, stillbirth or low birth weight with associated risk of neonatal death.[11] Proguanil and chloroquine at normal doses can be used with daily folic acid 5 mg, but pregnant women should be strongly advised against travelling to an area with chloroquine-resistant falciparum malaria.

Travel with children

Special care is needed when travelling with young children. Dehydration and sun exposure should be avoided. Skin care is important because young skin is delicate and easily damaged by the sun.[12]

All routine childhood immunisations should be up to date. BCG and hepatitis B can be given at birth and an accelerated course of hepatitis B given if necessary, with a booster dose 12 months later. Travel vaccinations, except yellow fever, are not normally given to children under one year of age; typhoid vaccine is less effective before 18 months of age. Exposure to hepatitis A in early childhood, whilst not causing severe symptoms in most children, will confer life-long immunity. Immunisation would be given mainly as a public health measure aimed at the prevention of spread of the disease in the community upon their return. Immunisation is recommended for children of immigrant parents, born in Western Europe, before visiting countries where hepatitis A is endemic.[13]

Children are particularly susceptible to malaria and every effort should be made to protect them from bites if parents cannot be deterred from taking them to a malarious area. The dosage of antimalarials suitable for children is usually calculated according to their weight.

Travel for patients with respiratory diseases

Travellers with preexisting respiratory problems may find they are more at risk of contracting respiratory illnesses whilst abroad. A respiratory health check is advisable before departure to ensure that the patient is fit to travel and knows what to do if unwell.

Care should be taken to:

- Plan the trip to avoid known trigger factors
- Ensure health insurance is adequate
- Consider vaccination against influenza and pneumococcal disease if appropriate
- Carry sufficient inhalers for the trip – some in hand luggage and some in main luggage
- Be aware of the signs of deterioration of his/her condition and know when to commence emergency treatment
- Have a standby course of emergency medication
- Carry a spacer device and MDI (metered dose inhaler) of a reliever for medical emergencies.

Travel for patients with diabetes

Patients with diabetes should obtain advice before long journeys, especially if crossing time zones. These points should be considered when advising on foreign travel.

- Make sure that travel insurance is adequate and that the insurer knows about the diabetes. Diabetes UK will advise patients.
- Carry a doctor's letter to outline current treatment and the need to carry insulin, if appropriate. An Insulin User's Identity Card can be purchased from Diabetes UK.[14]
- Carry a European Health Insurance Card if travelling within the European Union. These have replaced the E111 cards.[15]
- Ensure you have sufficient medication, etc. for the entire trip.
- Carry a blood-monitoring kit in the hand luggage and carry emergency carbohydrates, such as glucose tablets or Lucozade. Carry a snack in case of unexpected delays.

- Carry all insulin in the hand luggage (in case baggage gets mislaid and because the insulin could freeze in the hold if travelling by air). Use an insulated bag to keep the insulin cool. Airlines have imposed stringent rules about hand luggage in response to international terrorism and patients may be requested to hand insulin to the cabin crew for storage during a flight. Such items should be placed in a carrier bag. It would be sensible to contact the airline in advance to check on their regulations.
- Take medication, if needed, to prevent travel sickness.
- Follow the normal sickness advice if vomiting or diarrhoea occurs (see Chapter 16).
- Pay particular attention to foot care while away.

Responsible travel

There is a danger that the explosion in world tourism will lead to the destruction of the places being visited, especially in developing countries. The effect is not totally negative because the money brought by tourism can help in the conservation of the environment as well as development of the infrastructure, but fragile ecosystems may be subjected to intolerable strain. There are websites devoted to ethical tourism, which patients could be encouraged to access so that they can be sure that their holiday will not have an adverse effect on the place being visited.

IMMUNISATION FOR TRAVELLERS

Practice nurses usually work out the schedules and administer immunisations for travellers under Patient Group Directions (PGDs). The choice of database for deciding which vaccines are needed is a matter for practice policy. Each nurse should maintain an up-to-date and signed PGD for each vaccine and should know when to consult a doctor regarding travel health issues. Many surgeries now purchase the vaccines and claim reimbursement and dispensing fees. The storage of vaccines needs special care and temperature control (see Chapter 4).

Immunisation serves two purposes: to prevent the spread of diseases and to protect the individual from infection. Proof of immunisation may be mandatory in some countries and entry can be denied without a valid certificate of immunisation. Yellow fever is the only disease for which an International Certificate of Immunisation may be required. Pilgrims travelling to Saudi Arabia require proof of meningitis immunisation before a visa will be granted.

Individual schedules of immunisation will depend on:

- The injections previously received
- The length and type of journey
- The time available before departure.

Accelerated schedules are possible sometimes but it is best to start 6–8 weeks before departure (14 weeks if a full course of tetanus, diphtheria and polio is needed). Some diseases are seasonal, so up-to-date information is necessary.

The safeguards and emergency procedures should be specified in the PGDs. All the specific advice given and the vaccines administered must be recorded accurately in the patient's records. Computer records of immunisation save time when planning vaccination schedules and are also valuable for administration and audit purposes. Item-of-service fees are no longer paid but patients who are not registered at a practice may be asked to pay for travel immunisations. Vaccines such as yellow fever are not available on prescription and must be given privately. Ideally there should be a fixed scale of charges for immunisation but in reality, practices are able to specify their own rates. This can cause problems if people planning to travel together attend different practices in a locality and have to pay different amounts.

Contraindications to immunisation

A checklist helps to ensure that no essential questions are omitted (Table 11.3).

The manufacturer's instructions for administration and contraindications to immunisation must always be observed.

Table 11.3 Checklist for contraindications to immunisation

Questions	Rationale
Are you well today? (if the answer is 'no', check what the problem is)	Postpone immunisation if acute or febrile illness
Are you taking steroids or have you any condition that affects your immune system?	Live viruses should not be given to immunosuppressed patients
Is there any chance that you might be pregnant? (female patients)	Vaccines should not be administered unless risk of disease outweighs possible risk to the fetus; consult the GP
Have you reacted badly to any previous vaccine?	Medical advice needed before the vaccine is given
Are you allergic to eggs?	Previous anaphylactic reaction to eggs may contraindicate vaccines such as yellow fever made from viruses cultured in eggs

Tetanus

The risk of tetanus occurs throughout the world. Spores of the bacillus are found in the soil and can thus be transmitted to humans through wounds. The faeces of domestic animals may also contain the spores. A primary course or booster is recommended for anyone not already protected (see Chapter 10). The combined vaccine Td/IPV should be used (see below).

Poliomyelitis

Polio is still prevalent in many developing countries. A primary course or booster is recommended for anyone who is not fully immunised and planning to travel to areas where polio is still endemic. Children should be protected by their routine immunisations. Oral polio drops have been discontinued; the combined Td/IPV vaccine should be used for adults.

Diphtheria

Diphtheria reemerged as a risk for long-term travellers following the decimation of the healthcare system in the Soviet Union after the collapse of communism. Low-dose diphtheria vaccine is recommended for all adults who need immunisation against this disease. The combined vaccine against diphtheria, tetanus and polio (Td/IPV) is recommended.

Typhoid

Typhoid fever is a salmonella infection transmitted by food or water contaminated by the faeces either of a person suffering from the disease or a chronic carrier who has recovered from the disease but still excretes the bacterium. The infection causes a systemic disease, which can be fatal if untreated. The food and drink precautions given above are important but immunisation is also recommended for many areas.

- Vi capsular polysaccharide vaccine: one dose gives protection for three years.
- Attenuated live oral vaccine consists of three capsules, one to be taken on alternate days. Three capsules give protection for three years, but the instructions for storing the capsules and timing the doses must be followed. It is not recommended for children under six years old.

Hepatitis A

Hepatitis A is a viral infection usually caused by faecal contamination of food and water. The disease is usually mild in young children and may not be recognised but they can still transmit the infection. Vaccines for active immunisation have been available for many years. Two doses give protection for up to ten years. Passive immunisation with immunoglobulin is no longer recommended because of the risk of transmitting other infection from the donor. Blood can be taken beforehand to test for hepatitis A antibodies, if previous infection is thought likely to have occurred. Laboratories in some areas may charge a private fee for such tests.

Hepatitis B

Immunisation against the hepatitis B virus is not routinely recommended for short-term travel but it may be offered to people planning to spend long periods in an endemic area and to travellers likely to be at special risk through their work or lifestyle. Patients should know that hepatitis B is spread through contact with blood and other bodily fluids and the measures to take to avoid that contact.

Combined vaccines

Newer vaccines are available which combine hepatitis A and typhoid vaccines and hepatitis A and B vaccines. These may be useful for reducing the number of injections for patients who are afraid of needles or when time is limited before departure. Immunisation against hepatitis A will require a separate booster if the first dose is combined with typhoid vaccine.

Yellow fever

Yellow fever is a viral infection transmitted by mosquito bites in tropical Africa and South America. The incubation period is 3–6 days. Immunisation is given only at designated centres but with the increase in foreign travel, many practices have now been accepted as yellow fever centres by the Department of Health. From January 2005, all existing yellow fever vaccination centres must reapply for designation. At least one member of staff must attend a training seminar (see NaTHNaC website for details and registration form). At times when only unlicensed vaccine is available, the GP must decide if it is to be offered and must prescribe the vaccine for individual patients. Unlicensed vaccine cannot be given under a PGD. An International Certificate of Immunisation against yellow fever is issued after immunisation and becomes valid ten days after immunisation. One dose conveys immunity for ten years, so patients should be advised to take care of their certificates during that time. A private fee can be charged because the vaccine has to be purchased and is not reimbursable. Patients from other surgeries may be seen privately for yellow fever immunisation. Suitable paper records must be kept of these immunisations if the patient is not entered on the practice computer.

Meningococcal meningitis

Meningococcal meningitis usually occurs in epidemics. It is a bacterial infection spread by droplets, so is most common in areas where people are crowded together. Some visitors to the 'meningitis belt' of Africa, northern India and the lowlands of Nepal during the dry seasons could be at risk of meningitis. One dose of meningitis $ACW_{135}Y$ vaccine provides immunity for three years for adults and children over two years of age. A certificate will be needed for pilgrims travelling to the Hajj or Umrah.[16] The certificate is valid for three years from ten days after immunisation and must be issued within two years of immunisation. The vaccine is not licensed for patients under two, so the doctor should authorise immunisation of a patient younger than that; there is likely to be suboptimal response to the vaccine and two doses will be needed for patients aged between three months to two years.[17] ACWY vaccine should be given to patients at risk abroad even if they have had meningitis C vaccine previously.

Rabies

Rabies is a viral infection, usually transmitted by the bite or saliva of an infected animal. Preexposure immunisation may be offered to travellers to rabies-endemic areas. The 'Green Book' specifies the patients for whom rabies immunisation is recommended. Travellers have to pay privately but patients at occupational risk can have the vaccine through the NHS; 1 ml of vaccine should be given on day 0, day 7 and day 28. The third dose may be given from day 21 if time is limited. Postexposure treatment is still needed if exposed to rabies but patients who have had preexposure immunisation do not need to have rabies-specific immunoglobulin or so many postexposure injections; the immunoglobulin might not be available or be safe in some countries.

A patient who is scratched or bitten by an animal that could have rabies should also be advised:

- To cleanse the wound thoroughly with soap and water, followed by a disinfectant and non-occlusive dressing
- To avoid primary suturing of a wound
- To get the name and address of the animal's owner (if known), so the animal can be observed for signs of rabies
- To get advice from a local doctor about the risk of rabies in that area and to get postexposure treatment even if immunised beforehand.

Japanese B encephalitis

Japanese B encephalitis is a viral disease spread by mosquitoes, most commonly found in rural areas of Asian countries during the monsoon season, where there are concentrations of pigs and birds near rice fields. The prevention of mosquito bites is the best preventive measure. An inactivated vaccine is available on a named-patient basis only on a private prescription. Severe allergic reactions can occur after immunisation and delayed reactions are possible. The need for the vaccine must be weighed against possible risks of the disease, with further advice being sought if necessary.

Tick-borne encephalitis

A virus transmitted by the bite of an infected animal tick, mainly during the spring and summer, causes tick-borne encephalitis. Ticks are picked up from the undergrowth in warm, forested areas of Europe and Scandinavia. Hikers and campers are most at risk. People planning trips to those areas should be advised not to walk with bare legs and to use an insect repellent. A full course of vaccine to last three years requires three injections. Two injections give protection for one year. Half the adult dose is recommended for the first dose for children aged 3–15 years.[18] The vaccine must be shaken well to ensure that the volume given actually contains half the antigen.

Cholera

Cholera is spread by faecal contamination of water, so patients can be advised that the way to avoid the disease is to adopt sensible food and water precautions. A certificate of vaccination is no longer necessary but travellers who will be crossing borders in remote areas may choose to carry a statement on official paper to say that cholera vaccination is not required.

Cholera vaccine is not recommended for routine travel. Patients may be advised to be immunised if they are going to work in disaster areas or travelling to remote areas where cholera is epidemic and access to medical care is limited. The only licensed vaccine available in the UK is an oral preparation, *Dukoral*. A second dose is needed 1–6 weeks after the first.

Suggestions for reflection on practice

- How effective is your travel health service?
- Are appointment times long enough to provide comprehensive advice?
- Are your knowledge and reference materials up to date?

REFERENCES

1. Health Protection Agency (Undated) *Mortality in Travellers*. www.hpa.org.uk (accessed 26/12/05).
2. Royal College of Nursing Travel Health Forum (2005) *Delivering Travel Health Services: RCN guidance for nursing staff*. Royal College of Nursing, London.
3. Curtis, V. & Cairncross, S. (2003) Effect of washing hands with soap on diarrhoea risk in the community: a systematic review. *Lancet Infectious Diseases*, 3(5), 275–81.

4. Prodigy Guidance (2003) *Gastroenteritis.* www.prodigy.nhs.uk/guidance.asp? Gastroenteritis (accessed 29/12/05).
5. Al-Abri, S.S., Beeching, N.J. & Nye, F.J. (2005) Traveller's diarrhoea. *Lancet Infectious Diseases,* **5** (6), 349–60.
6. National Travel Health Network and Centre (2005) Malaria. *The Yellow Book* 6.1. www.nathnac.org/yellow_book/06.htm (accessed 30/12/05).
7. Prodigy Guidance (2004) *Malaria.* www.prodigy.nhs.uk/guidance.asp? Malariaprophylaxis (accessed 30/12/05).
8. Dawood, R. (2002) Effects of climatic extremes. In: *Travellers' Health: how to stay healthy abroad,* 4th edn. Oxford University Press, Oxford.
9. Bagshaw, M. (2004) *BMA Hot Topic: traveller's thrombosis.* www.bma.org.uk/ap.nsf/ Content/LIBTravellersThrombosis (accessed 6/1/06).
10. Loke, Y.K. & Derry, S. (2002) Air travel and venous thrombosis: how much help might aspirin be? *Medscape General Medicine,* **4** (3), 4.
11. World Health Organisation (2005) Malaria. In: *International Travel and Health.* World Health Organisation, Geneva.
12. Cancer Research UK (undated) *Sunsmart – Children.* www.cancerresearchuk.org/ sunsmart/staysafe/children/?version=2 (accessed 7/1/06).
13. Kassionos, G. (2001) *Immunization, Childhood and Travel Health.* Blackwell Science, Oxford.
14. Diabetes UK (2002) *Air Travel and Insulin.* www.diabetes.org.uk/infocentre/ inform/airtravel.htm (accessed 8/1/06).
15. Department of Health (2005) *Important Information for People using E111 Forms.* www.dh.gov.uk/PolicyAndGuidance/HealthAdviceForTravellers/GettingTreat mentAroundTheWorld/ (accessed 8/1/06).
16. Department of Health (2005) *Going to Hajj or Umrah? Protect yourself and your family, guard against meningitis and save lives.* Department of Health Publications, London.
17. Department of Health (2005) *Immunisation Against Infectious Disease 1996,* Draft replacement chapter 23 – Meningococcal. www.dh.gov.uk Search under Green Book (accessed 9/1/06).
18. Department of Health (2005) *Immunisation Against Infectious Disease 1996,* Draft replacement chapter 32 – Tick-borne encephalitis. www.dh.gov.uk Search under Green Book (accessed 9/1/06).

FURTHER READING

British Medical Association and Royal Pharmaceutical Society of Great Britain (2005) *British National Formulary 50.* BMA and RPSGB, London.

Dawood, R. (2002) *Travellers' Health: how to stay healthy abroad,* 4th edn. Oxford University Press, Oxford.

Department of Health (2005) *Immunisation Against Infectious Disease 1996,* new draft chapters. www.dh.gov.uk Policy and Guidance, Green Book.

Jones, N. (2004) *The Rough Guide to Travel Health,* 2nd edn. Rough Guides, London.

World Health Organisation (2005) *International Travel and Health.* World Health Organisation, Geneva.

USEFUL ADDRESSES AND WEBSITES

Medical Advisory Service for Travellers Abroad (MASTA), Keppel Street, London WC1E 7HT
Telephone Travellers Healthline: 09068 224 100
Website: www.masta.org.uk
IV Telecom hotline: 09068 44 4546

PHLS Malaria Reference Laboratory, London School of Hygiene and Tropical Medicine, Keppel Street, London WC1E 7HT
Telephone: 0207 636 3924 (for advice for health professionals)
Premium line telephone: 09065 508 908 (advice line for the general public)
Website: www.lsthm.ac.uk/itd/units/pmbbu/malaria/malariaref

Health Protection Scotland, Clifton House, Clifton Place, Glasgow G3 7LN
Telephone: 0141 300 1100
Website: www.hps.scot.nhs.uk

Aventis Pasteur MSD Vaccine Information Service
Telephone: 07000 766 73847
Website: www.apmsd.co.uk

Department of Health Travel Advice (for the general public)
Website: www.doh.gov.uk/traveladvice

TRAVAX
Website: www.show.scot.nhs.uk

Fit for Travel
Website: www.fitfortravel.scot.nhs.uk

World Health Organisation
Website: www.who.int

Updates for *International Travel and Health*
Website: www.who.int/ith

National Travel Health Network and Centre (NaTHNaC)
Website: www.nathnac.org

Travel Health Information Services
Website: www.travelhealth.co.uk

Ethical tourism
www.responsible-travel.org
www.tourismconcern.org.uk

Chapter 12
Sexual Health

Patients have the added advantage of continuity of care when a practice provides a comprehensive range of services. Practice nurses see patients of all ages and have the opportunity to promote sexual health as a part of healthy living. There are several aspects to sexual health.

- Having a positive sense of sexual identity and self-worth
- Being able to sustain mutually satisfying relationships in which both partners feel secure enough to express personal needs or wishes
- Preventing unwanted pregnancies
- Avoiding sexually transmitted diseases.

SEXUAL IDENTITY

Sexual identity involves more than male or female gender (which is usually decided *in utero*). Practice nurses need to be aware of cultural differences and the variety of ways in which sexuality can be expressed. Ideas of masculinity and femininity undergo periodic changes. In areas of high male unemployment, men who previously had a dominant role in the household may lose their sense of self-worth as their wives find employment instead. In other areas, women expect equality as a right but this change in the balance of power can cause anxiety for men. Some women can be frustrated in their attempts to achieve their full potential, while some men feel inadequate when faced by assertive females.

Conflict can occur in immigrant families, when young people brought up in the West rebel against the cultural expectations of their families. Forced marriages and different attitudes to divorce can cause problems within families. Female genital mutilation is still practised in some African and Middle Eastern countries. It has been illegal in the UK since 1985; a new law was passed in 2003 in England and in 2005 in Scotland.[1] Female genital mutilation could pose child protection issues for doctors and nurses working with refugees and asylum seekers who still adopt this custom. Risk of female genital mutilation should be recognised as legitimate grounds for refugee or asylum status.[2]

In a predominantly heterosexual society, minority groups have had to campaign hard for equality. Attitudes to homosexuality have been changing gradually but a great deal of homophobia still exists. Anybody who feels uncomfortable dealing with gay men or lesbians should examine the reasons and find ways to ensure that homosexual patients are not disadvantaged.

The need for sexual health education and advice for patients with learning disabilities has only been recognised relatively recently and attempts have been made in some areas to tailor services to those needs.

Sexuality has been a neglected area of nurse education and many nurses do not feel comfortable discussing issues relating to sex. Every nurse needs to have come to terms with her/his own feelings before being able to help patients. The degree of involvement in sexual health issues will vary with the knowledge and expertise of individual nurses.

RELATIONSHIPS

Nurses should be aware of the many ways in which patients can experience problems:

- Ignorance about the way the body functions or how the emotions can affect sexual functioning
- Lack of self-esteem – not being able to say 'no' or to refuse unsafe sex
- Conflict between personal desires and the pressures to conform to the cultural norm
- The effects of illness, drugs or disability. Carers can experience a role conflict when expected to be both nurse and lover. Medication such as beta blockers can cause impotence. Patients recovering from a heart attack may fear a recurrence with any exertion. Patients with severe arthritis, paraplegia or other disabilities may have practical problems with sexual performance
- Loneliness in patients without a partner can lead to depression and a lack of purpose in life
- Ageism – when people over a certain age are no longer thought to need a sexual relationship.

Patients with some of these problems may need specialised help but a practice nurse who recognises the existence of the problem can offer appropriate information, counselling or referral elsewhere as appropriate.

EDUCATION FOR NURSES

Practice nurses who do not wish to specialise in family planning are advised to obtain a foundation-level qualification in sexual and reproductive health. Most universities with a healthcare faculty run such courses. Some areas also provide a foundation course in sexually transmitted infections (STIF), which all practice nurses should attend. Information can be obtained from the local PCO or the internet. The Royal College of Nursing runs a distance-learning foundation course that is open to all nurses, not just College members. The FPA (formerly the Family Planning Association) produces a wide range of useful literature, runs courses for health and social care professionals and provides advice and information.

A fertility and fertility control qualification (ENB 900, 901, A08 or equivalent) is required to work autonomously in this field. Courses are not easy to access and advice, if needed, should be sought from the primary care organisation nurse with responsibility for family planning.

FERTILITY AND FERTILITY CONTROL

Fertility control should not be considered as an exclusively female concern. Couples may attend the surgery together to discuss contraception, preparation for pregnancy, infertility or sterilisation. Some patients prefer to visit a family planning clinic because it offers anonymity. Family planning nurses, who can prescribe or work within the terms of Patient Group Directions, now run many clinics. Adolescents often fear that the GP will tell their parents about the con-sultation. In many areas, special under-18 centres have been developed for young people at suitable venues, in order to address this concern. However, some Area Child Protection Committees have issued protocols with regard to underage sex, which could undermine the patient's right to confidentiality. Health professionals have expressed their concern over this development.[3]

In the main, practice nurses can offer reassurance that their service is confidential and will not be discussed with anyone without the consent of the patient. The Department of Health guidance stresses that the Sexual Offences Act 2003 does not affect the duty of care and confidentiality of health profes-sionals to young people under 16.[4] However, the guidance also states that the overriding objective must be to safeguard the young person and the duty of confidentiality is not absolute. Except in the most exceptional circumstances, disclosure should only take place after consulting the young person. The law on the provision of contraceptive advice to children under 16 was clarified in 1985, as a result of the judgement by Lord Fraser in the Gillick case.[5] Parental respons-ibility should not be undermined and whenever possible, the young person should be persuaded to tell a parent or guardian but if, for example, family rela-tionships have broken down, a doctor or nurse would not be acting unlawfully if the young person:

- Was sufficiently mature to understand all the implications
- Would not allow a parent to know that contraceptive advice was being sought
- Would be very likely to have sexual intercourse without contraception
- Would be likely to suffer physical or mental ill health if not given contracept-ive advice or treatment.

Since that time, young people have been assessed for what has become known as Gillick competence.

Assessment of the patient

A number of aspects need to be considered when a doctor or nurse first sees any patient for sexual health advice and contraception.

- General medical history – to identify any contraindications to specific methods of contraception.
- Obstetric and gynaecological history – including menses, pregnancies, rubella status, cervical screening.
- Social history – because smoking, lifestyle or relationships may influence the choice of method.
- Family history – in case the patient may have an inherited susceptibility to cardiovascular disease, diabetes or cancer.
- Measurement of BP, weight and height as part of the general health assessment (also because hormone contraception can cause weight gain and elevation of the blood pressure).
- Cervical screening as appropriate if aged 25 or over.
- Pelvic and breast examination if clinically indicated.

Criteria for choice of contraceptive

There is no perfect method of contraception. The points to consider when choosing a method include:

- The safety of the method and any potential health risks
- The efficacy and reliability of the method
- The acceptability to both partners
- The availability – where and how easily it can be obtained
- The cost, if any.

Counselling

Patients should be able to make their own decisions after receiving adequate information and having the chance to explore any fears or anxieties. It is important not to impose one's own values and judgements. *Your Guide to Contraception*, a leaflet produced by the FPA, explains all the methods currently available, how they work, their reliability, advantages and disadvantages and other relevant information. The leaflet can be used as a basis for discussion when helping patients to compare the different methods.

Methods of contraception available

Oral contraception

There are many formulations of the pill but they can be grouped into two distinct types:

- The combined oral contraceptive pill
- The progestogen-only pill.

The doctor or FP nurse will prescribe the appropriate type of pill after a discussion with the patient and consideration of any contraindications.

The combined oral contraceptive pill (COC)

COCs contain oestrogen and progestogen and act by inhibiting ovulation. A pill is taken daily for 21 days followed by seven pill-free days. A withdrawal bleed usually occurs during this week. If any pills are missed, especially at the beginning or end of a packet, to lengthen the number of pill-free days, then ovulation and pregnancy could occur (see Box 12.1). The combined pill is often the first choice of younger women, for whom convenience and reliability rate highly. COCs can increase the risk of thromboembolism, so may be contraindicated for some patients. The risk is higher in women with some inherited clotting factor defects. Thrombophilia screening is no longer recommended for asymptomatic women with a history of DVT in first-degree relatives.[6] Women with a personal history of thrombosis should not take COCs.

Phasic pills contain varying hormone strengths, which are intended to mimic the natural cycle. They have been thought to give a better bleeding pattern but more pill-taking errors can occur and the evidence for their use is inconclusive. Every Day (ED) pill packets contain seven placebo pills to be taken after the 21 active pills. They are useful for patients who forget to restart a packet after a week's break but the pills must be taken in the correct order. Mistakes can happen more easily if two packets need to be taken without a pill-free break.

The progestogen-only pill (POP)

POPs work mainly in three ways: by thickening the cervical mucus to make it impenetrable to sperm, inhibiting transportation in the Fallopian tubes, and by making the endometrium unsuitable for implantation. POPs may also inhibit ovulation in some women but this is not the main mode of action. Therefore, the pills must be taken at the same time (or within three hours) every day, without a break, in order to maintain these physiological effects. A newer POP (*Cerazette*) acts by suppressing ovulation, so has a 12-hour window and may thus be more suitable for patients with a disorganised lifestyle. The bleeding pattern with POPs may be more erratic than with the COC pill and weight gain or mood changes may make the method less well tolerated. POPs do not carry a thromboembolic

Box 12.1   Missed pill guidelines

COC pills

- If less than 12 hours late, take the pill as usual and continue normal pill taking
- If more than 12 hours late and not more than two pills missed (one if low-strength pills, i.e. Loestrin 20, Mercilon or Femodette), take the most recently missed pill and continue normal pill taking
- If three or more pills missed (two if low-strength pills), take the most recently missed pill, ignore other missed pills, continue normal pill taking but use extra precautions (abstain from sex or use a condom) for seven days. Emergency contraception might be needed if unprotected intercourse within the past few days
- If less than seven pills left in the packet, omit the pill-free week and start the next packet without a break. Omit any placebo pills if using an ED preparation
- Emergency contraception is recommended if two or more pills missed in the first seven days of a packet or four or more consecutive pills missed in mid-packet

POPs

- Should be regarded as 'missed' if more than three hours late (12 hours if taking *Cerazette*) or pills not taken at all
- If more than three hours late (12 hours for *Cerazette*), take the most recently missed pill, ignore any others missed and continue normal pill taking, even if it means taking two pills in one day. Use extra precautions (abstain from sex or use a condom) for two days
- Emergency contraception is recommended if one or more pills are 'missed' and sexual intercourse occurs before two pills have been taken correctly

risk so are more suitable for older women, heavy smokers and others who cannot take the combined pill (see *BNF* 7.3.2). POPs can also be taken by breast-feeding mothers.

Oral contraceptive routines

Each practice should have agreed guidelines for working with both patients who need oral contraception for the first time and those having follow-up appointments.

First-time pill users

New pill users require education about:

- How the pill works and affects the body
- How to take the pill and when to start (day 1 of cycle will give immediate contraceptive protection)

- What to do if a pill is missed (see Box 12.1)
- How diarrhoea and vomiting or some medicines and antibiotics can prevent the pill from being absorbed so extra precautions, such as condoms, are needed for seven days after recovery for patients taking COCs or two days after recovery for POP users
- How to recognise any abnormal effects and when to contact the surgery
- The risk of sexually transmitted diseases and the use of condoms for protection
- When to return for a 'pill' check.

There is too much information for a patient to remember after being told once, so appropriate instruction sheets are needed as well. The doctor or nurse must check that the patient understands the information given. The FPA leaflets are excellent and it is recommended that a stock is kept for each method.

Patients already taking the pill

New pill users should return after three months, when BP, weight and bleeding can be recorded and any problems or worries discussed. Established pill users require a pill check every six months to one year, depending on the practice policy. Regular cervical smears should be offered once a woman has reached 25 years of age. The patient's knowledge and understanding of her pill use should be checked to ensure that no essential information has been forgotten or misunderstood.

Emergency contraception

Emergency hormonal contraception can be prescribed up to 72 hours after unprotected intercourse, but it is likely to be most effective if taken within 24 hours of the accident.[7] The patient needs to understand why she should be honest about any other unprotected sexual intercourse during that menstrual cycle; she could already be pregnant, in which case hormone emergency contraception would not work. Some nurses may supply the tablets under a Patient Group Direction, but it is essential to adhere to the terms of the PGD and to ensure there are no contraindications to the treatment.

A single tablet of levonorgestrel 1500 mcg has replaced the two-tablet regimen used previously. This can also be purchased by women over 16 from a pharmacy. The tablet will not cause a withdrawal bleed but the patient should be warned that the next period could be earlier or later than expected. Other information and advice should cover the need:

- To use a barrier method until the next period
- To contact the surgery if vomiting occurs within three hours of taking the tablet (the dose may be repeated and domperidone given as an antiemetic)
- To consider suitable methods of contraception for the longer term or, if already using oral contraception, to continue taking their pills as usual

- To return to the surgery if low abdominal pain develops, which could indicate an ectopic pregnancy
- To attend for follow-up after 3–4 weeks if the period is abnormally light, heavy or does not start at all.

A written information sheet would help to reinforce any verbal advice given. Patients who attend for emergency contraception could also be at increased risk of sexually transmitted infections. A sexual history should be taken and testing offered if appropriate.[8]

Postcoital intrauterine device (IUD)

A copper-bearing intrauterine device may be fitted as an alternative to hormone emergency contraception, if more than 72 hours have elapsed since unprotected intercourse, but may also be inserted up to five days after the likeliest date of ovulation, if calculable. The method is considered to be more reliable than hormone emergency contraception and should be considered if the avoidance of pregnancy is essential. However, it is an invasive procedure that carries other risks. The contraindications and side effects are the same as for IUDs fitted for regular contraception (see below, IUDs). Tests for sexually transmitted infections, especially chlamydia, should be carried out before insertion. Routine antibiotic prophylaxis is not recommended but should be considered in patients under 25 or women older than that with a new partner or who have had sex with more than two partners in the previous year.[9]

The intrauterine device (IUD)

This method, also known as the 'coil', involves the insertion of a small plastic and copper device into the uterus where it acts by inhibiting the passage of sperm and preventing the implantation of a fertilised ovum in the endometrium. An IUD, which has a surface area of over 300 mm^2 of copper, can stay in place from five to eight years or until one year after the last period if inserted in women over 40 years, in the absence of any problems.[10] Fine nylon threads, attached to the end of the IUD, pass through the cervix to aid removal of the device.

The method is considered suitable for the majority of women.[11] It was traditionally thought to be more suitable for multiparous women because the slightly increased risk of pelvic infection could threaten the fertility of women without children. Moreover, insertion could be more difficult when the cervix has never been dilated in labour. It is good practice to take swabs from all patients before inserting an IUD in order to rule out any infection. A family planning trained doctor or a specially trained FP nurse must insert the device. The ideal time for insertion is at the end of a menstrual period. The practice nurse will usually prepare the equipment, assist as needed and look after the patient throughout the procedure (see Chapter 5). Patients can imagine tremendous horrors, so it is worth keeping some unsterile IUDs and a model to demonstrate to patients what the coil looks like, where it is put and how it works.

The patient needs to have clear information about the possible immediate and later effects and when to consult the doctor. Any slight abdominal discomfort usually settles within a day or two but an urgent appointment is needed if there is persistent pain in the three weeks following insertion. If low abdominal pain, fever or vaginal discharge occurs there may be some pelvic infection, which requires treatment.

An IUD should not be removed when a woman is mid-cycle unless pregnancy is desired or extra precautions were taken for seven days beforehand. Sperm can survive for that length of time and postcoital contraception might be needed if it is essential to remove the device urgently at that time.

Gynefix

Unlike the rigid IUDs, Gynefix is a flexible device consisting of six copper beads strung on a suture, which is attached to the fundus of the uterus. Special training is needed to insert and remove the device, which can stay in place for five years.

The intrauterine system (IUS, Mirena)

The IUS looks like a conventional IUD but instead of copper wound around the stem, it has a sleeve containing levonorgestrel, which is released in minute quantities every day. Levonorgestrel acts locally to thicken the cervical mucus and to prevent proliferation of the endometrium. This, in turn, can make bleeding so light that the IUS can be used to control menorrhagia.[12] Patients can experience spotting and irregular bleeding when the IUS is first inserted but bleeding may eventually become non-existent as the progestogen inhibits ovulation. The device may also be used to oppose the effect of oestrogen on the endometrium in women taking hormone replacement therapy. The IUS obviates the need for oral or transdermal progestogen monthly.

Contraceptive hormone injections

Injectable contraceptives have become popular with some patients. Depot medroxyprogesterone acetate (DMPA) is most commonly used. It is given as *Depo-Provera* 150 mg by deep intramuscular injection every 12 weeks and provides immediate contraceptive cover if started before day five of the cycle. The injection can also be given within five days of a miscarriage or abortion or 5–6 weeks after childbirth. *Depo-Provera* suppresses ovulation and, as with other progestogens, makes the cervical mucus impenetrable to sperm and prevents proliferation of the endometrium.

Norethisterone enanthate (*Noristerat*) is an oily injection licensed for short-term contraception. It lasts for eight weeks and may be repeated once only.

There are few indications for its use in general practice; perhaps when a patient needs to avoid pregnancy following immunisation against MMR or is waiting for a negative sperm count after a partner's vasectomy.

Nurses giving depot contraception under a Patient Group Direction must observe the exclusions to administration and seek medical advice when necessary. Nurses who give injections prescribed by a GP should have a practice procedure to follow. The hormone cannot be removed once it has been injected, so patients must be made aware of possible side effects so they know what to expect and can give informed consent to the procedure. The following points need to be remembered.

- Weight gain can be a problem for some patients. Advice can be given about eating sensibly.
- Mood swings or depression akin to premenstrual syndrome may occur.
- Heavy, prolonged or irregular bleeding in the months after the first injection will usually settle and amenorrhoea occurs frequently, as a result of the suppression of ovulation.
- Delay in return to fertility can occur. It can take up to a year for periods to recommence once injections are stopped.
- Bone mineral density may be affected if adolescent women are given DMPA injections. Maximum bone density is normally achieved during the teenage years. More research is needed into the long-term effects but to date, the evidence suggests that for most patients, the residual effects of DMPA on postmenopausal bone density are small and unlikely to increase the risk of fractures in the postmenopausal years. Women who continue using DMPA until the time of the menopause may not have sufficient time to regain their bone density. The current guidance is that there should be no restriction on using DMPA by women aged 18–45, who are otherwise eligible to use the method.[13]

Patients should be made aware that the effect of the *Depo-Provera* injection starts to wear off after 12 weeks and should be repeated then but that it can be given earlier if the patient will be away on the due date. A recall date should be arranged at the time of injection. Advice should be sought if a patient presents more than 12 weeks and five days after her last injection. Emergency contraception may be necessary. Pregnancy must be excluded before giving another depot injection.

Progestogen implant

Implanon is the only implant available in the UK now. It consists of a single rod inserted subdermally, which releases etonogestrel over a three-year period. At the end of three years the rod should be removed and replaced. Insertion and removal must be done by a trained practitioner. The implant has been found to be a reliable method of long-term contraception but weight gain and irregular bleeding have been common side effects. Counselling of the patient before insertion can help to ensure perseverance with the method.

Transdermal contraceptive patch (Evra)

This is a newer contraceptive method, which might be suitable for patients who comply poorly with oral contraception. One patch is applied weekly for three weeks, followed by a patch-free week. A withdrawal bleed usually occurs during this time. Contraceptive cover is immediate if the first patch is applied on day 1 of the menstrual cycle. The method has been shown to be as effective as the combined pill in preventing pregnancy.[14] Possible side effects include headache, breast tenderness and skin reactions. The patient information leaflet explains how to apply the patch and what to do if it becomes dislodged.

Barrier methods

The diaphragm

The diaphragm is a fairly commonly prescribed barrier method. Diaphragms are made of thin latex rubber, in a range of sizes from 60 mm to 90 mm in diameter. Each one has a flexible wire inside the rim to make it fit comfortably in the vagina. The diaphragm covers the cervix with the rim positioned in the posterior fornix and behind the pubic rim in the vagina. Flat spring, coil spring and arcing spring diaphragms are available on prescription.

Some practices choose to purchase a supply of diaphragms and to claim reimbursement for them on prescription as personally administered items.

The cervical cap

These fit over the cervix and are held in place by suction. Although caps are less commonly prescribed in general practice, they can be useful for patients with lax pelvic floor muscles or women prone to cystitis when using a diaphragm.

Diaphragms and caps should be used in conjunction with a spermicide, which has to be supplied on prescription or bought OTC. The patient needs to be fitted and taught how to use the method by a family planning trained nurse or doctor. A plastic model of the female reproductive tract, specially designed to receive a diaphragm, is an excellent visual aid. The teaching should cover:

- How to locate the cervix
- How and when to insert the diaphragm or cap and to check that the cervix is covered
- To use extra spermicide if more than three hours have elapsed since the device was inserted, or intercourse last occurred
- How and when to remove the device (six hours but not more than 30 hours must have elapsed after intercourse)

- How to look after the cap and check for any damage or perishing
- To avoid any contact with oil-based products, including vaginal medication and massage oils, which will cause the rubber to perish
- When to return for a check or refitting (annual checks or if a significant weight change or pregnancy occurs)
- How to obtain emergency contraception if needed.

A diaphragm or cervical cap is a popular method with many women for whom the pill is unacceptable or contraindicated. The method may not be suitable for a woman who is unhappy about feeling her cervix or inserting the device. Some patients may develop an allergy to the spermicide or to latex and may have to use an alternative method.

Male and female condoms

Condoms have had significant publicity since the advent of HIV and AIDS. Free condoms are issued at family planning and GUM clinics but, unfortunately, too few general practices are able to provide them. They can be obtained free from FP or GUM clinics or can be purchased easily. Patients need to be reminded about the protection condoms can offer against sexually transmitted diseases as well as pregnancy and of the correct way to apply a condom. The following points are essential when using a male condom.

- Make sure the condom has been stored properly, has a British Standard kite mark and is not past its expiry date
- Use a non-spermicide lubricated condom
- Use a non-latex condom if either partner is allergic to latex
- Open the foil wrap carefully so the condom is not damaged
- Expel the air from the teat at the end of the condom to allow room for the ejaculate
- Avoid contact with oil-based products, which would perish latex
- Roll the condom onto the erect penis before any contact with the partner's genital area
- Hold the condom in place and withdraw the penis before it becomes flaccid after ejaculation
- Dispose of used condoms safely (wrap it in a tissue and place in a bin; do not flush it down the toilet)
- Make sure a female partner knows about emergency contraception if a condom fails.

The female condom (Femidon) is a more recent innovation that has not achieved widespread popularity. The condom is a polyurethane sac with a polythene ring inside to help the insertion of the condom into the vagina and a fixed ring around the opening, which lies over the labia. It provides some protection against genital herpes and other sexually transmitted diseases. Unlike the male condom, the

Femidon can be inserted at any time and so should not affect spontaneity. The condom is not affected by oil-based products and is less likely to tear. However, the rings can cause discomfort and there is a risk of the condom being pushed into the vagina or of the penis being inserted between the condom and the vaginal wall.

Natural methods (fertility awareness)

Religious or personal reasons may lead some couples to opt for natural family planning. A high level of motivation is required and special teaching is essential. Couples can avoid intercourse once they have learned to identify the fertile time each month. Various methods may be used, often in combination.

- Calendar – keeping records of the menstrual cycle. Ovulation occurs about 14 days before the menstrual period starts but cannot be predicted accurately in advance, even with a regular cycle.
- Temperature – very careful recordings of the body temperature each day, using a special fertility thermometer, to identify the slight temperature rise which occurs at ovulation (febrile illness will nullify the readings).
- Cervical mucus can be used to recognise the fertile time because the consistency and amount of the mucus changes around the time of ovulation to facilitate the entry of sperm.

Commercially available test kits detect ovulation by the surge in luteinising hormone, but do not yet predict ovulation early enough to be reliable for contraception because sperm can survive for up to seven days.

The success or failure of natural methods relies on being able to predict ovulation accurately so that intercourse is avoided for at least seven days before and three days afterwards.

Male and female sterilisation

Sterilisation is the ultimate contraception. It should be regarded as permanent even though advances in microsurgery might make reversal possible. Couples who have completed their families may opt for this method, but with divorce and second marriages now so common, they need to consider all the possible eventualities before reaching a decision about sterilisation. The advantages and disadvantages of alternative long-term methods of contraception should be discussed because informed consent is essential. Information should be supplemented with written material and supplied in translation if possible for those that need it.

Vasectomy

Sterilisation for the male entails cutting the spermatic cord just as it enters the inguinal canal after leaving the scrotum. It is an easy operation that can be performed under local anaesthetic as an outpatient. Some specially trained GPs will perform vasectomies in the surgery. The patient should be advised not to undertake strenuous physical activity for a few days, in order to minimise any possibility of bruising around the operation site. The following points should be emphasised when discussing this method of sterilisation with patients.

- It is permanent, but not until two consecutive sperm counts are negative
- There will be no adverse effect on erection, sexual performance or ejaculation
- The patient will notice little change after the operation as the majority of the ejaculate is made up of secretions from the prostate and other glands
- There is no proven link between vasectomy and prostate cancer and heart disease[15]
- Semen samples are required monthly for 3–4 months after the operation. Contraceptive precautions must be continued until two consecutive samples contain no sperm.

Female sterilisation

A woman is sterilised by occluding the Fallopian tubes so that the ovum cannot pass down them into the uterus. The vast majority of female sterilisations are carried out under general anaesthetic using a laparoscope in a day surgery unit. Patients may experience some discomfort after the procedure but this rarely lasts more than a few days. The practice nurse may be required to remove the sutures from the small abdominal incision sites. Women should be aware that the failure rate could be higher than for vasectomy and that if conception does occur, it could result in an ectopic pregnancy.

Education about contraception

Any method of contraception can fail if the user does not learn everything he or she needs to know about using the method safely. Doctors and nurses who provide family planning services need to have enough time, appropriate visual aids and be able to choose suitable teaching styles for each patient.

Administrative aspects

Patients who receive contraceptive advice or treatment by a GP or family planning nurse must also have regular reviews. This means that the patient's record must show what method is being used and when the next check is due. Items of service are no longer paid for providing contraceptive services in general practice because they form part of the Additional Services under the 2004 GP Contract. It is essential for staff to be able to refer patients to the appropriate place when a practice does not provide the full range of contraceptive services patients may need. For example, the PCO may have commissioned some practices in a locality to provide IUD fitting for the patients of doctors in practices that do not fit them. The NICE guidance on contraception recommends that patients are given the choice of long-term reversible contraception.

TERMINATION OF PREGNANCY

It is vital that nobody enters a sexual relationship with the attitude that 'if anything goes wrong an abortion can be arranged'. Apart from the undesirability of using termination as a form of contraception, there are health risks that include:

- A higher incidence of pelvic inflammatory disease
- Cervical incompetence in future wanted pregnancies
- The usual operative risks of anaesthesia and of haemorrhage.

The psychological consequences

The decision to refer a woman for a termination will depend on a number of factors that can only be taken into account after careful discussion and counselling. The law requires that a statement be completed by two doctors (preferably the GP and the gynaecologist) who have to state that the patient falls into one of five categories.

- The continuance of the pregnancy would involve risk of injury to the physical or mental health of the pregnant woman greater than if the pregnancy was terminated.
- The continuance of the pregnancy would involve risk of injury to the physical or mental health of the pregnant woman or any existing child(ren) of her family greater than if the pregnancy was terminated.
- The continuation of the pregnancy would involve risk to the life of the pregnant woman greater than if the pregnancy was terminated.
- There is substantial risk that if the child were born it would suffer from such physical and mental abnormalities as to be severely handicapped.
- Termination is necessary to save the life or prevent grave permanent injury to the physical or mental health of the pregnant woman.[16]

The time limit for abortions for the first two reasons given above was reduced to 24 weeks gestation in 1990 as a result of the Human Fertilisation and Embryology Act. A termination may be performed within the NHS or privately. The legislation does not apply to Northern Ireland. Abortion is only available there in very exceptional circumstances.

All patients who have a termination must be encouraged to undertake ways of preventing further unwanted pregnancies. The moral and ethical aspects of termination have not been considered here because each reader will have his or her own opinion on this emotive subject. However, the NMC requires all nurses to promote the interest of their patients and clients. This includes helping them to gain access to health and social care, information and support relevant to their needs. A nurse must report to a relevant person, at the earliest possible time, any conscientious objection that may be relevant to professional practice but continue to provide care until alternative arrangements are implemented.[17]

SEXUALLY TRANSMITTED DISEASES

The risks of acquiring a sexually transmitted disease (STD) should be explained when discussing contraception or sexual health issues. Chlamydia, genital warts, herpes, HIV and hepatitis B can all be transmitted sexually, not just syphilis and gonorrhoea. A patient with symptoms of a sexually transmitted disease might be advised to attend the genitourinary medicine (GUM) clinic, where the facilities exist for prompt diagnosis and treatment, as well as counselling and contact tracing. However, in many areas this work is being undertaken in primary care. It is not uncommon for patients to have more than one sexually transmitted infection at the same time, which makes a full sexual health screen so important. Doctors and nurses must have had the appropriate education and training in order to provide a sexual health service in general practice comparable with that provided by a GUM clinic.

Chlamydia

Chlamydia is a disease caused by the bacterium *Chlamydia trachomatis*, which is primarily transmitted through sexual intercourse. The urethra and rectum may be infected and transmission of genital discharge to the eyes can cause conjunctivitis. The infant of a mother with chlamydia may be born prematurely, have a chlamydial eye infection or develop pneumonia after delivery.

Symptoms

Both men and women can be asymptomatic and thus be unaware of the problem. Pelvic inflammatory disease, leading to infertility, is a serious consequence of chlamydia infection. For this reason, a programme is being developed for screening young sexually active men and women for chlamydia.[18] Plans have been made for a national screening programme but not all areas are covered yet, so local policies should be followed if necessary. Screening will be offered to all patients aged 16–24 by March 2007.

Symptomatic men may experience burning during micturition or discharge from the penis. In the longer term, they may develop epididymitis, Reiter's syndrome (an autoimmune condition affecting the joints and the eyes) or fertility problems. Women could experience burning on micturition, an abnormal vaginal discharge, intermenstrual or postcoital bleeding.

Genital warts

Genital warts, caused by the human papilloma virus (HPV), are usually transmitted sexually and may have a long incubation period from infection to the development of warts. They may be difficult to see or be flat or cauliflower-shaped in appearance. They are not usually painful but can cause intense irritation. They may be found on the shaft of the penis, on or under the foreskin in males or around the vulva or in the vagina in females. Patients of either sex may have warts around the anus and the mouth may be infected through oral sex. Treatment may be by the application of podophyllin, cryocautery, laser or surgical excision. HPV is recognised as a cause of cervical neoplasia. Women with genital warts must be advised to have regular smear tests. Research is ongoing into an effective vaccine against HPV.[19]

Genital herpes

Genital herpes is caused by the herpes simplex virus (HSV). There are two types. HSV-1 usually causes cold sores on the mouth (see Chapter 8), although cold sores can also be transmitted to the genital areas through oral sex. HSV-2, which causes the typical blisters of genital herpes, is primarily transmitted sexually and usually affects the genital areas. HSV-2 can be transmitted to the mouth and throat through oral sex. Patients need to be aware of how the virus is spread so they can:

- Adopt good hygiene practices to avoid spread to other parts of the body
- Practise safer sex and also avoid the risk of infection through oral sex
- Avoid sex when the herpes is present or developing.

Topical or systemic antivirals may be helpful in the very early stage of herpes. The most severe symptoms usually occur with the first outbreak but recurrent attacks can occur when the dormant virus is reactivated in response to stress or other factors. Immunocompromised patients may develop very severe herpes.

Hepatitis B (see Chapter 4)

Patients at risk of contracting hepatitis B through sexual activity should be offered immunisation in addition to information about the disease and the need to practise safe or safer sex.

Human immunodeficiency virus infection (HIV)

HIV infection, like hepatitis B, can be transmitted through blood or body fluids. This may be via an infected needle, contact with mucous membranes or through unprotected sexual intercourse. The majority of people with HIV infection are asymptomatic. The progression of the disease to acquired immune deficiency syndrome (AIDS) varies from person to person. Persistent generalised lymphadenopathy, or generalised symptoms related to immune deficiency, such as severe diarrhoea and weight loss, fatigue, night sweats, candidiasis and herpes, might first point to a diagnosis of HIV infection. Opportunistic diseases that would normally be overcome by the T4 cells can become life threatening. *Pneumocystis carinii* pneumonia (PCP), cytomegalovirus infection, tuberculosis and Kaposi's sarcoma are diagnostic of AIDS in HIV-positive patients. Neurological involvement can lead to loss of motor or sensory function and dementia.

Better drugs and technology are allowing many patients to live for years with HIV infection but they still require support and kindness. Voluntary organisations exist for HIV-positive men, women, children and partners, as well as members of ethnic groups and religions. Practice nurses can assist by treating patients with HIV as any other patients who need help or advice and by educating other people about the disease. The local HIV/AIDS adviser will provide any extra training needed.

The spread of HIV infection is linked to the incidence of other sexually transmitted diseases like syphilis and gonorrhoea. When the number of cases increases, it shows that the message about safe sex is not getting through or is being ignored. Practice nurses may have the opportunity to spread the message when discussing contraception with patients or when giving travel advice. The terms 'safe sex' and 'safer sex' tend to be used interchangeably. However, safe sex is said to relate to activities such as kissing, fondling, massaging and masturbation that do not involve contact with body fluids, while safer sex is the term used to describe vaginal, oral or anal sex protected by an appropriate condom. There are a wide variety of condoms available. Extra strong ones are necessary for anal intercourse.

Suggestions for reflection on practice

- How good is your sexual health service?
- Is your knowledge up to date?
- Do all patient groups access the service?
- Can patients get emergency contraception promptly?
- How do you know what patients have understood from a consultation?
- How do you know if the patients are satisfied with the service?

REFERENCES

1. HM Government (2003) *Female Genital Mutilation Act 2003*. Scottish Parliament (2005) *Female Genital Mutilation (Scotland) Act 2005*. Stationery Office, London.
2. British Medical Association (2004) *Female Genital Mutilation – caring for patients and child protection*. www.bma.org.uk/ap.nsf/Content/FGM (accessed 10/1/06).
3. Faculty of Family Planning and Reproductive Health Care (2005) *Confidentiality of Adolescent Sexual Health Services: joint statement*. www.ffprhc.org.uk/admin/uploads/FinalSignedDJTStatement.pdf (accessed 10/1/06).
4. Department of Health (2004) *Best Practice Guidance for Doctors and Other Health Professionals on the Provision of Advice and Treatment to Young People under 16 on Contraception, Sexual and Reproductive Health*. www.dh.gov.uk (accessed 11/1/06).
5. House of Lords (1985) *Gillick v. West Norfolk and Wisbech Area Health Authority*. HMSO, London.
6. National Screening Committee Policy Position (2005) *National Screening Committee – thrombophilia screening*. www.nelh.nhs.uk/screening (accessed 12/1/06).
7. Prodigy Guidance (2005) *Contraception – emergency*. www.prodigy.nhs.uk/guidance. asp?gt=contraception%20-%20emergency
8. Faculty of Family Planning and Reproductive Health Care Clinical Effectiveness Unit (2003) FFPRHC guidance: emergency contraception. *Journal of Family Planning and Reproductive Health Care*, **29** (2), 9–15.
9. Prodigy Guidance (2005) *Contraception – emergency*. www.prodigy.nhs.uk/guidance. asp?gt=contraception%20-%20emergency
10. Faculty of Family Planning and Reproductive Health Care Clinical Effectiveness Unit (2004) FFPRHC guidance: the copper intrauterine device as long-term contraception. *Journal of Family Planning and Reproductive Health Care*, **30** (1), 43–5.
11. World Health Organisation (2000) *Medical Eligibility Criteria for Contraceptive Use*. World Health Organisation, Geneva.
12. Faculty of Family Planning and Reproductive Health Care Clinical Effectiveness Unit (2004) FFPRHC guidance: the levonorgestrel-releasing intrauterine system (LNG-IUS) in contraception and reproductive health. *Journal of Family Planning and Reproductive Health Care*, **30** (2), 99–109.
13. World Health Organisation (2005) *WHO Statement on Hormonal Contraception and Bone Health*. World Health Organisation, Geneva. www.who.int/reproductive-health/family_planning/docs/hormonal_contraception_none_health.pdf (accessed 12/1/06).
14. Faculty of Family Planning and Reproductive Health Care Clinical Effectiveness Unit (2003) *New Product Review: Norelgestron/ethinyl oestradiol transdermal contraceptive system (Evra)*. www.ffprhc.org.uk/admin/uploads/EVRA%20Final.pdf (accessed 13/1/06).
15. Royal College of Obstetricians and Gynaecologists (2004) *Male and Female Sterilisation*. Evidence Based Clinical Guidelines No. 4. Royal College of Obstetricians and Gynaecologists, London.
16. HM Government (1967) *The Abortion Act 1967*. HMSO, London.
17. Nursing and Midwifery Council (2004) *Code of Professional Conduct*, Para 2. Nursing and Midwifery Council, London.

18. Department of Health (2004) *National Chlamydia Screening Programme(NSCP) in England*, 2nd edn. www.dh.gov.uk Policy and guidance, Sexual health general information (accessed 13/1/06).
19. Stanley, M. (2005) *HPV Vaccines*. www.gateway.nlm.nih.gov (accessed 13/1/06).

FURTHER READING

Andrews, G. (ed.) (2005) *Women's Sexual Health*, 3rd edn. Elsevier, Edinburgh.
British Medical Association and Royal Pharmaceutical Society of Great Britain (2005) *British National Formulary 50*, 7.3. BMA and RPSGB, London.
Guillebaud, J. (2003) *Contraception: your questions answered*, 4th edn. Churchill Livingstone, Edinburgh.
National Institute for Health and Clinical Excellence (2005) *NICE Guidance – long-acting reversible contraception*. www.nice.org.uk/catgd.aspx?o=33918
Royal College of Nursing (2004) *Sexual Health Competencies: an integrated career and competency framework for sexual and reproductive health nursing*. Royal College of Nursing, London.

USEFUL ADDRESSES AND WEBSITES

FPA (formerly the Family Planning Association)
Website: www.fpa.org.uk

National AIDS Helpline (24 hours)
Telephone: 0800 567123

National AIDS Trust
www.nat.org.uk

Chapter 13
Women's Health

Society's expectation that women should care for others, such as partners, children and elderly parents, can mean that in some situations they have little time left to care for themselves. A practice nurse who shows a friendly concern can allow women to put their own interests first, for a while. Regular well-woman checks have been offered since the National Cervical Screening Programme was established. However, this relies on the postal system so travellers, homeless women or those not registered with the NHS may not receive an invitation to attend. Well-woman screening involves factors related to the female reproductive function, in addition to the general health screening outlined in Chapter 9, and should involve much more than cervical cytology. A thorough history is needed to ensure that every patient receives the appropriate care and advice.

MENSTRUATION

Nurses should be aware of the range of normal menstrual cycles for different women in order to recognise any abnormalities of menstruation. There may be considerable variations in cycle length and menstrual flow but an average normal pattern can be considered as:

- The start of menstrual periods (menarche) at age 10–13 years. They may be irregular at first but settle into a regular cycle by about age 16
- A menstrual cycle of approximately 28 days, with bleeding over 4–5 days (the first day of bleeding is calculated as day 1 of the cycle)
- The cessation of menstrual periods (menopause) between about 48 and 54 years. However, some women could have a normal menopause at an earlier or a later age. Premature menopause is the term used when it occurs before the age of 40.

A practice nurse can help a woman with concerns about menstruation by:

- Getting the patient to give a clear outline of the problem
- Checking on the patient's knowledge and understanding of menstruation

- Showing her how to keep a menstrual chart and encouraging her to consult the GP with it, if necessary
- Giving practical advice for dealing with discomfort, and using appropriate sanitary protection
- Referring the patient to the GP for any problem needing medical investigation or treatment.

Young women should be taught why menstruation is a normal event rather than a curse but women who do have problems with menstruation deserve sympathetic understanding.

Dysmenorrhoea

Painful periods cause misery for some women each month. Exercise can often relieve the cramp-like pain of normal periods, and mild analgesics may help. Mefanamic acid or the contraceptive pill may be prescribed for more severe pain. An IUD, pelvic inflammatory disease, endometriosis or fibroids can cause secondary dysmenorrhoea, requiring medical investigation.

Menorrhagia

Heavy, regular menstrual bleeding over several consecutive cycles can be distressing and embarrassing to the patient and lead to iron deficiency anaemia. The extent of the problem needs to be assessed and abnormal pathology ruled out. Patients can be asked to record the number of pads or tampons used, the frequency of change and any clots passed. Heavy, irregular bleeding may develop in the perimenopausal years but postcoital or intermenstrual bleeding could be indicative of more serious problems. A haemoglobin estimation is needed to check for anaemia but a patient with menorrhagia should be examined by a GP. A levonorgestrel-releasing intrauterine system might be inserted to control menorrhagia as an alternative to hysterectomy.[1]

Amenorrhoea

Primary amenorrhoea – delay in the onset of periods – may be the result of:

- A congenital physiological factor, such as the absence of a uterus or vagina
- An endocrine disturbance
- An eating disorder.

Secondary amenorrhoea – the absence of menstruation for six months in a woman who has previously had periods – is most commonly caused by pregnancy, a cause which should always be considered and tested for if pregnancy is feasible. Breastfeeding may delay the return of menstruation after pregnancy.

Secondary amenorrhoea can result from hormone contraceptive use and patients should be made aware of this when it is prescribed. Other factors include:

- Anxiety
- Moving to a new environment
- Examination stress
- Strenuous exercise
- An eating disorder
- Endocrine problems.

Premenstrual syndrome (PMS)

Most women experience some physiological changes during the latter half of the menstrual cycle (luteal phase). Breast tenderness or mood changes are a response to the changing hormone levels. More extreme physical or psychological symptoms are termed premenstrual syndrome. The cause is not fully understood and therapy is therefore focused more on the management of symptoms than on the underlying cause.[2] Practice nurses can help patients to talk about their problems and encourage them to keep a diary of their symptoms in relation to the menstrual cycle.

The symptoms may be eased by a healthy diet and aerobic exercise. Coffee should be restricted because the caffeine may increase irritability. A low salt intake might reduce fluid retention and diuretics can be prescribed by the GP if necessary. Pyridoxine (vitamin B6), in a dose not exceeding 100 mg daily, might be beneficial.[3] The contraceptive pill may also help some patients but there is no proof of the efficacy of evening primrose oil.[4] The capsules are no longer available on prescription but can still be purchased in some health food shops.

CERVICAL CYTOLOGY (SEE ALSO CHAPTER 6 UNDER DIAGNOSTIC TESTS AND INVESTIGATIONS)

Cervical smears are taken to detect any premalignant changes in the cells of the cervix; cervical intraepithelial neoplasia (CIN), which might develop into invasive cancer if not treated. The cytology report will indicate the severity of any changes and suggest when the test should be repeated or if the patient should be referred for colposcopy. The reduction of death from cancer is one of the targets in *Saving Lives: our healthier nation*.[5]

Targets

GPs are paid for meeting a target of 70%, or a lower target of 50%, for cervical screening for women aged from 25 to 64 years. As with many screening activities, those most at risk can be the least likely to attend. Opportunistic screening is needed in addition to an effective call and recall system. A good administration system will help to maintain the practice income, but the prime concern should be the welfare of women. Younger women are not included in the smear targets. However, there may be local variations in the policy on screening patients who are under 25 and women in the target group who have never been sexually active. The risks may be lower for the latter group of patients but they do still face some risk. In addition, lesbian women may contract the human papilloma virus and thus develop cervical neoplasia.[6]

Practice nurses can help to reduce the anxiety associated with cervical screening, but any nurse involved must have had the necessary theoretical and practical experience and be accountable for her practice. The degree of nurse involvement will depend on the level of knowledge and expertise. Nurses who take cervical smears must have been taught correctly and have been assessed as competent by a qualified cytology trainer. Routine bimanual pelvic examination as a screening test for ovarian cancer in asymptomatic women is not recommended.[7] Bimanual pelvic examination should only be carried out for symptomatic women by nurses with advanced qualifications, such as nurse practitioners or advanced family planning nurse specialists.

Nurses may be involved at any of three levels.

- *Level 1*
  - Administration – checking when smears are due and reminding patients to make an appointment when they are seen for other purposes.
  - Educating patients about cervical screening and providing appropriate literature for them to read.
- *Level 2* as for level 1 and in addition:
  - Taking an appropriate history and completing the smear form with all the relevant personal details, and comprehensive information about previous smears.
  - Taking a satisfactory cervical smear.
  - Recognising any abnormality of the genital tract and referring to a GP if necessary.
  - Making sure the patient knows how to get the result of the test and that a contact address is known.
  - Interpreting an abnormal smear result for a patient.
- *Level 3* as for levels 1 and 2 and in addition:
  - Performing a bimanual pelvic examination to detect any tenderness or palpable masses in the pelvic organs, if appropriate.

Laboratories vary in the terminology used to describe cervical cell changes. Nurses should ask for clarification from their local department of cytology. Smears may be described as:

- *Inadequate, due to insufficient cells* – the number of inadequate smears is likely to be reduced by the use of liquid-based cytology
- *Negative* – no abnormality detected

- *Negative with an incidental finding* – commonly candida or another type of organism
- *Transformation cells not seen* – the sample may not have contained cells from the squamocolumnar junction (the transformation zone), where premalignant changes most commonly occur
- *Inflammatory* – cell changes due to infection or irritation of the cervix
- *Borderline dyskaryosis* – some atypical cells seen
- *Mild dyskaryosis or CIN 1* – changes in the nuclei of some cells
- *Moderate dyskaryosis or CIN 2* – more marked changes in the nuclei
- *Severe dyskaryosis or CIN 3* – a larger number of cells with grossly abnormal nuclei
- *Malignant cells present* – suggestive of invasive cancer.

Patients with borderline squamous cell changes or mild dyskaryosis will usually be recalled for repeat smears after six months. After one borderline endocervical cells result, three inadequate smears, three borderline squamous cells results or if CIN 2 or 3 is found, the patient will be referred to a gynaecology clinic for colposcopy.[8] A Department of Health leaflet supplied by the local health promotion department explains to patients the procedure of colposcopy and the treatment of abnormal cells.

Colposcopy entails examining the cervix with a special microscope attached to a vaginal speculum. The cervix is stained with iodine or acetic acid to delineate any areas of abnormality and a biopsy can be taken. Abnormal cells can be destroyed by laser cautery or cryosurgery. Sometimes a cone biopsy may be performed under general anaesthetic to remove abnormal cells that extend into the cervical canal. Patients who have had treatment for CIN must have regular smear tests and follow-up.

BREAST AWARENESS

Breast cancer is the largest single cause of death of women in the UK. The government's Cancer Plan includes the target to reduce deaths from breast cancer.[9] Patients with several close female relatives who have had the disease may be referred to a breast unit for regular screening.

Since a CNO letter in 1998 advised against the routine examination of patients' breasts, practice nurses have been encouraged to concentrate on teaching breast awareness to their patients. Obsessive self-examination should not be encouraged; a relaxed attitude to the process is needed. There is little evidence that self-examination affects the mortality figures for breast cancer but that is not to say that it is ineffective at an individual level. Patients should learn what is normal for them so that they can seek early medical advice if anything seems amiss.[10] The principles include:

- Looking at the breasts to detect anything unusual (change in the outline, dimpling of the skin, retraction or change in a nipple). A patient should do this in front of a mirror with her arms at her side, then raised above the head, and finally with her hands pressed onto the hips, to accentuate the breast contours

- Feeling the breast tissue. The patient may do this in the bath or shower. Alternatively, she should lie flat with her head on a pillow and a towel or small pillow under the shoulder to centralise the nipple of the side to be examined. Using the flat of the fingers together and working systematically around all the breast tissue and into the axilla, the breast tissue should be compressed firmly but gently against the chest wall. The nipple should be squeezed gently to see if any blood or discharge is expressed
- Consulting a doctor without delay if anything abnormal is found. The patient must be seen within two weeks if cancer is suspected, although it should be emphasised that many breast lumps are benign.

NHS Breast Screening Service

Women aged 50–70 are offered mammography every three years. Women over 70 will not receive routine recall letters but may request to continue to have mammography screening. The screening programme has been in operation since 1990 and a significant number of early cancers have been detected. Nurses can encourage their patients to attend and reassure them that the procedure only takes a few moments. It entails stripping to the waist and standing next to an X-ray machine while the breast is compressed between two special plates. This can be rather uncomfortable but only lasts for a few seconds while the X-ray is taken. If further tests are needed the patient will be invited to see the specialist at her local breast unit. Explanatory leaflets are available from regional breast screening centres, local health promotion departments and the NHS Cancer Screening website.

Women under 50 years are not currently eligible for the programme. Women of any age who have symptoms should consult their GP because the national screening programme is only intended for asymptomatic women. Although breast screening may ultimately save lives, the unexpected diagnosis of cancer can be devastating. Such patients require skilled counselling and support.

PRECONCEPTUAL CARE

Patients may ask for advice about the best ways to prepare for pregnancy. Such advice for both partners should cover lifestyle factors and the avoidance of known hazards. Healthy living means not smoking tobacco, sensible alcohol intake, having regular exercise and adequate sleep, and eating a well-balanced diet (see Chapter 9). Folic acid is important because a deficiency is thought to contribute to neural tube defects.[11] Foods rich in folic acid include dark leafy vegetables, oranges, beans, fortified bread and breakfast cereals, beef and yeast extracts. However, increased dietary folate alone may not prevent neural tube defects. Women are advised to take 0.4 mg folic acid daily while trying to conceive and during the first trimester of pregnancy. Patients on medication for epilepsy should consult their doctor before starting folic acid because it can affect the blood levels of some antiepileptic drugs.

Blood should be taken to test for rubella antibodies if a woman's immunity has not been confirmed. If a patient needs to be immunised against rubella with MMR vaccine, she must be warned to avoid becoming pregnant for a minimum of one month after immunisation. A smear test should be offered if due. Any occupational hazards to pregnant women should be identified and a transfer may have to be considered at work. Radiation and anaesthetic gases, for example, are known to be hazardous. Any medicines a patient takes should be checked to ensure they would not harm the fetus. Some changes to medication may be necessary, so the patient should see her GP or hospital specialist. Patients who are planning to travel abroad should be made aware of any health risks, especially from malaria (see Chapter 11).

It may be necessary to check the patient's understanding of the menstrual cycle and when ovulation is most likely to occur. The natural methods of contraception (see Chapter 12) can also help patients who want to conceive to recognise their fertile time. Ovulation kits can also be purchased, which detect the LH surge prior to ovulation and thus help women to discover their fertile period. Patients with any family or personal history of a hereditary condition may need to be referred for genetic counselling.

INFERTILITY

Patients who are unable to have children may consult their GP for help. Initial investigations will probably include an assessment of lifestyle factors that could affect fertility and a physical examination of both partners as well as a semen analysis and blood test to detect ovulation. A progesterone level should be done at day 21 of the cycle or seven days before the period is due if the patient has a longer cycle. The patients are likely to be referred to an assisted conception specialist according to the local protocol. Patients who embark on the stressful process of investigation and treatment of infertility will require patience and commitment. A sense of humour also helps. Specialist infertility centres must ensure that patients are adequately counselled before consenting to treatment.[12] Practice nurses can also help by listening to patients' concerns, being sympathetic to their needs and making sure they have received all the information they require.

In vitro fertilisation (IVF) and embryo transfer

IVF was first done successfully in 1978 and has hardly been out of the news since then. Multiple births have been the most significant complication but concern is also growing about the possible increase in birth defects.[13]

Drugs are used to stimulate several ova to ripen at once. This is carefully monitored by blood tests and ultrasound and at the appropriate time, the mature eggs are collected via a laparoscope and placed in a culture medium. Specially prepared sperm collected from the partner's semen are added to the ova in the containers. Once fertilisation has occurred, the selected embryos are introduced through the cervix into the patient's uterus. Only two embryos may be introduced to women under 40 years, in order to reduce the problems of multiple births. Women over 40 may have three of their own embryos transferred.[14] Progesterone injections or pessaries may be given to assist the implantation. Extra embryos may be deep frozen for future use in case the pregnancy does not become established. Intracytoplasmic sperm injection (ICSI) is a method developed to help couples where a man has a low sperm count, in preference to sperm donation. Ova are matured and harvested from the woman as for IVF and sperm are aspirated from the epididymis from the partner. A single sperm is injected into each egg and after two days, the embryos can be inserted into the woman.

PREGNANCY

A practice nurse may be the first person to confirm a pregnancy after performing the pregnancy test. First-time parents will welcome some information about what to expect. The pregnancy is counted from the first day of the last menstrual period, so the expected date of delivery can be calculated as 40 weeks from then. Special calculator discs are available for this purpose. Smoking and a high alcohol intake in pregnancy are known to be harmful so the opportunity should be taken to advise on their avoidance. Help may be offered to quit smoking. Food poisoning during pregnancy can be harmful to the fetus so unpasteurised soft cheeses, paté and undercooked meat should be avoided because of the risk of listeria infection. Raw or undercooked eggs and raw shellfish can also be a source of infection. A high intake of vitamin A can be dangerous, so pregnant women should be advised not to eat liver or take vitamin A supplements, including fish liver oils, without medical advice.[15]

Maternity care

The arrangements for maternity care can differ from area to area, so it is useful for a practice nurse to familiarise herself with the arrangements locally. Shared care between the GP, the community midwife and the obstetrician is often popular. Some GPs may provide medical cover for home confinements. Patients with uncomplicated pregnancies should be managed by their GP or midwife and only those who may need additional care should be managed by an obstetrician.[16]

Antenatal care

A patient will attend the first antenatal clinic when she is approximately 11 weeks pregnant. The midwife obtains a full medical and obstetric history, which is summarised in the obstetric record. The patient will be given her own record to take to clinic appointments and to the hospital during the rest of the pregnancy. The height, weight and blood pressure are recorded, and the urine is tested for albumin. A urine sample may be sent for microscopy and culture to detect asymptomatic bacteriuria. Routine screening for diabetes mellitus is no longer recommended. Blood tests are taken for full blood count, blood group and rhesus status, rubella antibodies, hepatitis B, HIV and syphilis. The GP or midwife may perform a physical examination. The appropriate booking is made for home, GP unit or hospital confinement, and the patient is given a certificate of eligibility for free dental care and prescriptions.

A patient with an uncomplicated pregnancy will return for further antenatal checks as deemed necessary. Nulliparous women will usually have ten antenatal visits and women who have had previous uncomplicated pregnancies will be seen seven times. There may be local variations in the clinic intervals and investigations performed, but the following is a guide to the tests offered.

- 12–14 weeks: ultrasound scan to confirm due date and to check for multiple pregnancies and nuchal translucency screening for Down's syndrome (if the patient gives informed consent to be screened).
- 18–20 weeks: routine ultrasound scan to confirm normal growth and development of the fetus. Another scan at 36 weeks will be offered to women with placenta praevia extending over the cervical os.
- 28 weeks: FBC, blood group and antibodies. Rhesus-negative women will be offered anti-D immunoglobulin.
- 34 weeks: FBC, blood group and antibodies, if a rhesus-negative mother. A second dose of anti-D may be given.

After 20 weeks pregnancy, a certificate (MatB1) is issued, which entitles a woman to maternity benefits. Fathers may need to supply a copy of this form when applying for paternity leave from work. Since 2003, fathers have been entitled to two weeks paid paternity leave and up to 13 weeks unpaid leave.[17]

Most patients have antenatal checks fortnightly until their expected date of delivery. Women who have not given birth by 41 weeks may have their labour induced.

Postnatal care

The patient attends for a full postnatal examination about six weeks after confinement. The haemoglobin may be checked and MMR immunisation given, if not immune to rubella and not immunised before leaving hospital. If a cervical smear is due, it should be postponed until at least 12 weeks post partum. Contraception should be discussed at the postnatal check and appropriate arrangements made. Oral contraception can be started right away, but the progestogen-only pill must be used while the patient is breastfeeding. An IUD or diaphragm can be fitted, if preferred.

Lax pelvic floor muscles contribute to urinary incontinence and uterine prolapse. The patient should be encouraged to continue postnatal exercises to regain muscle tone and to practise pelvic floor exercises every day. Patients need to learn how to contract the pelvic floor muscles by squeezing and drawing in the muscles around the anus and vagina without tightening the buttock or abdominal muscles. The patient should aim to do this ten times slowly to strengthen the pelvic floor muscles and ten times quickly to help the muscles react to stresses such as coughing that put pressure on the bladder. The exercises should be performed up to six times a day, even when performing household chores. Information can be found on the Continence Foundation website.[18] It is a good idea for all women to learn to practise pelvic floor exercises to prevent stress incontinence, not only women after childbirth.

Practice nurses usually have a peripheral role in ante- and postnatal care but such contacts offer the chance to establish a good relationship so the parent will be less anxious about bringing the baby for immunisation.

Miscarriage and stillbirth

The loss of a pregnancy up to 24 weeks gestation is termed a miscarriage. After that time, the term stillbirth is used. A live birth between weeks 24 and 37 is termed a premature or preterm birth.

There can be many mishaps between conception and the delivery of a healthy infant. An anxious patient could telephone the surgery for advice. Bleeding in the early months of pregnancy might settle down but patients need support while they wait to see what happens. Although rest probably will not affect the outcome, it can help a woman to feel she did everything possible if the pregnancy is lost. The doctor will usually arrange an urgent ultrasound scan but admission to hospital will be needed if the bleeding is severe. It may be necessary to perform a dilatation and curettage to remove retained products of conception. The Miscarriage Association is one of several groups that provide information and support for parents who have suffered a miscarriage, including an ectopic or molar pregnancy and recurrent miscarriages.

The Stillbirth and Neonatal Death Society (SANDS) provides information and support for bereaved parents as well as information on the topic for professionals. The parents need the chance to grieve when a stillbirth or a neonatal death occurs. The importance of acknowledging the loss is now recognised and parents are encouraged to collect mementos of the infant and to arrange a funeral ceremony.[19]

HYSTERECTOMY

The reaction of a woman after hysterectomy may range from relief at the end of miserable symptoms or the fear of pregnancy, to severe depression and grief at the supposed loss of her femininity. Physical problems, such as pain, wound infection and urinary incontinence, are not uncommon and can cause distress. A patient who has had a hysterectomy because of a malignancy will continue to need vaginal vault smears. Those who have a subtotal hysterectomy retain the cervix and thus need to continue routine smear tests. Opinions differ about the value of preserving the ovaries when performing a hysterectomy.[20] However, premenopausal women whose ovaries are removed may experience a sudden menopause. Oestrogen replacement therapy may be offered after careful assessment of all the risks. Extra care must be taken if giving unopposed oestrogen to women with a history of endometriosis because proliferation can occur outside the womb, even after hysterectomy. Women who have a menopause before the age of 45, whether natural or as a result of oophorectomy, have a high risk of developing osteoporosis.

THE MENOPAUSE

The menopause marks the end of fertility for women as the ovaries cease to function. The decrease in oestrogen production causes physical and emotional changes; the type and severity of symptoms can vary from one woman to another. Common symptoms include hot flushes and night sweats although the causes are not well established. The temperature-regulating centre in the hypothalamus is believed to be stimulated by the increased production of gonadotrophic hormones in the adjacent region of the brain, in response to the reduced oestrogen in the circulation. Vaginal dryness and atrophy as well as urgency and urinary leakage are also caused by the reduction of oestrogen. Palpitations, depression, irritability and lack of concentration are other common complaints, but caution should prevail before attributing every problem to the menopause. An unsatisfactory relationship with a partner, children leaving home, business worries or unfulfilled ambitions can also lead to depression or sexual difficulties in middle age. A thorough history and medical examination are needed for each patient.

Among the conditions that can occur after the menopause are an increased risk of coronary heart disease and osteoporosis. Practice nurses are able to help women at the menopause by:

- Listening to their concerns
- Providing factual information about the menopause and the treatments available for symptoms
- Assessing their general health and risk factors for heart disease and osteoporosis

- Referring them to the GP for medical assessment and treatment
- Monitoring the effects of any treatment.

Management of menopausal symptoms

Practice nurses should be aware of the treatments available and encourage patients to consult their doctor when necessary. The available local treatments to relieve vaginal dryness and dyspareunia caused by vaginal atrophy include:

- Vaginal lubricants (*KY Jelly*)
- Vaginal rehydrating gel (*Feminesse, Replens*)
- Topical oestrogen as estriol pessaries or cream (*Ortho-Gynest, Ovestrin*), estradiol vaginal tablets (*Vagifem*) or estradiol vaginal ring (*Estring*).

Topical oestrogen is not suitable to be used alone for more than a few weeks by women who still have a uterus because it may cause a proliferation of the endometrium. The treatment may be repeated after some weeks or months if necessary.

Systemic treatment for the relief of symptoms includes:

- Hormone replacement therapy – tablets, patches, gels or implants
- Synthetic steroids (tibolone).

Hormone replacement therapy (HRT)

Practice nurses who advise patients about the menopause need to be familiar with the arguments for and against HRT. The popularity of HRT has declined in recent years since research showed an increased risk of breast cancer and other adverse affects such as stroke, coronary heart disease and venous thromboembolism. The Committee on the Safety of Medicines recommends that if HRT is prescribed, its use is reappraised at least once a year. HRT can relieve many of the distressing symptoms of the menopause and the benefits may outweigh the risks for short-term use. Unopposed oestrogen is appropriate for women without a uterus. Oestrogen and progestogen, either sequential or combined, have traditionally been given to patients with an intact uterus because unopposed proliferation of the endometrium could lead to endometrial cancer. However, difficult decisions have to be made by patients and their doctors, since this type of HRT was shown to pose an even greater risk of breast cancer than oestrogen alone. All HRT, including tibolone, showed an increased risk within 1–2 years of starting treatment.[21]

Absolute contraindications to HRT are:

- Undiagnosed vaginal bleeding
- Pregnancy or lactation

- Cancer of the breast, of the endometrium or other oestrogen-dependent tumours
- Current or previous deep vein thrombosis or other thromboembolic disorder
- Severe renal or liver disease
- Dubin-Johnson or Rotor syndromes (congenital diseases affecting the transport of bilirubin from the liver)
- Acute intermittent porphyria.

Relative contraindications, which must be considered carefully by the prescriber, include:

- Family history of thromboembolic disease
- Otosclerosis
- Malignant melanoma
- Systemic lupus erythematosus
- Obesity
- Hypertension
- Mild chronic liver disease or renal impairment
- Diabetes, asthma, epilepsy, migraine or multiple sclerosis
- Prolonged immobility, trauma or surgery
- Sickle cell disease
- Endometriosis.

All patients over 50 on HRT should be encouraged to attend for routine mammography and should have been taught breast awareness. HRT does not act as a contraceptive and perimenopausal women need to be aware that they could still be fertile. A barrier method or alternative form of contraception may be needed. HRT injections are not available in the UK but sometimes patients may bring them from other countries and ask the nurse to administer them. In such cases, authorisation for administration must be obtained in writing from the GP and the patient must have been counselled about the risks.

Tibolone is a synthetic steroid used to control menopausal symptoms and as a second-line drug for the prevention of osteoporosis. It can also be helpful for patients with decreased libido but carries similar risks to HRT and so long-term use is not recommended.

OSTEOPOROSIS

Lack of oestrogen affects the density of bone with the consequent risk of fractures of the hip, wrist and spine in later life. The prevention of falls and subsequent fractures is one of the standards in the National Service Framework for Older People. Particular risk factors include an early menopause or a history of infrequent periods but up to one in three women may develop osteoporosis in their lifetime. Yet this is not exclusively a female problem because one in 12 men may also develop the condition.[22] Osteoporosis in men may be linked to low testosterone levels. Other factors known to contribute to osteoporosis include:

- Heavy smoking
- Long-term corticosteroid use
- High alcohol intake
- Physical inactivity
- Malnutrition
- Family history of osteoporosis.

The main problem arises from the loss of the protein matrix of the bone, although a reasonable calcium intake also helps to preserve the bone mass. Patients should understand the importance of a healthy lifestyle. Regular weight-bearing exercise, e.g. walking or dancing, and exposure to sunlight for vitamin D synthesis can help to delay osteoporosis. Some hospitals undertake bone densitometry to identify patients at risk of developing osteoporosis. There are mixed views about the value of HRT for preventing osteoporosis in women over 50 at high risk. The drugs used for the treatment of osteoporosis may not be suitable for long-term use to prevent fractures at a later age.[23] The National Osteoporosis Society campaigns to raise awareness of the condition, funds research and provides advice and support for the public and professionals.

Treatment for osteoporosis includes:

- Analgesia for pain
- Physiotherapy to achieve maximum mobility and prevent falls; weight-bearing exercise can help to maintain bone density
- Hip protectors if at risk from falls and hip fracture
- Calcium and vitamin D supplementation, if dietary intake is insufficient
- Biphosphonate drugs (alendronate, etidronate and risedronate) which inhibit bone resorption and increase bone mass
- Calcitonin to regulate bone turnover
- Selective oestrogen receptor modulator (SERM) (Raloxifene).

Fractures due to osteoporosis cost the NHS millions of pounds every year as well as causing pain and suffering to countless people. Practice nurses are well placed to educate patients about the risks and to encourage them to adopt preventive measures or seek help if needed.

BLADDER PROBLEMS

Women of all ages may experience problems with the urinary bladder. The start of sexual activity or the atrophic changes after the menopause can both contribute to cystitis (see Chapter 8).

Incontinence of urine

The control of bladder function depends on:

- Intact neurological pathways
- Competent pelvic muscles
- The ability to get to the toilet in time.

Childbirth, obesity, lack of exercise and pelvic surgery can all weaken the muscles of the pelvic floor. Chronic constipation can create pressure on the bladder and diuretics pose a particular problem for elderly people when their mobility is restricted. An assessment of the patient should include an MSU to exclude an infection, testing for diabetes and a full history, to identify the factors contributing to incontinence. Urodynamic studies may be arranged for patients with severe problems.

Management of urinary incontinence

The GP or practice nurse can make referrals as appropriate to the district nurse, physiotherapist, occupational therapist or local continence adviser. Prime consideration should be given to helping incontinent patients to preserve their dignity. Adaptation of the patient's clothing or the home may make access to the toilet easier for people with reduced mobility or urgency. Patients with dementia may need to be taken to the toilet and encouraged to pass urine at regular intervals. Impacted faeces can cause retention of urine with overflow. Treatment of the underlying problem may relieve the urinary symptoms.

Stress incontinence

This occurs when the abdominal pressure is raised, as in coughing, sneezing or laughing, and the urethral sphincter muscles are unable to prevent the leakage of urine. The degree of urine loss can vary. Treatments include regaining a normal weight and regular pelvic floor exercises. The exercises involve tightening the muscles around the anus, as if trying to avoid passing wind, and around the urethra, as if trying to stop the stream of urine. Instruction leaflets can be obtained from the health promotion department or from the Continence Foundation. The physiotherapist may be asked to ensure that the patient understands how to perform pelvic floor exercises or to improve pelvic muscle tone by electrical stimulation. Patients can obtain special cone-shaped weights to insert into the vagina; muscle tone is improved through the effort needed to keep the cone in situ. Cones of a heavier weight can be used as the muscle tone increases. Surgery may be needed to treat severe stress incontinence.

Urge incontinence

This occurs when the patient feels an overwhelming need to pass urine before the bladder is full and is unable to get to the toilet in time. The bladder muscle starts to contract too soon (detrusor instability). Treatments include:

- Topical oestrogen replacement therapy which may help with atrophic changes in older women.
- The replacement of drinks containing caffeine such as tea, coffee and cola with plain water to reduce bladder irritability.
- Bladder training programmes, which involve learning to ignore the urge to pass urine for longer and longer periods of time until control of bladder function is regained.
- Oxybutynin or tolterodine tartrate, which may be prescribed to control unstable detrusor contractions.

Some patients may have a combination of stress and urge incontinence. Patients with neurological disorders can also have problems with bladder function and some patients may be taught to empty their bladders by intermittent self-catheterisation. A specialist continence adviser or a district nurse usually does such teaching. Indwelling catheters are avoided as much as possible in the management of bladder problems because of the risk of infection but they are still used at times in the community.

Primary care organisations will have their own procedures for the assessment and supply of incontinence products for patients who need them. The Department of Health issued guidelines in the year 2000 on the provision of continence care.[24] Urinary incontinence can pose specific problems for women from some minority ethnic groups. The ability to perform ritual cleansing before prayers has been shown to be seriously affected by incontinence, with detrimental effects on the self-esteem and marital relationships of some Muslim women.[25] The Continence Foundation produces leaflets in many minority ethnic languages. Patients who have any communication difficulties, either through language or speech problems, may need help to express their concerns and to receive the service they need.

INFORMATION FOR PATIENTS

Leaflets and fact sheets are available on a wide range of topics, but patients may be too embarrassed to pick some of them up in a public waiting area. Careful attention should be given to siting potentially embarrassing information about continence services, family planning or genitourinary medicine clinics in appropriate places. People with access to the internet may prefer to get information that way.

Suggestions for reflection on practice

Consider your service for women in your practice.

- Are any improvements needed to the facilities, equipment or information material?
- Do you need to increase or update any of your knowledge or skills in order to provide a comprehensive service?
- How do you know whether patients are satisfied with the service provided?

REFERENCES

1. Prodigy Guidance (2005) Menorrhagia. www.ProdigyGuidance.nhs.uk/guidance.asp?gt=Menorrhagia (accessed 14/1/06).
2. Owen, P. (2005) Premenstrual syndrome (PMS or PMT). www.netdoctor.co.uk/diseases/facts/pms.htm (accessed 14/1/06).
3. British Medical Association and Royal Pharmaceutical Society of Great Britain (2005) Vitamin B Group. *British National Formulary 50*, 9.6.2. BMA and RPSGB, London.
4. Wyatt, K. (2002) *Premenstrual Syndrome Interventions: clinical evidence.* www.clinicalevidence.com.
5. Department of Health (1999) *Saving Lives: our healthier nation.* Department of Health, London.
6. Marrazzo, J.M., Koutsky, L.A., Kiviat, N.B., Kuypers, J.M. & Stine, K. (2001) Papanicolaou test screening and prevalence of genital human papillomavirus among women who have sex with women. *American Journal of Public Health*, **91** (6), 947–52.
7. National Library for Health Primary Care Answering Service (28/1/05) Is there any guideline regarding whether pelvic examination should be done simultaneously when women have their routine cervical smear? www.clinicalanswers.nhs.uk/index.cfm?question=177.
8. NHS Cancer Screening Programmes (2004) *Colposcopy and Programme Management: guidelines for the NHD Cervical Screening Programme.* www.cancerscreening.org.uk/cervical/publications/nhscsp20.html.
9. Department of Health (2000) *The NHS Cancer Plan: a plan for investment, a plan for reform.* www.dh.gov.uk Publications policy and guidance (accessed 15/1/06).
10. NHS Cancer Screening Programme (2004) *Breast Awareness.* www.cancerscreening.nhs.uk/breastscreen/breastawareness.html (accessed 15/1/06).
11. Hasan, B. & Bhutta, Z.A. (2005) Periconceptional folate supplementation to prevent neural tube defects: RHL commentary. WHO RHL Library, No 8. www.rhlibrary.com/commentaries/htm/Bhcom.htm (accessed 15/1/06).
12. Royal College of Obstetrics and Gynaecology Clinical Effectiveness Support Unit (2000) *Management of Infertility in Tertiary Care: counselling and support.* NeLH Guidelines. www.nelh.nhs.uk/guidelinesdb/html/fulltext-guidelines/InfertilityInTertiaryCare.html (accessed 16/1/06).
13. Van Hoorhis, B.J. (2006) Outcomes from assisted reproductive technology. *Journal of Obstetrics and Gynaecology*, **107** (1), 183–200.

14. Human Fertility and Embryology Authority (2003) *Code of Practice*, 6th edn. pp 8.18–8.22. www.hfea.gov.uk/HFEAPublications/CodeofPractice (accessed 16/1/08).
15. British Medical Association and the Royal Pharmaceutical Society of Great Britain (2005) *British National Formulary 50*, 9.6.1. BMA and RPSGB, London.
16. National Collaborating Centre for Women's and Children's Health (2003) *Antenatal Care: routine care for the healthy pregnant woman*. RCOG Press, London.
17. Department of Trade and Industry (2005) *Paternity – leave and pay*. www.dti.gov.uk/er/individual/paternity-pl514.htm (accessed 16/1/0).
18. Continence Foundation (2001) *Pelvic Floor Exercises for Women*. www.continence-foundation.org.uk/docs/pelvwom.htm (accessed 16/1/06).
19. Kohner, N. (2002) *Pregnancy Loss and the Death of a Baby: guidelines for professionals*. www.uk-sands.org/.
20. Reich, H. (2001) Issues surrounding surgical menopause. Indications and procedures. *Journal of Reproductive Medicine*, **46** (3 suppl), 297–306.
21. Committee on Safety of Medicines (2003) Hormone replacement therapy (HRT) and breast cancer – results of the UK Million Women Study. www.mhra.gov.uk/home CSM (accessed 17/1/06).
22. National Osteoporosis Society (2004) *Men Ignoring Increased Risk of Osteoporosis*. www.nos.org.uk/newsshow.asp?ID=19 (accessed 19/1/06).
23. Stevenson, J. & Rees, M. (2003) *Further Confusion in Postmenopausal Health*. Women's Health Concern and the British Menopause Society. www.the-bms.org/furconf.html (accessed 19/1/06).
24. Department of Health (2000) *Good Practice in Continence Services*. Department of Health, London.
25. Wilkinson, K. (2001) Pakistani women's perceptions and experience of incontinence. *Nursing Standard*, **16** (5), 33–9.

FURTHER READING

Andrews, G. (ed.) (2005) *Women's Sexual Health*. Elsevier, Edinburgh.
Bankhead, C., Austoker, J. & Davey, C. (2003) *Cervical Smear Results Explained: a guide for primary care*. NHS Cancer Screening Programme and Cancer Research UK, London.
Royal College of Nursing (2002) *Improving Continence Care for Patients: the role of the nurse*. Royal College of Nursing, London.

USEFUL ADDRESSES AND WEBSITES

Cancer BACUP – cancer information service
Website: www.cancerbacup.org.uk

Infertility Network
Website: www.infertilitynetworkuk.com

Stillbirth and Neonatal Death Society, 28 Portland Place, London W1N 4DE
Telephone: 020 7436 7940
Helpline: 020 7436 5881
Website: www.uk-sands.org/

British Menopause Society
Website: www.the-bms.org

National Osteoporosis Society
Website: www.nos.org.uk

Continence Foundation
Website: www.continence-foundation.org.uk/

Chapter 14
Men's Health

The specific health needs of women have been recognised for many years and well-woman clinics and screening programmes have been developed. Men's health has generally received less attention, although there are several valid reasons for targeting men's health issues.

MORBIDITY AND MORTALITY

While the life expectancy for both men and women continues to rise and the gap between the sexes in the older age groups is narrowing, the life expectancy of men is still lower than that for women.[1] Moreover, there are still class differences in health. By 2001 in England and Wales, life expectancy at birth for men in professional work was 79.4 years, while it was only 71 years for unskilled men.[2]

Mortality rates vary with age and gender but more males than females died in England and Wales in every age group in 2002. The following were the most common causes of death.

- Age 15–29 – injury and poisoning (41:100 000 men and 10:100 000 women)
- Age 30–44 – the highest causes of death differed between the sexes in this age group: injury and poisoning (45:100 000 men), cancers (32:100 000 women)
- Age 45–64 – cancers (245:100 000 men and 218:100 000 women)
- Age 65–84 – circulatory diseases (1861:100 000 men and 1269:100 000 women)
- Age 85 and over – circulatory diseases (7982:100 000 men and 7016:100 000 women). Figures for respiratory diseases and cancers were also high in both sexes.[3]

Most of the above conditions are included in the targets for reducing mortality in *Saving Lives: our healthier nation*.[4]

Suicide

The incidence of depression is usually described as being higher in women but depression in men may not be so recognisable. Women are more likely to seek help from primary care. However, men with depression may resort to other means; some may mask their distress by violent behaviour or alcohol abuse. The traditional idea of masculinity requires men to be strong, so that accepting help can make them feel unmanly. Boys learn at an early age not to cry or show emotion.

Suicide is much more common in men than women. In 2003, three-quarters of all suicides were by men although the total number of suicides was the lowest for nearly 30 years.[5] Various factors are thought to contribute to the incidence of suicide in men.

- Teenage problems – bullying, sexuality or body image. Problems may be exacerbated by substance abuse.
- Unemployment – affecting sense of self-worth.
- Mental illness – particularly schizophrenia.
- Previous self-harm – increases risk of successful suicide.
- Prisoners (especially those on remand) – criminal activity may also be linked to underachievement at school, lack of parenting and suitable role models, drug or alcohol abuse or violence.
- Farmers – especially during crises in the rural economy.
- Occupational groups (doctors, dentists, veterinary surgeons, pharmacists) – may reflect greater knowledge and access to drugs for suicide.
- Older men – possibly due to social isolation, loss of a partner or hopelessness.

The assessment of the risk for suicide is fraught with difficulty but practice nurses who are alert to the possibility and who are able to establish a rapport with patients may be able to identify some warning signs when talking to them. Has the patient:

- Recently felt depressed?
- Been uncharacteristically religious?
- Made a will or been unusually extravagant?
- Talked of self-harm or made plans to self-harm?
- Been unusually elated? (Can occur once the decision to end it all has been reached.)

Gentle questioning about how the patient sees the future can lead to more direct questions about suicidal intent.

The needs of the family and those close to patients who commit suicide must also be considered. Guilt, anger and depression are all part of the grieving process; financial problems or behaviour problems in children can also occur. Whatever the situation, it would be useful to know how to help patients who need support or where to refer them.

Accidents

Some men are socialised to engage in high-risk activities. Even though the value of exercise is strongly promoted, sports injuries are common; they range from musculoskeletal injuries to permanent disability or death. Contact sports carry a risk of serious injury. The desire to impress others or the adrenaline rush from extreme sports can lead men, in particular, to place their lives in danger. Motorbike and car accidents, through reckless driving, are sadly all too common.

Occupational hazards

Despite moves towards sex equality, men are still generally exposed to greater health hazards at work. Men have traditionally been employed in heavy industry, with its attendant risks of accidents. Work-related health problems also include:

- Occupational asthma, from working with dust or fumes
- Dermatitis, from allergy to chemicals or substances in the workplace
- Cancer linked to the work environment, e.g. mesothelioma from asbestos[6]
- Skin cancers from prolonged exposure to the sun
- Stress – long working hours and the competitive nature of some jobs, combined with the ever-present fear of redundancy, can be detrimental to mental health
- Post-traumatic stress disorder (see Chapter 15). Some occupations such as the fire brigade, police and ambulance services expose employees to horrifying experiences. Although not the exclusive province of men, women in such occupations may be more able to use the support offered and to express their feelings and show emotion. Men, however, may feel unable to use the counselling services provided for fear of being thought weak or unable to cope.

Health and safety regulations are designed to minimise work-related injuries but some men choose to flout the regulations in order to appear macho. Giving information or providing protective clothing may not be enough – the whole culture may need to be changed. Efforts are being made in this respect; lunchtime drinking is no longer considered acceptable in many companies and failure to wear the protective clothing provided is a dismissible offence on some building sites.

Coronary heart disease (see also Chapters 9 and 16)

Men have always been known to have a greater incidence of heart disease than women. Oestrogen protects women until the menopause but then their risk increases, especially in women with a history of smoking. The National Service Framework for Coronary Heart Disease sets national standards of care for preventing and treating CHD. Practice nurses are at the forefront of the efforts to meet the standards set for primary care. That is why an understanding of the different ways in which men view health issues is essential so that different approaches can be tried.

MALE PATIENTS IN GENERAL PRACTICE

Education for practice nurses on issues of men's health is usually patchy, with specific topics such as sexual health or testicular self-examination being covered in different courses. Obesity is a major problem nowadays in both sexes but many men consider weight to be a 'girl thing'. Central obesity contributes greatly to the risk of developing type 2 diabetes and cardiovascular disease. Innovative ways will have to be found to engage men in trying to lose wight.

One important fact to remember is that men are not all alike and any discussion of men's health must consider these differences.

- *Social background and employment* – there may be differences in attitude to health issues in relation to education and social class. The effect of unemployment on physical and mental health is well known. There may be role reversal, with men responsible for childcare while women go out to work. Some men may be happy with their new role, while others may feel resentful and undervalued.
- *Relationships* – men may have come from homes without a male role model or have been subjected to physical or mental abuse. Such men may have difficulty in making satisfactory relationships. Perpetrators of domestic violence can come from any social class but those from the higher social classes may not be recognised as abusers. Although some men can be the victims of violence by women, it should not be forgotten that most domestic violence is perpetrated by men.[7]
- *Cultural background* – men from different ethnic backgrounds may have particular health risks but be reluctant to attend for a health check. The practice profile should help to identify the specific health risks of men in the local population.
- *Sexual health* – some gay men may be more aware of their own health needs and have a support network to contact but many younger gay men still need advice and information. The statistics for HIV and STD infections over time partly reflect the way the message about safe sex is, or is not, getting through to young men of all sexual persuasions.[8] Male rape has been a criminal offence since 1994. Although still relatively rare compared to the rape of women, the effect on some men can be totally devastating and victims will need referral for specialised help and support. Leaflets are available in several languages for patients in Greater London giving information and contact addresses for men who have been the victims of sexual assault.[9] Nurses in other areas should familiarise themselves with local rape support services.
- *Disability* – any form of disability that results in dependence on others may challenge the concept of masculinity and male dominance.

- *Knowledge* – some men are ignorant about how their bodies work and what contributes to good health. They may be amenable to information about ways of increasing their fitness. Other men may have a good knowledge of physiology and may, or may not, take care of their health.

Valuing diversity entails accepting people as they are and tailoring the nursing approach to suit their needs.

Women generally have more contact with general practice than men do – especially young men. There could be several reasons why women feel more comfortable in the practice setting.

- A higher proportion of the staff are usually female – receptionists, nurses and, often, doctors.
- Women are accustomed to personal consultations for contraception, well-woman screening, pregnancy or consultations for their children with childhood illnesses or for immunisations.

Surgery times could also deter men from attending well-man clinics because they are unwilling to take time off work when they are not ill. Some men equate visiting the doctor with being sick and they may feel anxious about being amongst ill people. They may have had a bad experience in the past and wish to avoid being told off about their eating, drinking or smoking habits. Moreover, when men do have something wrong with them, they may put off seeing the doctor for a longer period.[10]

Traditionally there has been less investment in men's health. In 1999, the RCN Men's Health Forum reported that for every pound spent on men's health, eight pounds were spent on women. This inequality is being addressed with new approaches to health services for men. Enlightened individuals have shown how this can be done. One excellent example is the Health of Men Group (HOM) in Bradford and Airedale where drop-in centres and a website for men of all ages are run. Research is currently in progress in that area to study men's awareness of their health needs and their access to and opinion of the services available to them.[10] The nursing journals publish details of these and other ventures; often their success depends on the skills and efforts of charismatic leaders, with good management support. It is hoped that by learning from their successes and setbacks, primary care staff in other areas will be inspired to adopt similar methods. Primary care organisations can incorporate schemes for improving men's health in their local health plans.

WELL-MAN CHECKS

Given the constraints mentioned above, some men will come to see the practice nurse for a new-patient health check (see Chapter 9). Others may request a general check-up; this may be triggered by a landmark birthday, ill health in a family member or work colleague, or pressure from a partner. It is always worth finding out what prompted the patient to attend, in order to elicit any particular health concerns. Younger men are more likely to attend for travel advice and immunisations. There would not usually be enough time in a consultation to discuss many general health issues, but safer sex, the risk of accidents and sunburn, especially when associated with alcohol excess, should be included.

In older men there is an increased risk of osteoporosis, as discussed in Chapter 13. The andropause, or age-related hypogonadism, has received more attention recently; it is a condition associated with the decline in the circulating levels of testosterone. The diagnosis must be supported by biochemical blood tests and assessment of other symptoms such as depression, fatigue, decreased libido, decreased muscle volume or body hair, decreased bone mineral density or increased visceral fat. If the diagnosis is confirmed, then treatment may be instituted by testosterone replacement, providing there are no contraindications.[11]

Sexual health (see Chapter 12)

Sexual risk taking is common amongst young men. Peer pressure and the need to save face exert significant influence. Yet many of them do not perceive themselves as having access to the sexual health services available to young women. Young male patients will be unlikely to attend the surgery to discuss their concerns unless they can be guaranteed confidentiality and ease of access. Yet there is a great need for services for this group of patients and some practice nurses feel confident enough to provide such a service. Alternatively, there should be easily accessible information about services in the local area, discreetly placed for young people to pick up.

TESTICULAR CANCER

Cancer of the testes occurs most commonly in men aged between 20 and 40 years. Nearly 2000 men were affected in the UK in 2001.[12] The condition is rare in non-Caucasian men. The incidence of testicular cancer has doubled since the 1970s but early detection allows a 90% cure rate. Hence the need for men to be aware of the disease and for them to know how to examine their testicles. Just as women are taught breast awareness, so men need to know how to perform testicular self-examination. Leaflets can be obtained from health promotion departments to back up this education. The earlier the disease is detected and treated, the better the chance of a cure.

Many sexual health courses include testicular self-examination (TSE) in their curricula. Men should be taught to be familiar with the normal weight, texture and consistency of their testes and to examine themselves regularly after a warm bath or shower, when the scrotum is relaxed. The epididymis could be mistaken for a lump if the patient is not aware of the normal anatomy of the testes. It is normal for the testicles to be different in size and for one to be lower than the other.[13]

The cause of testicular cancer is not fully understood but factors known to be associated with the condition include an undescended testicle. There is also a greater risk if a close relative (father or a brother) had testicular cancer.

Treatment

Removal of the diseased testicle is usually performed. If the remaining testicle is healthy, the patient may still be able to father children but when fertility is at risk, semen can be collected and frozen for future use. Radiotherapy and chemotherapy may be used after surgery, depending on the type of tumour. The prognosis is usually very good for the majority of men. More than 90% of tumours are treatable.

The diagnosis of testicular cancer can have a devastating effect on the self-esteem and body image of the individual. Patients can benefit from a self-help group for men with the same condition. Nurses can provide information about any local group or encourage the setting up of a group if none exists.

Testicular cancer usually affects young men and despite the relatively small number of cases nationally each year, each case can be particularly poignant. Information about the importance of TSE can be given to mothers, girlfriends and partners when they attend for well-woman screening, so that they can pass the message on to their menfolk. This is one way of reaching men who are not likely to visit the surgery.

PROSTATE DISEASE

Benign prostatic hyperplasia (BPH)

BPH is a common disease of men over 50 years of age which, if left untreated, can lead to recurrent bladder infections, bladder calculi and acute urinary retention. The prostate gland, which is the shape and size of a chestnut, is situated around the urethra at the neck of the bladder. Enlargement of the prostate gland happens gradually, so symptoms tend to develop slowly and patients may accept them as part of the ageing process. Typically there may be:

- Hesitancy – difficulty or delay in starting micturition
- A poor or intermittent urinary stream
- A feeling of not completely emptying the bladder
- Terminal dribbling
- Nocturia.

All of these symptoms can affect the quality of life of men with BPH. Renal function can be adversely affected and acute retention of urine, apart from causing extreme discomfort, can necessitate surgical removal of the prostate.

Opportunistic questioning during new-patient, well-man and over-75 health checks can help in identifying patients with prostatic symptoms. Ask such questions as:

- Do you have any trouble passing urine?
- Do you have to get up at night to pass water?

If the answer to either of the questions is 'yes', further enquiry may elicit the extent of the problem and the effect on the patient's quality of life. The International Prostate Symptom Score (IPSS) questionnaire is available on the Prodigy website to help in assessing the impact of BPH on the patient.[14] Patients with urinary symptoms should be offered an assessment and examination to rule out prostate cancer and to identify ways of relieving the symptoms. A detailed history is necessary, covering:

- An account of any symptoms
- Usual daily fluid intake
- Medication (including diuretics)
- Bowel habit (constipation can cause or exacerbate urinary obstruction)
- Any history of urinary infections or surgery to the urinary tract.

Investigations

Urinalysis is necessary to identify any infection, haematuria or glycosuria. A specimen may be sent for microscopy and culture if an infection is suspected. A blood glucose test may be needed if diabetes is a possibility. A blood test for serum creatinine will determine if the renal function is impaired. The test for prostate-specific antigen (PSA) is also likely to be requested, but this test can be raised with BPH as well as prostate cancer, so can cause difficulties with interpretation of the result. Digital rectal examination is usually performed by a GP but some nurses are specially trained to undertake the examination. The patient may also be referred for a transrectal ultrasound examination.

Treatment

The following can be used.

- *Watchful waiting* – men with mild to moderate symptoms, which cause them little inconvenience, may opt to delay treatment. They should be monitored annually.
- *Drug treatment* may be offered – alpha-blockers, e.g. alfuzosin, tamsulosin and terazosin, relax smooth muscle and so may improve urinary flow. These drugs

can also cause hypotension so careful monitoring of the blood pressure is necessary. Alpha-blockers are contraindicated for patients who have a history of orthostatic hypotension or micturition syncope. Antiandrogens, e.g. finasteride and dutasteride, inhibit testosterone metabolism, leading to a reduction in prostate size, with subsequent improvement in urinary flow. They are most suitable for men with a prostate volume of more than 40 ml. Decreased libido, erectile dysfunction and ejaculation disorders are some of the possible side effects of finasteride. Men taking these tablets are advised to use a condom when having sexual intercourse with a woman of childbearing age and women who are pregnant or could become pregnant should not handle finasteride tablets if they are crushed or broken or leaking dutasteride capsules.[15]

- *Herbal remedies* – American saw palmetto (*Serenoa repens*) has been shown to be as effective as finasteride in relieving mild to moderate symptoms of BPH.[16]
- *Surgical treatments*, usually transurethral resection of the prostate (TURP), are more effective in relieving symptoms but have a higher rate of complications such as retrograde ejaculation, erectile dysfunction and urinary incontinence or death.
- *Minimally invasive treatments* carry fewer risks and can sometimes be performed as day cases.[17,18]

Prostate cancer

Prostate cancer accounts for 1:8 of all male cancer deaths. The condition is more common in men over the age of 50 and the risk of developing it rises with age. In men aged 85 and over, 26% of all cancer deaths are due to prostate cancer.[19] The symptoms can be similar to those of BPH, although some men may be asymptomatic or else present with haematuria.

Apart from age, other risk factors for developing prostate cancer include a family history of the disease and possibly a diet high in fat. African and Afro-Caribbean men have a higher risk of developing prostate cancer than white men; Asian men have the lowest incidence of the disease.[20] The increased incidence may partly relate to improved detection rates through PSA tests, digital rectal examination and transrectal ultrasound. However, the earlier diagnosis of the disease could result in the patient undergoing many unpleasant investigations and treatments, when the disease might not have caused serious problems or affected the patient's mortality. The debate about PSA testing relates to this dilemma: the challenge for researchers is to devise a test that can differentiate aggressive tumours, that require immediate treatment, from those that can be safely managed by watchful waiting.

Prostate-specific antigen

PSA is a glycoprotein produced by the prostate and released into the bloodstream. Raised levels of PSA in a blood sample may indicate the presence of prostate cancer, but the test is not specific for cancer because prostatitis and BPH can also cause the PSA level to be elevated. Patients may request PSA tests in response to media interest in the subject or government pronouncements. The NHS Cancer Plan stated that PSA testing to detect prostate cancer would be made available, supported by information about the risks and benefits, to empower men to make their own choices.[21] Patients must be counselled about the implications of the test so that they can make an informed decision. Leaflets have been supplied to all surgeries explaining the benefits and drawbacks of PSA tests. Practice nurses have also been identified as being ideally placed to advise older male patients.

A PSA test should not be performed if the patient:

- Has a urinary infection
- Ejaculated in the previous 48 hours
- Exercised vigorously in the previous 48 hours
- Had a digital rectal examination in the past week
- Had a prostate biopsy in the previous six weeks.

Digital rectal examination should be performed after a PSA test.[22]

Gleason score

There are several systems around the world used for grading tumours within the prostate but the one most commonly used in the UK is Gleason grading. This uses a score from 1 to 5, with 1 being the most well differentiated, through to 5 being the most poorly differentiated tumour. Each tissue sample is graded and the scores of the two highest graded samples are added together. Therefore a score of 8 or more indicates a poor prognosis. While such knowledge can be empowering and help patients to make decisions about their treatment, it can also engender anxiety when levels rise. Practice nurses should be able to provide information about cancer support groups and helplines for patients who wish to use them.

Metastases

A magnetic resonance imaging (MRI) or computed tomography (CT) scan may be ordered if a tumour is thought to have spread outside the prostate gland. Pain in the lower back, hips or pelvis could indicate metastases. Adequate analgesia will be needed but sometimes this can be tailed off if the tumours respond to drug treatment or radiotherapy.

Treatment

The statistics for the long-term survival of men with prostate cancer, unlike those with testicular cancer, do not appear to change significantly whether they are treated or not. Active surveillance has replaced 'watchful waiting' as the term for describing the process of monitoring patients whose tumour is unlikely to cause problems before the end of their natural life.[23] Treatment of aggressive tumours is likely to be more successful if the tumour is localised within the capsule of the prostate. Possible treatments include the following.

- *Radical prostatectomy* – this can reduce the risk of metastases but, in addition to the usual dangers of surgery, carries the risk of sexual dysfunction and urinary incontinence.
- *Radiotherapy and interstitial irradiation (brachytherapy)* – this can cause diarrhoea and proctitis as side effects of the treatment, as well as erectile dysfunction.
- *Cryotherapy* – freezing of the cancer cells through a probe or needle inserted into the prostate. Can cause damage to the rectum or urethra and, possibly, irritation of the bladder. This treatment may be useful if the cancer recurs after radiotherapy.
- *Drug treatments* – prostate tumours are generally dependent on testosterone. Orchidectomy is the most radical way of reducing testosterone but, as few men are willing to be castrated, this is usually achieved chemically by the use of luteinising hormone-releasing hormone antagonists in order to suppress the release of LHRH by the pituitary gland. Practice nurses may be asked to administer these drugs. They are usually prescribed for men with advanced prostate cancer, in a slow-release preparation, either as an injection, e.g. leuprorelin, or as an implant, e.g. goserelin. The drug company that manufactures goserelin will provide training for nurses and a video on the insertion technique. The manufacturers do not recommend the use of local anaesthetic before insertion of the implant, but some doctors and nurses prefer to anaesthetise the skin first. Anaesthetic cream and an occlusive dressing can be prescribed for the patient to apply one hour before coming to the surgery.

The implant technique is not difficult but should not be attempted before training. The procedure is as follows.

- Clean the skin with an alcohol swab or povidone iodine to minimise the risk of introducing infection.
- Instil local anaesthetic to the injection site if needed or use ethyl chloride spray.
- Check that the pellet can be seen in the neck of the syringe and carefully remove the guard from the plunger to avoid accidentally expelling the pellet.
- Pinch up and hold a fold of skin and subcutaneous tissue of the patient's abdomen with the non-dominant hand.
- Insert the needle subcutaneously into the fold of skin and depress the plunger to insert the implant.
- Withdraw the needle; it will automatically retract after insertion.
- Check the insertion site and apply a small sterile dressing.

Warn the patient that there may be some bruising after the procedure.

The side effects can be troublesome for some men. They include hot flushes, sweating, gynaecomastia and weight gain. The suppression of testosterone also causes loss of libido and erectile dysfunction. Other side effects are listed in the *BNF*. Nurses administering the drugs should enquire about side effects and if the side effects are troublesome for the patient, either refer him to the GP or suggest that he discusses them with the urologist. Hormone treatment may be used to shrink a tumour prior to prostatectomy or radiotherapy.

Whatever treatment the patient is undergoing, the practice nurse can offer support to him and his family. No nurse can be expected to be knowledgeable on every subject but it is essential to know where to find the information needed.

ERECTILE DYSFUNCTION (ED)

Erectile dysfunction, previously called impotence, can be described as the persistent inability to obtain or maintain sufficient rigidity of the penis to allow satisfactory sexual activity. The condition is often associated with ageing but should not be dismissed as such until other causes have been ruled out. The portrayal of sex by the media and the pressures on men related to changes in their role in society can undermine the sexual confidence of many men. The inability to achieve or maintain an erection can affect a man's self-esteem and damage the relationship with a partner. Some men, if unable to discuss the problem, may avoid physical contact altogether, with the result that their partner feels unloved and rejected.

Erectile dysfunction is not a disease; it is a complication of other conditions. Thus the causes of ED may be physical, psychological or a combination of both.

- Endocrine disorders – diabetes mellitus is a common cause. Testosterone insufficiency, abnormal thyroid function, hyperprolactinaemia and excess growth hormone may all cause ED.
- Vascular disease – arteriosclerosis can affect the blood flow through the penis. Cardiovascular disease and hypertension are associated disorders.
- Surgery and radiotherapy – these can cause damage to the cavernous nerves or the pelvic plexus. Altered body image after surgery can also be a psychogenic cause.
- Drugs – both prescribed and illicit drugs may affect erectile function, e.g. antidepressants, antipsychotics, antihypertensives, diuretics, anticholinergics, some hormones, antiandrogens, anticonvulsants, antiparkinson drugs, fibrates, H_2 antagonists and psychotropic drugs, including alcohol.
- Sedentary lifestyle – lack of exercise has been shown to be a modifiable risk factor for ED.[24]
- Neurodegenerative disorders.
- Anatomical deformities of the penis – Peyronie's disease is characterised by fibrosis in the shaft of the penis, which may require surgical correction.

- Psychogenic causes – depression, anxiety, stress disorders and psychoses may be primary causes. Performance anxiety and fear of failure or rejection can compound the situation, whatever the primary cause.

Patients would not usually consult the practice nurse primarily to discuss ED, unless the nurse is known to have a specialist qualification in this field of sexual health. However, up to one in ten men experiences the problem at some time, so nurses are likely to encounter men with ED in any clinical setting. The possibility should be borne in mind at any health check or consultation for chronic disease management. It may be necessary to explain that many drugs and illnesses are known to have an effect on sexual functioning and that help is available if it is ever needed. Open-ended questions may help some patients to articulate any worries about sexual matters.

Assessment and investigations

A full medical, social and sexual history is needed, together with the patient's view of the problem and that of the sexual partner. It is important to establish how and when the problem started and to understand what happens when the patient anticipates making love and whether erections occur at night or when waking up. Any medication being taken should be checked for known effects on erectile function. Whether a nurse or a doctor carries out this interview will depend on individual practice circumstances. A patient would quickly sense any embarrassment by the practitioner, with a detrimental effect on the consultation and any future progress. Blood pressure should always be measured. A physical examination should identify any anatomical abnormalities of the penis or testes as well as signs of peripheral vascular or neurological disease. Other blood tests will depend on individual circumstances but could include the following.

- Blood glucose – if undiagnosed diabetes is a possibility.
- Serum lipids – if dyslipidaemia suspected.
- Haemoglobinopathies – if sickle cell disease is a possibility.
- Thyroid function – especially if loss of libido.
- Hormone profile – these tests are more controversial but should be considered in young men, especially if they also have loss of libido: testosterone, prolactin, follicle-stimulating hormone and luteinising hormone.

Treatment

Any underlying physical cause should be addressed and any medication reviewed. Alternative drugs may be prescribed in some instances. Psychosexual counselling may be appropriate for some patients and their partners.

Drug treatments

The licensing of sildenafil brought erectile dysfunction into the public arena for a while, when the topic was discussed freely in the press and on prime-time television. Drug treatments for ED may only be prescribed on NHS prescriptions for men with specific medical conditions (see *BNF*). Such prescriptions must be endorsed SLS to be valid. The following drugs may be prescribed.

- Sildenafil (*Viagra*) 50 or 100 mg tablet taken one hour before expected sexual activity. It is contraindicated for patients taking nitrates, because it can potentiate their hypotensive effect, and when vasodilation or sexual activity is inadvised, because of a recent stroke or myocardial infarction.
- Alprostadil (prostaglandin E_1) may be given as a tablet inserted by an applicator into the male urethra (*MUSE*) or by intracavernous injection (*Caverject*, *Virida*). A condom should be used if there is any possibility of pregnancy in the partner. Priapism can be a serious side effect and patients should be advised to seek medical help if an erection lasts longer than six hours.

Yohimbine (not available on prescription) is derived from the bark of the African yohimbine tree. It may be more effective than placebo, without having serious side effects, but some of the trials reviewed were of questionable validity.[25]

Vacuum constriction devices

Various devices are available. Vacuum pumps draw blood into the penis and a constriction ring is then placed over the base of the penis to maintain rigidity. The penis can feel cold because of the restricted blood flow and the constricting ring should not be left on for longer than 30 minutes because of the risk of ischaemia. Patients taking anticoagulants should not use this method, owing to the risk of haemorrhage within the penis.

Prostheses

As a last resort, some men may have a prosthesis implanted surgically. This can entail destruction of the patient's own cavernous tissue to accommodate the implant. Infection occurred in 2–7% of cases in one study reviewed.[26]

CONCLUSION

Practice nurses have the opportunity to ensure that the health needs of male patients receive equal attention to those of women. The Men's Health Forum organises Men's Health Week every June. Details can be found on the website.

Suggestions for reflection on practice

How friendly is your surgery towards men?

- Are appointment times appropriate?
- Are there magazines for men in the waiting area?

How prepared are you to deal with men's health issues?

- Could any changes be made?
- Do you need any further training or resources?

REFERENCES

1. National Statistics Online (2004) *Life Expectancy: more aged 70 and 80 than ever before.* www.statistics.gov.uk/cci/nugget.asp?id=881 (accessed 19/1/06).
2. National Statistics Online (undated) *Trends in Life Expectancy by Social Class 1972–2001.* www.statistics.gov.uk/STATBASE/Product.asp?vlnk=8460 (accessed 19/1/06).
3. National Statistics Online (2004) *Mortality Rates for England and Wales.* www.statistics.gov.uk/cci/nugget.asp?id=919 (accessed 19/1/06).
4. Department of Health (1999) *Saving Lives: our healthier nation.* Department of Health, London.
5. National Statistics Online (2005) *Suicides: UK Numbers Reach 30 Year Low in 2003.* www.statistics.gov.uk/cci/nugget.asp?id=1092 (accessed 20/1/06).
6. Health and Safety Executive (2005) Cancers. www.hse.gov.uk/statistics/causdis/cancer.htm (accessed 21/1/06).
7. Department of Health (2005) *Responding to Domestic Abuse: a handbook for health professionals.* Department of Health, London.
8. Health Protection Agency (2005) *HIV and other Sexually Transmitted Infections in the United Kingdom: 2005.* www.hpa.org.uk/hpa/publications/hiv_sti_2005/default.htm (accessed 20/1/06).
9. Metropolitan Police/Sapphire (undated) *Male Victims of Sexual Assault.* www.met.police.uk/sapphire (accessed 21/1/06).
10. Leeds Metropolitan University (2005) *Report of the First Phase of the Study on Men's Usage of the Bradford Health of Men Services.* www.healthofmen.com/documents/BradfordinterimreportFeb2005.pdf (accessed 22/1/06).
11. Morales, A. & Lunenfeld, B. (2002) *Standards, Guidelines and Recommendations of the International Society for the Study of the Aging Male (ISSAM): investigations, treatment and monitoring of late-onset hypogonadism in males.* www.andropause.org.uk/training/issam.pdf (accessed 22/1/06).
12. Cancer Research UK (2004) *Testicular Cancer Incidence Statistics for the UK.* www.cancerresearchuk.org/cancerstats/types/testis/incidence/ (accessed 22/1/06).
13. Lowson, P. (2005) Encouraging testicular self-examination by men. *Practice Nursing,* **16** (3), 115–20.

14. Prodigy Guidance (2005) *Prostate – benign hyperplasia.* www.prodigy.nhs.uk/guidance. asp?gt=prostate (accessed 22/1/06).
15. British Medical Association and Pharmaceutical Society of Great Britain (2005) Dutasteride and finasteride. *British National Formulary 50*, 6.4.2. BMA and RPSGB, London.
16. Wilt, T., Ishani, A. & MacDonald, R. (2002) Serenoa repens for benign prostatic hyperplasia. Cochrane Database of Systematic Reviews. www.mrw.interscience. wiley.com/cochrane/clsysrev/articles/CD001423/abstract.html (accessed 23/1/06).
17. National Institute for Clinical Excellence (2003) *Transurethral Electrovaporisation of the Prostate.* www.nice.org.uk/page.aspx?o=64414 (accessed 23/1/06).
18. National Institute for Clinical Excellence (2003) *KTP Laser Vaporisation of the Prostate for Benign Prostatic Obstruction.* www.nice.org.uk/page.aspx?o=76546 (accessed 23/1/06).
19. Cancer Research UK (2002) *Prostate Cancer Mortality Statistics for the UK.* www. cancerresearckuk.co.uk.
20. NHS Cancer Screening Programme (undated) *Prostate Cancer Risk Factors.* www. cancerscreening.nhs.uk/prostate/statistics.html (accessed 23/1/06).
21. Department of Health (2000) *The NHS Cancer Screening Plan: a plan for investment, a plan for reform.* Extending cancer screening, Executive Summary, para 25. p 10. Department of Health, London.
22. Department of Health (2004) *Making Progress on Prostate Cancer.* Department of Health Publications, London.
23. Harris, G. (2005) Prostate cancer: grading and staging, screening and treatment. *Practice Nurse*, **29** (9), 72–8.
24. Rosen, R.C., Friedman, M. & Kostis, J.B. (2005) Lifestyle management of erectile dysfunction: the role of cardiovascular and concomitant risk factors. *American Journal of Cardiology*, **96** (12b), 76M–79M.
25. Webber, R. (2003) *Erectile Dysfunction: yohimbine.* Clinical Evidence. www.clinicalevidence.com/ceweb/conditions/msh/1803/1803_19.jsp (accessed 23/1/06).
26. Webber, R. (2003) *Erectile Dysfunction: penile prostheses.* Clinical Evidence. www. clinicalevidence.com/ceweb/conditions/msh/1803/1803_16.jsp (accessed 23/1/06).

FURTHER READING

Mitchell Beazley (2004) *The Complete Book of Men's Health: everything a man needs to know.* Mitchell Beazley Publishing, London.
Wilkins, D. (2005) Hazardous waist? *Practice Nurse*, **29** (11), 43–8.

USEFUL ADDRESSES AND WEBSITES

Men's Health Forum,
Tavistock House, Tavistock Square, London WC1H 9QB
Telephone: 020 7388 4449
Website: www.menshealthforum.org.uk

CancerBACUP
3 Bath Place, Rivington Street, London EC2A 3JR
Telephone: 020 7696 9003
Helpline: 0808 800 1234
Website: www.cancerbacup.org.uk

Prostate Cancer Charity,
3 Angel Walk, London W6 9HX
Telephone: 020 8222 7622
Helpline: 0845 300 8383
Website: www.prostate-cancer.org.uk

Patient UK – list of self-help groups
Website: www.patient.co.uk/selfhelp.asp

Chapter 15
Mental Health

Holistic care grew from the recognition that physical, mental, social and spiritual wellbeing are all closely interlinked. Modern nursing courses place emphasis on caring for the whole person within the community but this concept has been challenged recently as possibly being too intrusive for some patients or costly for the health service.[1] Holism is derived from the ancient Greek word *holos*, meaning whole. It has been accepted by most nurses as being fundamental to nursing.

The pace and competitiveness of modern life mean that more people are seeking help for stress-related illnesses while at the same time, the closure of psychiatric institutions has shifted the focus of mental healthcare to the community. There are as many adults who are likely to have some form of mental illness at any one time as there are people with asthma, according to the foreword to the National Service Framework for Mental Health. The NSF specifies the standards expected for adults up to the age of 65. The National Service Framework for Older People includes mental health standards for people aged over 65 years. The staff in general practice must be able to contribute to new flexible mental health services.

Mental health nursing has always been a separate specialty and only a small proportion of practice nurses had been educated as mental health nurses at the time of the last national survey. Concern has been expressed about practice nurses' knowledge and preparedness for dealing with patients' mental health needs.[2] It is essential for nurses in general practice to obtain the training needed to be competent in this field.

THE HISTORICAL BACKGROUND TO THE DEVELOPMENT OF MENTAL HEALTH SERVICES

In the eighteenth century mentally ill people whose families could not afford to confine them in private madhouses usually ended up in prison or the workhouse. During the nineteenth century the state assumed responsibility for the care of lunatics by building huge county asylums in sparsely populated areas. Social reformers campaigned for a more humane treatment of the inmates.

The asylums continued to expand during the first quarter of the twentieth century but there was also a move towards alternative management. Voluntary patients and outpatients began to be treated. The county asylums came under the control of the regional hospital boards when the NHS was founded, but the provision of aftercare was in the hands of the local authorities.

The development of phenothiazine drugs in the 1950s and 1960s revolutionised the treatment of patients with schizophrenia and reduced the time they needed to be in hospital. A series of scandals, enquiries and reports brought the services for mentally ill and mentally handicapped people into public focus in the 1960s and 1970s.[3,4] At the same time there was a growth in new care facilities, such as day centres, hostels and psychiatric units in general hospitals. Community psychiatric nurses grew in numbers and the first CPN postregistration course began in 1974.

The move towards care in the community led to the National Health Service and Community Care Act (1990). The closure of the Victorian institutions, which had begun in the preceding decades, was not matched by adequate facilities for community care. There were success stories of people rehabilitated after years of confinement, but a huge burden was also placed on many families and carers. The acute psychiatric units in some inner-city areas were unable to cope adequately with the demand for acute admissions.

The Care Programme Approach (CPA) was introduced in 1991 with the aim of improving community care services for all people with a mental health problem through:

- An assessment of health and social care needs
- A detailed written care plan
- Appointment of a key worker (now called a care coordinator)
- Regular reviews of the plan and changes as necessary.

The lack of resources to meet this ambitious policy, and concerns that the available services would be overstretched, led to only those patients perceived as being vulnerable being selected for the CPA. Health authorities all developed their own criteria for deciding which patients should be selected. The NHS had responsibility for the CPA but care management was the responsibility of social services.

A change of government in 1997 resulted in ideas for radical changes to the NHS, with the stated intention of modernising the entire organisation. Mental health was accorded a high priority and additional funding was promised. The coordination of mental healthcare was decreed. The needs of carers were given prominence and public involvement at all levels began to be encouraged. The NHS Plan promised, among other things, hundreds of mental health teams to provide an immediate respond to crises, patient advocates to be set up in every hospital and improved primary care in deprived areas. The NSF expressed the government's intention of bringing mental health laws up to date to reflect modern treatments. The CPA and care management had already been found to be poorly coordinated; a review of the whole process was undertaken and a policy booklet was published, with the aim of achieving:

- Integration of the CPA and care management
- Consistency of implementation nationally
- A more streamlined process to reduce bureaucracy
- A proper focus on the needs of service users.[5]

Systems were required to demonstrate the quality of services provided, with joint auditing processes where different agencies were working together.

MENTAL HEALTHCARE IN GENERAL PRACTICE

Despite the way the term is used in the NSF, mental health should encompass much more than just dealing with mental illness. Health promotion is usually equated with physical health, with little attention paid to promoting mental health. Moreover, it should be remembered that people with mental health problems are entitled to expect the same screening and health promotion services as the rest of the population; the physical health needs of people with mental illnesses can easily be overlooked.[6] Conversely, people with physical illnesses have a higher rate of mental health problems than the general population. The Royal College of Psychiatrists website has a leaflet for patients that can be downloaded.[7] Depending on her/his previous experience and training, a practice nurse might become involved in some of the ways described below.

The promotion of mental health

Regular sleep, exercise, healthy food and secure relationships all contribute to physical and mental wellbeing. Nurses can provide practical help and advice as required on healthy living and also contribute to local and national initiatives to deter people of all ages from substance abuse.

Grief is a natural process in response to a loss, but it can turn into an abnormal reaction if it is not faced and worked through. Bereavement counselling or support groups may be needed to help a patient to deal with grief successfully. Hospices usually run training programmes for nurses on helping the bereaved. People need a chance to talk about the intense emotional and physical feelings they experience. Sometimes, when a person has died suddenly, the one left behind is burdened by a lot of things left unsaid or words spoken in haste that are regretted. Support groups are available in some areas for people bereaved in particular circumstances, such as parents who lose children or those bereaved through violence or major disasters. A practice nurse can help by providing information about local support services.

The difficulties of modern living, relationship problems or being the victim of crime can all cause their own problems. Acknowledgement of their existence can be the first step, so that help can be provided before a person's mental health is seriously affected.

The recognition and treatment of mental illness

The mental health NSF lists the people most vulnerable to mental health problems. Standard one requires all health and social services to work with individuals and communities, to combat discrimination and to promote social inclusion. Nurses working in areas with high unemployment or in rural communities affected by farming disasters like BSE and foot and mouth disease may encounter a higher than usual number of people with depressive illnesses. *Saving Lives: our healthier nation* has a target for reducing deaths from suicide by at least a fifth by 2010.

Short-term memory problems might alert the staff to a patient's impaired mental function when he/she telephones repeatedly to ask the same questions. Many patients are aware of their memory loss and become anxious about the future. Depression in older people may be masked by anxiety and impaired memory, but the onset of dementia should also be considered.

Practice nurses may be required to administer regular depot injections to patients with psychotic illnesses. An understanding of the possible side effects of the medication is required (see below). Drug treatments need to be well monitored. Patients with mental illnesses who request repeat prescriptions inappropriately may be missing medication, taking too much or stockpiling. The GP should be informed of any concerns.

Support and care for mentally ill patients and their carers

Carers may be under strain and require more support or help to manage at home. Standard six of the Mental Health NSF details the rights of carers to have their needs assessed and to agree a written care plan for the person being cared for. The needs of young carers must also be addressed. Staff in general practice are likely to know of children or young people who have a mentally ill relative at home. Standard three of the NSF expects people with common mental health problems to be able to access services at any time of the day or night.

The nurse might recognise when a patient's mood or behaviour has altered, if a patient is well known to a practice. A prompt referral to the GP or the community mental health nurse could prevent a further deterioration. When a crisis does occur, a crisis intervention team from the mental health unit might be able to provide an early intensive input within the patient's home. However, sometimes a patient will need acute admission to hospital. If the patient does not accept voluntary admission, compulsory admission is permitted under the Mental Health Act (1983) if he/she is considered to be a danger to him/herself or others. Serious efforts are made to safeguard the civil liberties of such patients. A new Mental Health Act is due to be passed soon. It is designed to be compatible with the Human Rights Act of 1998. An easy-to-read version of the draft Mental Health Bill is available.[8]

The Mental Capacity Act of 2005 is designed to empower and protect vulnerable people who are not able to make their own decisions.[9] Independent mental capacity advocates will safeguard the interests of patients who do not have family or friends to support them. A draft code of practice has been prepared, which should be finalised by 2007.

Dealing with aggression and violence

People who are aggressive or violent are not necessarily mentally ill, but mental illness can sometimes manifest itself in this way. Patients who are very anxious or who have never learned to control their emotions can become abusive if they have to wait to see a doctor. Others can become violent under the influence of alcohol or drugs. Practice nurses and receptionists may be in the front line. Prevention is better than cure; the time to consider staff safety is before an incident occurs.

Risk assessment

A survey of the practice layout and work arrangements should reveal anything that makes the staff vulnerable. Safety features should be incorporated in the design of practices and health centres. There must be a way of getting help quickly, as well as a practice policy specifying the action to be taken if an aggressive incident occurs. A member of staff could be at risk while alone in the building. In such instances the front door should be kept locked and a safety chain put on before opening the door to callers.

Nurses and doctors who undertake home visits need to consider the potential dangers and take appropriate precautions.

- Make sure someone knows where you have gone and when to expect you back. A mobile telephone is essential.
- Get all the relevant details of the patient's history and social situation beforehand. Report back after finishing the visit or if delayed.
- Arrange a coded message to be used if help is needed. All the staff must understand the significance of such a message.
- Be aware of any danger signs such as abusive language, strange behaviour or dangerous weapons on view. Do not enter if in doubt.
- Carry a personal alarm to attract attention if attacked in the street.
- Report any worrying incidents to the GP and to the police (if appropriate).

All staff should have access to training in ways of dealing with difficult situations. The Suzy Lamplugh Trust, a charity run for that specific purpose, provides guidance, resources and training in all matters of personal safety.

Some things to consider for avoiding incidents in the practice include the following.

- *Keep patients informed* of what is happening and offer alternative choices if a delay is inevitable.
- *Listen to what the patient is saying.* Allow frustrations to be expressed, without responding defensively. Acknowledge any legitimate cause for complaint and apologise.
- *Avoid confrontation.* Use a quiet, calm voice even if the patient is shouting. Adopt a non-threatening posture and do not fold the arms, as this can be interpreted as aggression. Avoid staring; this can be interpreted as provocation. Try to get the patient away from others in the vicinity.
- *Get someone to phone for the police* if a situation looks likely to get out of control.
- *Avoid being injured.* Stand just out of arm's reach, with the body at an angle so it is not square on to the patient. Have one foot slightly in front of the other to allow the body to tilt backwards. Endeavour to have a clear escape route and keep an eye out for anything that the patient might use as a weapon. Politely ask the patient to put down a weapon being held. Look out for something to use as a shield in case it is needed. Don't intervene if the patient breaks something; this can be a way of letting off steam.[10]

Reporting incidents

A report should be made of any aggressive incidents. Verbal abuse should be recorded in the patient's records. Any violence or injuries inflicted must be documented in an incident report, as well as in the records. Staff members who have been subjected to aggression require a debriefing session to discuss their feelings about the incident. Professional counselling may be needed in some instances. Analysis of a critical incident will allow people to learn from it. Most NHS premises now display notices to tell the public that verbal or physical abuse will not be tolerated.

Helping patients with mental health problems

It is beyond the scope of this book to discuss all the ways in which mental illness might be manifested. This chapter deals mainly with the situations which practice nurses are most likely to encounter.

Stress

The word stress is often used nowadays to indicate any situation in which a person feels unable to cope with life's demands. The problems of chronic habituation to tranquillisers have led to the search for safer ways to help. The distressing symptoms of stress derive from biological reactions that evolved to help our primitive ancestors to survive in the face of danger – the fight or flight response. There is usually a balance within the body between the parasympathetic and sympathetic nervous activity, but the outpouring of adrenaline in response to perceived danger stimulates the sympathetic nervous system. This is predominantly responsible for the effects associated with stress. At the same time, parasympathetic stimulation of the gastrointestinal tract can also result in nausea and diarrhoea.

A certain level of arousal is needed for normal social functioning and to avoid accidents. Long periods of understimulation will result in boredom, loss of concentration and apathy. Prolonged overstimulation can cause a breakdown in the body's ability to adapt, resulting in physical or mental illness. There may be a genetic link with the way individuals react to stress. Something that might overwhelm one person could seem an exciting challenge to another. Single major stressors such as bereavement, divorce or business failure may precipitate a stress-related illness or there may be multiple small events until a crisis point is reached.

Patients can consult the GP or nurse with a variety of symptoms that are ultimately attributed to stress: insomnia, depression, constant tiredness, panic attacks, muscular pains, indigestion, skin disorders or headaches. Counselling might help a patient to identify the problems and find an appropriate solution. A situation incapable of a solution is not really a problem – it's a fact of life. Sometimes people need help to differentiate between the two.

Depending on the circumstances, various strategies or support systems might be appropriate.

- *Developing self-awareness* – helping the individual to understand his/her behaviour; to learn to express powerful feelings, such as anger, grief, fear or guilt; and to accept the need for other people.
- *Assertiveness training* – learning to express personal needs or to refuse requests without giving offence.
- *Dealing with relationships*
  - Children. The health visitor can often advise on parenting skills, to minimise conflict with children. Childcare arrangements may allow parents some freedom. Referral for family therapy may be needed for disturbed children.
  - Partners. Advice about birth control can help in limiting the size of families. Counselling services such as Relate, or some churches, can help with relationship problems. Gay and lesbian self-help groups can provide specific support. Bereavement counselling services are available for bereaved partners.
  - Dependants. Community nurses and social services can provide help for carers. Respite care may be arranged and carers' associations can provide practical and emotional help.
- *Finance* – learning to live within an income or deal with debts (Citizens Advice Bureaux will advise). Ensuring benefits are being claimed (if applicable).

Leaflets about entitlement can be obtained from main post offices and social security offices.

- *Time management* – learning to identify priorities for action and to make time for recreation and rest.
- *Enjoying work* – learning to delegate, or even looking for alternative work if not happy.
- *Finding alternatives* – unemployment, retirement or children leaving home can leave a big gap in a patient's life. Part-time work, voluntary work, a hobby or study might help.
- *Relaxation* – learning to counteract the physical effects of stress by physical exercise, yoga, therapeutic massage, aromatherapy or relaxation exercises and tapes.

Post-traumatic stress disorder (PTSD) has been recognised in recent years as a particular type of stress-related illness. It was originally associated with major incidents like train crashes or fires but is now used to describe the range of psychological symptoms people may experience after any traumatic event, including witnessing or being involved in a car crash, violent crime or assault. The symptoms may emerge at any time after the event; they include night-mares, panic attacks, loss of memory and concentration, extreme tiredness and flashbacks. The National Institute for Health and Clinical Excellence has issued guidance on the treatment of adults and children with PTSD. People who have suffered severe PTSD should be offered trauma-focused cognitive behavioural therapy within the first month.[11]

Disorders of affect (disturbance of mood)

Depression

Depression is characterised by a low mood that affects the ability to carry out everyday activities. Women are twice as likely to be affected as men. The con-dition can sometimes be overlooked in a patient who presents with multiple physical symptoms. Other symptoms of depression can include:

- Sleep disturbance, often early-morning wakening and being unable to go back to sleep
- Feeling tired all the time
- Lack of concentration
- Loss of libido
- Agitation or irritability
- Feelings of worthlessness or guilt
- Thoughts of self-harm or suicide.

Possible physical causes for some of the symptoms (anaemia or hypothy-roidism) are usually ruled out through blood tests. The diagnosis of depression is made clinically. The use of screening and case-finding tools in general practice has not been shown to have much impact on the recognition, management or outcome of depression in primary care.[12]

The treatment of depression will usually depend on the severity of the condition. Mild to moderate depression will sometimes be helped by talking therapies, but severe depression is more likely to respond to antidepressant drug treatments.[13] St John's wort, available from health food shops, is popular and may be beneficial for treating mild depression. Patients should be warned of possible interaction with many other drugs, including the contraceptive pill, anti-epilepsy drugs, digoxin and warfarin.[14]

Depression in children and young people has received more attention recently. The use of some antidepressant drugs was found to increase the risk of suicide by young adults. The National Institute for Health and Clinical Excellence has issued specific guidelines on depression in children and young people.

Postpartum affective disorders

These may affect new mothers in the following ways.

- *Baby blues* affect a large number of new mothers. Emotional lability and tearfulness start within a week of childbirth and are usually self-limiting, but could progress to depression.
- *Postnatal depression* is a clinical depression that can affect about one in ten mothers. Health visitors may use a tool such as the Edinburgh Postnatal Depression Scale to help identify mothers with depression.[15] However, all primary care team members should be alert to the problem and refer if concerned.
- *Puerperal psychosis* is an acute psychotic illness, characterised by delusions and confusion, in the immediate postpartum period. Urgent psychiatric treatment is needed.

Bipolar affective disorder

Patients with this condition, also known as manic depression, experience extreme mood swings between deep depression and wild elation. There may be periods of normality in between. The condition tends to run in families but has a complex mode of inheritance that is not yet fully understood.[16]

Mania

The patient is overenergetic and enthusiastic, with rapid speech and thought processes. Grandiose schemes, flights of fancy and wild financial expenditure can cause great distress to the families affected. Sometimes the mania alternates with bouts of black depression, with periods of normality in between.

Treatment of mania

Antipsychotic drugs may be prescribed. Lithium carbonate is commonly used to control the mood swings. Blood levels need to be taken regularly to maintain a therapeutic dose and avoid toxicity. The blood sample should be obtained just before the next dose is due, so the residual blood level is established. The time elapsed since the last dose should be recorded on the pathology request form.

Psychotic disorders

Patients with psychotic disorders have a different way of viewing themselves and the world. Their behaviour may endanger themselves and cause distress or fear to others. Help is then needed to prevent injury and restore the patient's ability to function within society. The disordered thought processes and behaviour can be manifested in many ways.

Schizophrenia

Schizophrenia is a chronic illness characterised by disordered perceptions of reality. The speech pattern may be bizarre and emotions may either be dulled or wholly inappropriate to the situation. The person may be withdrawn or self-absorbed, or behave in ways that seem incongruous in their context; normal tasks cannot be completed. Hallucinations may affect any of the senses, but are most commonly auditory. There may be delusions of persecution or of grandeur. Patients with paranoid delusions may have bizarre ideas that neighbours are sending magnetic rays into their home or that they are receiving special messages through their television set. Delusions of grandeur may make the patient think that he or she is a famous person. Patients with schizophrenia have a higher risk of committing suicide.[17]

Treatment

Antipsychotic drugs are given to relieve the symptoms of schizophrenia. A psychiatrist usually makes the choice of drug which may be an oral or parenteral preparation. The main side effect is parkinsonism because antipsychotic drugs are thought to work by blocking dopamine receptors in the brain. Restlessness, abnormal face and body movements, intention tremor and muscle rigidity are parkinsonian symptoms, some of which may be mistaken for symptoms of schizophrenia. Patients with extrapyramidal symptoms are usually given anticholinergic drugs, e.g. procyclidine, to counteract the symptoms (see *BNF*). These drugs can, in turn, cause a dry mouth or gastrointestinal disturbance. They are also liable to abuse and can cause excitement, mental disturbance or confusion, especially in high doses.

Clozapine can cause agranulocytosis, so monitoring of the white cell count is a condition of the product licence. Regular blood samples are sent by post or courier to the *Clozaril* Patient Monitoring Service. All the equipment and postage material is supplied by the CPMS. Practice nurses who administer depot neuroleptic injections, e.g. flupenthixol (*Depixol*), haloperidol decanoate (*Haldol*), fluphenazine (*Modecate*) or zuclopenthixol (*Clopixol*), should be aware of the following points and seek advice if necessary.

- *Authorisation* – there must be a written prescription signed by the GP or hospital psychiatrist for each patient. The dose may need to be adjusted periodically and it is important that the nurse is aware of any changes.
- *Stock* – drugs for injection can either be obtained by each patient on individual prescriptions or be purchased by the practice and reimbursement claimed for personally administered items.
- *Administration* – depot injections should be administered by deep IM injection using a Z-track method. They should not be given if a patient is pregnant.
- *Side effects* – at each visit the patient should be asked how the injection is helping and if it is causing any problems. Some patients gain weight with the medication or develop parkinsonian side effects.
- *Records* – the injections given must be documented appropriately.
- *Monitoring* – annual blood tests for urea and electrolytes and liver function tests may be needed to detect any dysfunction.

The time intervals between injections can vary from weekly to monthly, according to the patient's needs. The patient should be encouraged to make the next appointment before leaving. Reminders may have to be arranged for patients who forget to attend.

Dementia

Dementia is a group of symptoms caused by a number of conditions that affect the brain. Loss of memory for recent events is an early sign of dementia. An inability to perform everyday tasks or to interact socially can follow, as all the higher mental functions become impaired. The degree and speed of impairment can vary between patients. The diagnosis is made clinically, once all the other causes of confusion have been eliminated. Computed tomography or magnetic resonance imaging can also be used.

Looking after a person with dementia can impose enormous strains on the carers. Practice nurses can offer a friendly ear as well as ensuring that carers receive information about all the services, benefits and support available. Many local authorities and voluntary services produce a directory of local services. The Alzheimer's Disease Society provides information and practical support.

Many of the volunteers have had personal experiences of caring for a relative with dementia. There are also support groups for people with other sorts of dementia, for example, Parkinson's disease, Huntington's chorea or AIDS.

A balance needs to be maintained between helping people with dementia as their faculties decline and making them unnecessarily dependent. Carers need help to identify realistic expectations and to take some risks.

Variant Creutzfeldt-Jakob disease (vCJD) is a brain disease, which could affect more people in the future. The symptoms of the early stages of the disease may be mistaken for other psychiatric conditions, such as depression, anxiety, panic attacks, delusions, paranoia or hallucinations. Other neurological symptoms soon develop, for example, forgetfulness, clumsiness and loss of balance, progressing to dementia and increasing immobility and helplessness. Young people are often affected, with devastating consequences for their families. A test is needed to identify carriers of the disease who could possibly transmit it to others.[18]

Substance abuse

Drugs have been used for their mind-altering properties for millennia. Taxes on tobacco and alcohol provide the Inland Revenue with vast sums of money every year and drug dealing is the only growth industry in some inner-city areas. Dependence on an addictive substance occurs when a person cannot cope without it. Physical or psychological dependence eventually causes the body to develop tolerance to the substance and ever greater amounts are needed to create the same effect. Severe physical or psychological withdrawal effects are experienced if the substance is not available for any reason.

Alcohol

Alcohol in small quantities is not usually harmful and there might even be some beneficial effects for older people. Alcohol is a central nervous system depressant, although initially it may create a sense of euphoria. Situations as diverse as accidents, suicide, hypertension and teenage pregnancy can often be linked to the abuse of alcohol. Binge drinking featured heavily in the news when the licensing law was changed in 2005 to allow longer opening hours. Regular alcohol use can result in dependence with a high cost to the patient, the family and society.[19] Deprivation of alcohol can then cause depression, anxiety, convulsions and terrifying hallucinations. Practice nurses may identify patients who already have or are in danger of developing a dependence on alcohol and provide help or refer for specialist advice (see Chapter 9).

Patients who seek help for alcohol dependence may be referred for detoxification. Long-term support will be needed to cope afterwards. Alcoholics Anonymous and other self-help groups provide peer support. Al-Anon and Al-Ateen provide support for the families of problem drinkers.

Other substances

The use of drugs and other substances depends to a certain extent on both their availability and on social pressures. Smokers may find themselves outnumbered at social gatherings now that smoking is less socially acceptable to many people. On the other hand, the peer pressure to experiment can be hard for young people to resist and alcohol, tobacco, drugs and solvents are readily available. Confusion has been created by the reclassification of cannabis as a Class C drug. Sixty five percent of young people under 18 years are likely to experiment with illegal drugs, the vast majority of them with cannabis.[20]

Illicit drugs have a large number of street names. Information about drugs and their effects can be obtained from the internet or from the local drug dependency unit.

Opiates

Heroin is an opium derivative with powerful analgesic properties that can also induce a sense of euphoria. The drug may be injected, smoked or inhaled. Tolerance quickly develops, so larger quantities are required. Self-neglect, weight loss, anaemia and infections can follow. The absence of quality control with illegal drugs means that they often contain impurities. However, accidental overdosing with unusually pure forms can result in death. Abscesses and septicaemia can develop from dirty needles; users who share equipment or who prostitute themselves to get money for drugs are at risk of developing and spreading HIV infection and hepatitis.

Cocaine is a powerful stimulant derived from the coca plant, which creates a psychological dependence. It is usually sniffed or smoked. Crack, a highly addictive concentrated form of cocaine, is readily available and posing a problem for the law enforcement agencies.

Amphetamines

Amphetamines are stimulants that create a feeling of increased energy and excitement. The user is restless and overactive but exhaustion can occur later, especially if the drug is injected. Sedatives may be taken in order to sleep. *Ecstasy* is an amphetamine drug, frequently taken for its stimulant effect by people at all-night clubs and parties. Deaths caused by cardiac arrhythmias and seizures have been reported.

Hallucinogens

Hallucinogens are taken for their mind-altering effects. Some are more dangerous than others.

Cannabis is obtained in dried leaf form, as resin or as concentrated oil. It is usually smoked but can be ingested with food. It can cause a mild euphoria and sense of wellbeing. It is not addictive but association with the illegal drug culture can encourage the move to more harmful substances. Some dealers have been known to mix crack with cannabis in order to create addiction. There is evidence that cannabis use is an independent risk factor for developing psychotic symptoms.[21]

Lysergic acid diethylamide (LSD) causes hallucinating effects that last for up to 12 hours. During that time the user may have a sense of disassociation from the body and be at risk from dangerous behaviour like trying to fly. LSD tablets are relatively cheap and readily available.

Solvents

The fumes from any volatile substance, such as glue, antifreeze, lighter fuel, nail varnish remover or aerosol propellants, can be inhaled from a plastic bag. The effects produced can look similar to intoxication with alcohol, but redness around the mouth and running eyes and nose can be a give-away. There may be a history of poor school performance and truancy. Respiratory and renal failure can be caused by solvent abuse, as well as accidents due to dangerous behaviour or death from asphyxia or inhaled vomit.

Role of the practice nurse

Substance abuse is a major health problem. Practice nurses can provide information about addictive substances to parents and young people in the practice. A nurse may detect signs of possible solvent abuse or note needle marks when taking a blood pressure or treating a wound. Patients may attend the surgery with physical complaints of weight loss, fatigue, gastric problems, blackouts or accidents. There may also be reports of relationship problems, altered behaviour, absenteeism, financial problems or self-neglect. Family members of people who misuse substances may be seen with frequent minor ailments which mask the true cause of their distress.

Eating disorders

Hunger is a physiological drive to eat in response to the body's needs for energy and nutrients. The appetite for certain foods can be indulged or overridden, irrespective of the feelings of hunger. Social and familial customs and beliefs associated with food can affect an individual person's eating behaviour.

Anorexia nervosa

Sufferers from anorexia nervosa have a distorted body image that makes them strive for an abnormally low weight because they mistakenly believe that they are fat. Calorie intakes are strictly regulated and induced vomiting may follow eating. Female sufferers usually develop amenorrhoea as a result of starvation. Death can result if the process is not reversed.

Bulimia nervosa

With bulimia, periods of binge eating are interspersed with vomiting, purging and violent exercise in an attempt to prevent weight gain. The shame and guilt associated with this loss of control reinforce the individual's poor self-image.

Role of the practice nurse

Practice nurses weigh patients during screening and well-person checks. Finding a very low BMI may identify patients with anorexia nervosa, but they are likely to deny having a problem. Patients with bulimia may have a normal weight/height ratio yet complain of being overweight. They may also have a past history of anorexia nervosa. The knuckles of patients with an eating disorder may be scarred by their teeth from persistently inducing vomiting. NICE guidance has been published on the treatment and management of eating disorders. Referral is needed for specialised help for patients identified with such a problem.

SELF-AWARENESS IN THE CARING PROFESSIONS

Nurses and doctors have to be able to deal with their own problems as human beings in order to provide empathic support and care for patients and their families. Many people in the caring professions seem to have a particular need to be admired and respected; emotional conflict can arise if patients appear demanding or ungrateful. The stress experienced by some doctors may be reflected in their higher than average suicide rate.[22]

All the members of the primary healthcare team should be encouraged to explore their own feelings and motivations. Clinical supervision and the review of critical incidents provide opportunities to discuss any matters of concern. The need for relaxation and stress-relieving activities applies as much to the professionals as to the patients. Co-counselling is a method whereby practitioners work in pairs to counsel each other. This is probably better done with a co-counsellor unconnected with the same GP practice. Other forms of counselling should be sought if they are needed.

Suggestions for reflection on practice

- How confident do you feel about looking after patients with mental health problems?
- Could the service they receive be improved?
- What system do you have for communicating with the community mental health team?

REFERENCES

1. Smart, F. (2005) The whole truth? *Nursing Management*, **11** (9), 17–19.
2. Gray, R., Parr, A-M., Plummer, S., Sandford, T., Ritter, S., Mundt-Leach, R., Goldberg, D. & Gournay, K. (1999) A national survey of practice nurse involvement in mental health interventions. *Journal of Advance Nursing*, **30** (4), 901–6.
3. Robb, B. (1967) *Sans Everything, A case to answer*. Nelson, London.
4. Secretary of State for Social Services (1978) *Report of the Committee of Enquiry into Normansfield Hospital*. HMSO, London.
5. Department of Health (1999) *Effective Care Co-ordination in Mental Health Servicse: Modernising the Care Programme Approach – a policy booklet*. Department of Health, London.
6. Hussain, A. (2005) People with severe mental illness receive sub-standard physical care. Regarding the launch of the report *Running on Empty*. www.psychminded.co.uk (accessed 24/1/06).
7. Royal College of Psychiatrists (2003) *Coping with Physical Illness*. www.rcpsych.ac.uk/info/help/pimh/index.asp (accessed 25/1/06).
8. Department of Health (2004) *Draft Mental Health Bill 2004: easy read version*. www.dh.gov.uk/PublicationsAndStatistics/ (accessed 25/1/06).
9. Department of Health (2005) *Mental Capacity Act 2005 – summary*. www.dh.gov.uk/PublicationsAndStatistics (accessed 25/1/06).
10. Walsh, M. & Kent, A. (2001) Violence and aggression. In: *Accident and Emergency Nursing*, 4th edn. Butterworth Heinemann, Oxford.
11. National Institute for Clinical Excellence (2005) *NICE Guideline – post-traumatic stress disorder (PTSD)*. www.nice.org.uk/pdf/CG026NICEguideline.pdf (accessed 25/1/06).
12. Gilbody, S., House, A.O. & Sheldon, T.A. (2005) Screening and case finding instruments for depression. Cochrane Database of Systematic Reviews, Issue 4, Art No.: CD002792.
13. National Institute for Clinical Excellence (2004) *NICE Guideline No 23. Depression: management of depression in primary and secondary care*. www.nice.org.uk/page.aspx?o=cg023niceguideline (accessed 25/1/06).
14. British Medical Association and Pharmaceutical Society of Great Britain (2005) *British National Formulary 50*, Appendix 1: Interactions. BMA and PSGB, London.
15. Dennis, C.L. (2004) Can we identify mothers at risk of postpartum depression in the postpartum period using the Edinburgh Postnatal Depression Scale? *Journal of Affective Disorders*, **78** (2), 163–9.
16. Shastry, B.S. (2005) Bipolar disorder: an update. *Neurochemistry International*, **46** (4), 273–9.
17. Montross, L.P., Zisook, S. & Kasckow, J. (2005) Suicide among patients with schizophrenia: a consideration of risk and protective factors. *Annals of Clinical Psychiatry*, **17** (3), 173–82.
18. Hilton, D.A. (2006) Pathogenesis and prevalence of variant Creutzfeldt-Jakob disease, *Journal of Pathology*, **208** (2), 134–41.
19. Simon, J., Patel, A. & Sleed, M. (2005) The costs of alcoholism. *Journal of Mental Health*, **14** (4), 321–30.
20. Jenkis, R. (2005) *Substance Misuse in Young People*. WHO–UK Collaborating Centre. www.nelh.nhs.uk/mentalhealth (accessed 26/1/06).

21. Semple, D.M., McIntosh, A.M. & Lawrie, S.M. (2005) Cannabis as a risk factor for psychosis: a systematic review. *Journal of Psychopharmacology*, **19** (2), 187–94.
22. Centre for Suicide Research (2006) *Suicide in High Risk Occupational Groups – doctors.* www.cebmh.warne.ox.ac.uk/csr/resdoctors.html (accessed 26/1/06).

FURTHER READING

Duffy, D. & Ryan, T. (eds) (2004) *New Approaches to Preventing Suicide: a manual for practitioners.* Jessica Kingsley Publishers, London.
NICE Clinical Guidance:
   (2005) Violence, No. 25
   (2005) Post-traumatic Stress Disorder, No. 26
   (2005) Obsessive-Compulsive Disorder, No. 8
   (2005) Depression in Children and Young People, No. 28
   (2004) Depression: management of depression in primary and secondary care, No. 23
   (2004) Anxiety, No. 22
   (2004) Eating Disorders, No. 9
   (2002) Schizophrenia, No. 1
Royal College of Nursing (2005) *Managing Your Stress: a guide for nurses.* Royal College of Nursing, London.
Ryan, T. & Pritchard, J. (eds) (2004) *Good Practice in Adult Mental Health.* Jessica Kingsley Publishers, London.

USEFUL ADDRESSES AND WEBSITES

National Institute for Health and Clinical Excellence
Website: www.nice.org.uk

Royal College of Psychiatrists
Website: www.rcpsych.ac.uk

Mind (mental health charity)
Website: www.mind.org.uk

Mental Health Alliance
Website: www.mentalhealthalliance.org.uk

Mental Health Foundation
Website: www.mentalhealth.org.uk

Suzy Lamplugh Trust
Website: www.suzylamplugh.org.uk

Chapter 16
Supporting Patients with Chronic Diseases

The 1990 GP Contract gave an impetus to the involvement of practice nurses in chronic disease management and nurses have demonstrated their ability in this field. Asthma, diabetes and hypertension were the first conditions with which large numbers of practice nurses developed expertise, followed by chronic obstructive pulmonary disease (COPD) and coronary heart disease (CHD). The Quality and Outcome Framework (QoF) under the new GMS Contract has often resulted in a concentration on those clinical areas that attract payments for meeting the specified quality points. Coronary heart disease, stroke, TIAs, hypertension, diabetes, COPD, epilepsy, cancer, mental health, hypothyroidism and asthma are the clinical areas that attract quality points.

No single nurse can expect to be sufficiently knowledgeable in all these subjects but many practices now employ more than one nurse, so there is nothing to stop each of them from specialising in different fields. In addition, a new course has been designed to help health professionals. The Diploma in Chronic Disease Management is awarded by the Educational Alliance for Long Term Conditions – a collaboration between the National Respiratory Training Centre, Heartsave and Warwick Diabetes Care.

Computers can be set up with reminders of what needs to be done before the end of the financial year and templates can be used to enter the necessary data but the reasons for doing this work should not be overlooked. The intention is to improve the care of patients with chronic diseases and, where possible, to encourage them to take control of their own medical conditions. The National Service Framework for Long-term Conditions deals specifically with patients with neurological conditions but much of the guidance will apply to any patient with a chronic disease.

THE EXPERT PATIENT

Anybody living with a long-term condition is encouraged to take part in an expert patient programme to teach them to manage the effects of their disease. The six-week courses do not deal with clinical or treatment issues but help people to develop the confidence to manage their own condition with less reliance on healthcare professionals. Bilingual tutors will run some courses and there may be specialist courses for children and their parents. Teenagers could be a difficult group to attract. Pilot studies are under way.[1]

CLINICS IN GENERAL PRACTICE

Although the word clinic is used for convenience throughout this chapter, patients do not necessarily need to be seen at special clinic times; they may be seen during normal surgery hours. However, some sessions may be more convenient for the patients if arranged when other health professionals, such as a dietitian and chiropodist, are working in the practice. In some instances, depending on the degree of autonomy of the nurse, it may be preferable to have a doctor available during nurse-run clinics in case a medical examination, prescription or hospital referral is needed.

Any patient who attends a clinic at a GP surgery or health centre has a right to expect a uniformly high standard of service. The following points should be considered when writing the protocol or guidelines.

Aims

Aims for each clinic should be clear. Most clinics for chronic diseases will have similar aims.

- To help the patients and their families to understand the disease and take responsibility for its control
- To minimise the number of critical incidents
- To help the patients to lead as normal a life as possible
- To maximise the quality points achieved towards the QoF.

Target groups may be all the patients who are known to have or suspected of having a particular disease, for example all patients with asthma, or a subgroup, such as patients with type 2 diabetes.

Organisation

This will include:

- The amount of time to be allocated to each consultation
- The equipment, teaching aids and resources needed
- The record system to be used
- Education (in order to comply with the NMC Code of Professional Conduct and to ensure that a patient receives the best possible standard of service, a

nurse must have acquired the appropriate knowledge and skills before attempting to run a clinic)
- A disease register and call/recall system
- Clerical support, necessary for contacting the patients and making appointments, so the nurse's time is used most effectively
- Outcome (how the achievements of the clinic will be audited).

Protocols for nurse-run clinics

A protocol can be tailored to minimum, moderate or maximum nursing input, in accordance with the practice nurse's knowledge and experience. Each protocol should specify the procedure to be followed at first and subsequent clinic appointments (see Chapter 3 for discussion on protocols, guidelines and clinical pathways).

ASTHMA

Asthma is an inflammatory disease of the airways, characterised by narrowing of the bronchioles due to:

- Inflammation and swelling of the mucosa
- Dysfunction of the smooth muscle in the walls of the bronchioles
- Thick mucus secretion.

The condition is intermittent and reversible, either spontaneously or when the correct treatment is given.

Incidence

The incidence of asthma has been rising over the past decades, although the reasons are not fully understood. One in 12 adults and one in ten children are currently estimated to have asthma in the UK.[2] Therefore, in a practice with 8000 patients, up to 700 of them could be expected to have asthma. Children have the highest incidence of asthma but the condition can begin at any age. Three-quarters of children with asthma may grow out of it, but unfortunately about 50% of those who do grow out of it can expect to develop asthma again in later life.

Causes

The trigger factors that precipitate asthma can be allergic or non-allergic. Anyone could have an asthma attack if exposed to a large enough trigger factor.

People with asthma differ in having hyperreactive airways, which react to even small contact with triggers. Allergic triggers include house dust mites, pollen, moulds and spores, animal dander and chemicals. Non-allergic triggers can be exercise, upper respiratory tract infections, cold air, cigarette smoke and emotional stress. The common cold is a very common trigger factor.

The British Thoracic Society and the Scottish Intercollegiate Guidelines Network (SIGN) have issued a revised national guideline on the management of asthma.[3] It is only available in electronic format but any nurse who deals with patients with asthma must be able to access the document.

Diagnosis

The diagnosis is likely to be more difficult in young children because they are unable to perform lung function tests such as peak flow recordings. Young children are prone to viral respiratory infections and wheezing is a common factor.

Tests that may be used to confirm the clinical diagnosis of asthma in adults include the following.

- Home monitoring of peak expiratory flow rate (PEFR) – a diary of readings can be kept. Readings that show more than a 20% diurnal variation on at least three days for two weeks are diagnostic of asthma.
- Reversibility test – perform spirometry and record FEV_1. Administer a short-acting bronchodilator – either two puffs salbutamol through a large-volume spacer or 250 mcg via a nebuliser. Repeat spirometry after 20 minutes. More than 15% (or 200 ml) increase in FEV_1 is diagnostic of asthma.
- Steroid reversibility test – spirometry should be recorded before and after a course of oral steroids. Oral prednisone 0.5 mg.kg for 8 days may be prescribed.[4] More than 15% (or 200 ml) increase in FEV_1 is diagnostic of asthma.
- Exercise tolerance test – this test is not often performed in general practice because of the risk of precipitating a severe asthma attack. The FEV_1 is recorded prior to six minutes of running. More than 15% decrease in FEV_1 is diagnostic of asthma.

Asthma treatments (see *British National Formulary*)

The aim of treatment is to suppress the bronchial hyperreactivity and the key to good control lies in concordance with the treatment. A patient who feels fit and well may be reluctant to continue with preventive therapy unless its importance is fully appreciated. Treatment is instituted at the step in the asthma guidelines considered necessary to control the asthma symptoms. Treatment at a higher or lower step should be given in accordance with the response. The patient's concordance and inhaler technique should be checked before any increase in treatment for poor control.

Short-acting bronchodilators

The commonly used drugs in this field are the short-acting beta$_2$ agonists salbutamol (*Ventolin*) and terbutaline (*Bricanyl*), which act mainly by relaxing bronchial smooth muscle, thus relieving bronchoconstriction. For this reason, bronchodilators are called 'reliever' drugs. They should be prescribed for use as needed, not as a regular dose. A spacer device, with a mask if necessary, should be used to administer the drug to children.

Corticosteroids

Patients who need to use a reliever drug three times a week or more usually require inhaled steroids to deal with the inflammation of the bronchial mucosa, e.g. beclomethasone dipropionate, budesonide or fluticasone. Patients may have confused ideas about steroids and be reluctant to use them long term. It is important to explain their action as 'preventers' and to ensure that patients know how to use them. Fungal infections of the mouth and throat are possible side effects. Patients can be advised to rinse the mouth after using the steroid inhaler. Children under five years and patients on high-dose steroids should use a large-volume spacer for steroid inhalations. Children on long-term inhaled corticosteroid treatment should have their growth measured regularly.[5]

A short course of oral steroids may be prescribed as treatment for acute asthma. Occasionally patients require daily doses of oral steroids to control chronic asthma symptoms. Patients on maintenance therapy should be given a steroid card to carry and be warned not to stop the drugs suddenly.

Add-on drugs

Any of the following additional drugs may be prescribed when asthma symptoms are not adequately controlled.

- Long-acting beta$_2$ agonists (LABA), e.g. formoterol and salmeterol, may be useful in some cases for night-time and exercise-induced asthma. They should not be used as a 'reliever' drug and should be used in conjunction with inhaled corticosteroids.
- Leukotriene receptor antagonists – montelukast and zafirlukast.
- Slow-release preparations of theophylline (*Slo-Phyllin, Uniphyllin Continus*) are bronchodilators that can be used to relieve nocturnal or early-morning asthma. The dose has to be carefully adjusted for each patient and the same brand of modified-release drugs should be ordered each time. Generic prescribing is not appropriate for these drugs. Regular blood tests are needed to maintain therapeutic drug levels.
- Cromones – sodium cromoglycate for adults, nedocromil sodium for children. Can be useful in allergic asthma.
- Oral modified-release long-acting beta$_2$ agonists. Caution is needed if the patient is already using a LABA inhaler.

Inhaler devices

These include the following.

- Pressurised metered dose inhalers (with or without spacer devices)
- Breath-actuated inhalers
- Dry powder devices.

Nurses should be familiar with the way all inhaler devices work. The NRTC sells a helpful video recording, *Devices in Detail*, which explains each system and how to teach patients to use them. Sales representatives will supply placebo inhalers for teaching purposes.

Asthma clinic

Nurse education

The National Respiratory Training Centre (NRTC) organises training for primary and secondary care nurses. The name and scope of the organisation have changed over the years. It began in 1986, in a small house in Stratford-upon-Avon, as the National Asthma Training Centre, later expanded into the National Asthma and Respiratory Training Centre, with larger premises in Warwick and then logically adopted its new name in 2001. Since then, the NRTC has joined forces with Heartsave as a single organisation called Education for Health. Both organisations still have their own websites.

The NRTC provides distance-learning modules at diploma and degree level in all aspects of respiratory diseases; 240 credits are needed for a diploma and 360 credits for a BSc (Honours) degree. The courses are validated by the Open University. Many practice nurses have studied for the NRTC Asthma Diploma, which is recommended as a minimum qualification for anyone who runs an asthma clinic.

Equipment

The equipment needed includes:

- Weighing scales and height chart
- Spirometer
- Peak flow meters (see Chapter 6 for discussion on EU scale and digital meters)
- Disposable mouthpieces for adults and children
- Spirometry and PEFR prediction calculator or charts, if not available on the computer
- Bronchodilator and spacer or nebuliser for reversibility tests
- Placebo inhalers for teaching inhaler techniques
- Blank asthma care plans
- Explanatory booklets for adults and children
- Instruction leaflets, diagrams and peak flow diaries
- Information about voluntary organisations and other services.

The practice computer may have an asthma clinic template. Many of the asthma drug companies provide useful materials for nurses and patients. Primary care organisations usually have guidelines for working with the pharmaceutical industry to ensure that undue pressure is not applied to promote particular products. Asthma UK funds asthma research, supplies literature and runs the Asthma Helpline telephone service. Information about asthma can also be obtained via the internet. The NRTC sells a range of literature and teaching aids.

Protocol

The amount of involvement in asthma management by a practice nurse will be governed by her/his knowledge and skills in this field. The protocol should specify how many of the following procedures will be undertaken by the nurse.

Procedure for a first consultation

For a patient with suspected or newly diagnosed asthma the following guidelines apply.

History

- Past medical history – including allergies or eczema
- Asthma history – age at onset, trigger factors, symptoms and treatments used
- Family history – including atopic conditions
- Social history – smoking and exercise, occupation and any relationship of the asthma to work
- Current medication – are inhalers used?

Tests and examination

- General health assessment, to identify any risk factors and establish a baseline (include BP, height, weight and urinalysis). Steroids can affect growth in children and precipitate diabetes in some patients.
- Peak expiratory flow rate (see Chapter 6). Compare with the predicted PEFR.
- Diagnostic tests (if asthma is not yet confirmed).

Asthma management and education

- Discussing the factors that may affect the asthma most.
- Encouraging smoking cessation, if applicable.
- Explaining the nature of asthma so that the patient can comprehend. Parents of children with asthma can have their lives severely disrupted. They need a chance to talk about their anxieties and to learn as much as possible about asthma. Asthma storybooks can be used for small children.

- Teaching the patient how to monitor and record his/her peak flow at home, if necessary and if the patient is able to use a peak flow meter.
- Explaining how the treatment works and how and when to use it.
- Identifying the trigger factors to be avoided.
- Inhaler technique – helping the patient or parent to select the most suitable device and teaching them how to use it.
- Providing a written asthma plan and ensuring that patients and parents understand the signs of worsening asthma and know what to do.
- Providing information about the voluntary societies.
- Offering immunisation against influenza (see Chapter 10).

Procedure for subsequent visits

Monitor progress using the following guidelines.

- Discuss the asthma diary and any significant entries.
- Discuss other lifestyle factors, e.g. smoking.
- Enquire about any work or schooling missed.
- Discuss any problems with the medication.
- Check the PEFR or FEV_1 and compare with the predicted or best-ever reading.
- Check the patient's inhaler technique, re-teach if necessary or consider an alternative delivery system. Give praise generously when it is due.
- Ask the patient or parent to explain what he/she understands about asthma and its treatment. Gently correct any misunderstandings. It is important to be sure that the patient really has understood. What seems very basic physiology to a nurse may be quite incomprehensible to a layperson.
- Check that the patient has a written self-management plan and knows what to do in given circumstances. Examples of action plans can be found on the Prodigy and National Asthma Campaign websites.

Records

Records need to be kept for several reasons. Patients who are able to do so, should keep their own asthma diaries of peak flow and symptoms. Computer records can make audit easier. The nurse's records must be kept in accordance with the NMC guidelines for Standards of Records and Record Keeping (see Chapter 2).

Audit

- Statistics can be collated about the number of patients on the asthma register, the percentage who attended a clinic in the past year and how many are receiving prophylactic therapy. Information will be needed on the achievement of the quality indicator points for the Quality and Outcomes Framework.

- The number and cost of repeat prescriptions for inhalers can be monitored: if requests are too frequent or infrequent, then patients may not be using their inhalers correctly or the treatment needs to be reviewed.
- Emergency hospital admissions or treatments for asthma can be analysed to see if they could have been prevented by better asthma management.

Anonymous questionnaires can help in discovering how many patients have asthma symptoms and how well they use the treatment. Patient satisfaction questionnaires will show whether services for patients with asthma need to be improved.

CHRONIC OBSTRUCTIVE PULMONARY DISEASE (COPD)

About 24 000 people died from COPD in 2002, as opposed to the 1400 people who died from asthma.[6,7] Yet only in the past decade has COPD begun to receive the same sort of attention as asthma. This could be because asthma often affects younger people and usually responds well to therapy and/or because COPD is closely linked with smoking, so the disease may be considered to be self-inflicted; also because treatment outcomes are often less certain. As yet, there is no National Service Framework on respiratory conditions but COPD is included in the Quality and Outcomes Framework of the nGMS Contract. All patients diagnosed with COPD should be on that disease register and be reviewed regularly.

The National Respiratory Training Centre runs a level 2 distance-learning module on COPD. The NHS Plan in the year 2000 expressed the intention to step up smoking cessation services and primary care organisations made help for smokers a priority in health improvement programmes around the country. NICE guidance on COPD was published in 2004.[8]

COPD is the term used for airflow obstruction, usually caused by chronic bronchitis and emphysema. It is a slowly progressive disorder of respiration, which commonly develops in later life. Smoking is the single most important cause, although not all smokers develop COPD. The symptoms of breathlessness, cough and increased sputum gradually affect the ability to perform the normal activities of daily living. The possibility of lung cancer should not be ruled out in patients with worsening symptoms. Chronic asthma can also result in COPD.

Chronic bronchitis

Chronic bronchitis is characterised by excessive mucus production – the 'smoker's cough'. Acute exacerbations, with infected sputum requiring antibiotics, are more common in the winter months, although not all exacerbations are caused by infection; there may be an increased airflow obstruction causing dyspnoea and wheeze.

Emphysema

The airspaces at the end of the terminal bronchioles become enlarged and their walls are destroyed, leaving less surface area for the exchange of gases. Destruction of lung tissue also decreases the elasticity of the lungs. This in turn leads to airway collapse, particularly during expiration. There is a reduction in airflow and the lungs may become overinflated. Breathlessness on exertion is a common symptom of this condition. The inelastic and overinflated lungs make inspiration more difficult for the patient. The inspiratory muscles become exhausted and inefficient.

Clinical signs may not be obvious in the earlier stages of COPD but as the disease progresses, the oxygenation of the blood can be affected. Compensation in the form of an increased red cell count causes increased viscosity of the blood, which carries the added risk of deep vein thrombosis and pulmonary embolism. Severe hypoxia causes cyanosis and mental confusion. Right heart failure develops as a result of pulmonary hypertension in COPD. The pulmonary capillaries become constricted and oxygenation of the blood is impaired. The right ventricle becomes hypertrophied from trying to pump blood through the damaged lungs and eventually fails, leading in turn to an increased systemic venous pressure and peripheral oedema. Respiratory failure may occur eventually.

Care is needed with oxygen therapy because the respiratory centre can sometimes be depressed further by oxygen. Hypoxia can become the stimulus to respiration in some people with COPD, rather than the build-up of carbon dioxide, which is the normal respiratory stimulus.

Diagnosis of COPD

The diagnosis should be made clinically in the light of the medical history and physical examination. All health professionals who assess and manage patients with COPD must have access to a reliable spirometer and have been trained how to interpret the results. Spirometry is the most important test of lung function. A forced expiratory volume in one second (FEV_1) of less than 80% of that predicted for that patient and a ratio of FEV_1 to forced vital capacity (FVC) of less than 0.7 will confirm airflow obstruction.

Routine reversibility testing is not recommended in the NICE guidance but there is a discrepancy with the quality indicators of the QoF. Reversibility testing for patients diagnosed after 1/4/2003 is a requirement and the diagnostic FEV_1 for COPD is less than 70% of the predicted level, instead of 80%. Patients who demonstrate reversibility should be placed on the asthma register. It is recognised that there is an element of reversibility in patients with COPD but the definition centres on a lack of reversibility.[9]

Treatment (see *British National Formulary*)

The aims of the early recognition and management of COPD are to:

- Alleviate the symptoms
- Prevent the more severe complications of the condition
- Improve the patient's quality of life
- Prevent premature death.

Smoking cessation (see Chapter 9)

Lung function reduces naturally with age and smoking can accelerate the rate of decline. The damage caused by smoking cannot be reversed but the rate of decline can be slowed significantly; hence the enthusiasm for helping people to quit smoking.

Bronchodilators

A short-acting $beta_2$ agonist or an anticholinergic may give a significant improvement in symptoms, even if the patient has a very limited degree of reversibility. A bronchodilator trial over 3–4 weeks is recommended. There is some evidence that the combination of a $beta_2$ agonist with an anticholinergic is more effective than either given singly.[10] Long-acting bronchodilators should be prescribed if a patient's symptoms persist.

Corticosteroids

The NICE guidelines for COPD recommend an inhaled steroid combined with a long-acting bronchodilator for symptomatic patients with moderate or severe COPD.

Therapy should be stopped after a reasonable trial if it is ineffective.

Pulmonary rehabilitation

A rehabilitation programme may help some patients with COPD. Physiotherapists can teach appropriate exercises to maximise lung function and retain mobility; occupational therapists can help with adaptations to the home and advise about ways to manage everyday activities. Local respiratory support groups may help patients to maintain the progress made through rehabilitation and reduce social isolation. A practice nurse needs to have information about the national and local services for patients with respiratory conditions.

The role of the practice nurse

The role of practice nurses in COPD will depend on the education and experience of each nurse. Where a practice owns a spirometer, the practice nurse should have training in how to use it. The NRTC trainers run spirometry essential skills workshops. Many patients with COPD may be wrongly diagnosed as having asthma. For this reason it might be better to run a combined respiratory clinic in general practice, although the diseases are separated in this chapter for convenience.

COPD clinic

Organisation

- Disease register of patients with COPD
- Call and recall system for appointments
- Recall system for annual influenza immunisation
- Spirometer and disposable mouthpieces
- Placebo inhalers
- Materials for teaching
- Appropriate record system.

Clinic procedure

- General health and respiratory history
- Spirometry
- Bronchodilator reversibility testing or possible steroid trial
- Smoking cessation advice and support (see Chapter 9)
- Pneumococcal immunisation
- Treatment as appropriate
- Referral as appropriate.

Outcomes

- Percentage of patients on the register who attended a COPD clinic in a year
- Improvements in lung function and/or quality of life in patients with COPD
- Number of patients who successfully stopped smoking
- Patient satisfaction with the service
- Number of emergency admissions with COPD.

Some of the data may be statistical, while other information, such as patient satisfaction or sense of wellbeing, will be more subjective. Both types of information can be used to demonstrate the value of a clinic. A reduction in the number of emergency admissions could demonstrate that the management of COPD is effective.

DIABETES MELLITUS

A practice with 8000 patients can expect to have about 160 known diabetic patients, but there may be almost as many again who are undiagnosed, hence the need for screening. The UK national average is between 2% and 3% of the population. Diabetes is a chronic metabolic condition caused by a deficiency of insulin, or resistance to its effect, classified as follows.

- Type 1 diabetes mellitus (previously called insulin-dependent diabetes). This is due to the destruction of beta cells in the pancreatic islets of Langerhans, resulting in the loss of insulin production. Children and adults under the age of 40 years are most commonly affected. The treatment is by regular injections of insulin. The aim is to maintain blood glucose levels as near to normal as possible.
- Type 2 diabetes (previously called non-insulin dependent diabetes or maturity-onset diabetes) results from either diminished insulin secretion or an increased peripheral resistance to the action of insulin. The cause is still uncertain. It usually occurs in later life and is often associated with obesity or a family history of diabetes. A recent phenomenon has been the increase of this form of diabetes in children.[11] Patients of Asian or Afro-Caribbean origin are known to be more susceptible to developing this condition. Women with a history of gestational diabetes are also in the risk group. The treatment may be by diet and exercise alone, or diet, exercise and hypoglycaemic drugs. Type 2 diabetes is not a mild form of the disease; the complications can be just as serious as those of type 1 diabetes so good metabolic control is equally important.

Diagnosis

A practice nurse might be the first person to discover that a patient has diabetes, either during routine screening or because the patient has particular risk factors or symptoms. Anyone complaining of thirst, polyuria or nocturia, who has recurrent boils or fungal infections, tiredness, paraesthesia, visual changes or ischaemic problems should be tested. A random blood glucose >11.1 mmol/l or a fasting glucose >7 mmol/l is indicative of diabetes.[12] The patient will need to be referred to the GP and the education process should be started. In some cases a glucose tolerance test may be needed to confirm the diagnosis.

Patients with type 1 diabetes are often referred to a diabetologist but the practice/PCO policy should determine which groups of patients are referred. Many practices now take full responsibility for the care of patients with type 2 diabetes. Diabetes care is included in the QoF and data need to be supplied to the practice when patients have tests and screening done at the hospital. Shared care between the hospital and the practice diabetic clinic can be a good way to make use of valuable resources and provide a consistently high level of service. The National Service Framework for Diabetes sets out standards for diabetes prevention, diagnosis and care. People with diabetes are encouraged to become expert patients and to take responsibility for managing their disease. Health professionals have to rethink their role and work in partnership with patients.

Initial patient education

Most patients will be shocked by the diagnosis of diabetes and will not retain very much information initially. A straightforward explanation about the condition can be backed up by written information to be read at home. The patient should be given verbal and written information on healthy eating and an appointment to see the dietitian. Special diet foods are not necessary. Healthy food for someone with diabetes is the same as healthy food for everyone else. The advice to patients should cover the following points.

- Eat regular meals containing starchy foods, e.g. potatoes, bread, cereals (foods high in fibre take longer to digest, so do not increase the blood sugar as much as rapidly digested refined carbohydrates)
- Have fewer sugary foods or drinks. Use sugar-reduced products instead
- Eat only small amounts of fried or fatty foods. Use reduced-fat products and skimmed or semi-skimmed milk
- Eat at least five portions of fruit and vegetables a day
- Use only a small amount of salt (to help avoid high blood pressure)
- Drink alcohol in moderation and avoid drinking on an empty stomach (alcohol can lower the blood glucose level).

Patients with polydipsia may have been compounding the problem by drinking large amounts of lemonade or sweetened fruit juice and squashes, in an attempt to quench their thirst, before the diagnosis of diabetes was made. A high blood glucose can also affect the lens of the eye, resulting in blurred vision. Patients should be advised not to buy new glasses until the diabetes has been controlled and reasonable glycaemic levels attained.

The patient should be offered another appointment as soon as possible after diagnosis for education about the nature of the condition and how to manage it. This should include:

- Reinforcement of the information about the nature of diabetes and how good glycaemic control can reduce the risk of complications
- Advice about healthy living (smoking, alcohol and exercise)
- The need to attain or maintain a normal body weight
- How to monitor and record blood glucose levels (diabetes is a life-long condition, which the patient needs to understand and take control of)
- The importance of a regular health check and an annual medical review and eye screening
- The importance of foot care
- Information about Diabetes UK, previously the British Diabetic Association (membership gives patients access to a lot of helpful information and

support). Diabetes UK also has a professional membership section, which anyone running a diabetic clinic would find useful.

Treatment

Diet

See above for general advice. A dietitian will make a full dietary assessment for each patient and advise accordingly.

Oral hypoglycaemic agents

Oral hypoglycaemic preparations may be prescribed once it has been shown that diet and exercise alone do not control the blood sugar level. NICE guidance has been published on the management of diabetes.[13]

Sulphonylurea drugs

Drugs such as glibenclamide, gliclazide, glipizide and tolbutamide act by stimulating the remaining insulin-secreting cells to perform more efficiently. All these drugs can cause weight gain and are therefore not the first choice for clinically obese patients.

Biguanides

Metformin acts by increasing the peripheral uptake of glucose. It can be added to the sulphonylurea treatment or used instead of it.

Glitazones

Rosiglitazone and pioglitazone act by reducing the peripheral resistance to insulin. The most recent NICE guidelines recommend that they are not used alone but as triple therapy in combination with metformin and a sulphonylurea drug or in combination with insulin. The exceptions are patients who cannot take a combination of metformin and a sulphonylurea, or if either is contraindicated.[14]

Other antidiabetic drugs

Acarbose may be used to delay carbohydrate absorption.

Insulin

This has to be administered parenterally because, being a protein, it would be digested if given orally. There are many different types of insulin, classified either according to their speed of action, or their source.

- Short-, medium- and long-acting insulins can be obtained individually or in various combinations.
- Insulins derived from pork or beef pancreas, or synthetically produced human insulins.

A patient's religious beliefs must be taken into account when prescribing insulin. Jewish and Muslim people cannot use porcine insulin and Hindus are forbidden to use insulin derived from beef.

Good glucose control has been said to reduce the risk of complications from diabetes.[15] However, the tighter the control, the greater is the risk of hypoglycaemia. Patients and the people close to them need to recognise the signs and symptoms of hypoglycaemia and know what action to take if it occurs.

Diabetic clinics

Practice nurse education

Nurses who run diabetic clinics should have adequate training. Information can be found on the internet about courses available. Warwick Diabetes Care run distance-learning courses that provide a sound grounding and qualification at certificate, diploma and degree levels. Diabetes nurse specialists often run updating sessions for practice nurses and will advise on setting up nurse-led diabetic clinics.

Resources

Diabetes UK has published guidelines for the management of diabetes in primary care.[16] Blood glucose monitoring is one important aspect of diabetes care, so it is essential that all healthcare professionals engaged in blood glucose monitoring have been trained adequately and understand how to use specific blood glucose meters correctly. Meters must be suitable for clinical use and be calibrated with each new batch of test strips. Appropriate quality control measures must be taken for each machine. Disposable finger-pricking devices should be used in a practice setting, to prevent the transmission of blood-borne diseases.

Services

There should be arrangements for prompt access to a dietitian and chiropodist. Local social services or district nursing may be required for patients with any disabilities associated with diabetes. All patients require an ophthalmic examination and retinal screening annually. Patients with severe visual problems may need to be referred to the social services sensory impairment team. Anyone with impaired mobility may require an occupational therapy assessment. Diabetes UK has information on its website telling patients of their rights and responsibilities and what diabetes care to expect from the NHS. Special holidays can be arranged to teach children how to lead a normal life with diabetes.

Procedure for initial consultations

A practice nurse will carry out the tests and investigations specified in the protocol. Apart from the immediate symptoms and reason for the consultation, the initial assessment should cover the following areas.

Social history

- Home situation and family support available.
- Lifestyle factors, such as smoking, alcohol consumption, diet and exercise.
- Occupation and driving – type 1 diabetes may preclude some occupations, such as driving heavy goods or public service vehicles. The licensing centre at Swansea must be notified about the diagnosis of diabetes and the motor insurers should also be informed.

Family history

Any history in the immediate family of diabetes, ischaemic conditions, eye problems or hypertension.

Medication

Ask about the contraceptive pill (female patients); a higher dose combined pill may be required if oral hypoglycaemic drugs are used.

Examination

Check the following.

- Weight, height and BMI – patients with type 1 diabetes may have lost weight. Patients with type 2 diabetes may be overweight.
- Urinalysis for:
  - Glucose
  - Protein
  - Ketones
  - Infection
  - Microalbuminuria.
- Blood pressure – because hypertension increases the risks for CHD and stroke. Hypertension may also be a sign of nephropathy. A postural drop may signify autonomic neuropathy.

- Feet – check the skin condition and circulation and need for chiropody. Peripheral neuropathy and microvascular damage can lead to gangrene if any traumatic lesions or ulcers are not detected early. Neuropathy testing and recording foot pulses are quality indicators for the QoF.
- Eyes – check visual acuity with spectacles, if worn. Patients must be referred for retinal screening annually.

Blood tests should include: full blood count, urea and electrolytes, serum creatinine, plasma glucose, liver function tests, fasting lipid profile, thyroid function tests.

Education for patients and management of diabetes

Discussions should take place to ensure that all the staff in general practice and the diabetic unit give consistent information and advice. The amount of information to be given at each visit needs to be judged carefully. More frequent appointments may be required during the initial period of adjustment. High-quality structured education has been shown to improve glycaemic control and reduce complications for patients with diabetes.[17]

- The patient and family need to understand the reasons for maintaining good blood sugar control, how to monitor the blood sugar levels and test the urine for ketones.
- Advice and information are needed on dietary management and lifestyle adjustments, such as dinner parties or business lunches. Stress the importance of not smoking and offer help to quit, if appropriate.
- A patient stabilised on insulin needs help to master the self-administration of injections and advice on care of the skin.
- Hypoglycaemia must be explained, so the patient knows how to recognise the symptoms and take appropriate action to raise the blood sugar level to normal limits.
- Patients must know what to do if they are ill (see Box 16.1).
- Preconceptual counselling and medical care during pregnancy are essential in order for patients to have a successful outcome of pregnancy.
- Ways of coping with travel might need to be discussed (see Chapter 11).
- A patient whose job is affected may need to be referred for specialist employment advice.
- Daily low-dose aspirin (75 mg) is recommended for patients aged over 30 in specified risk groups and who have a blood pressure between 130/80 and 150/90 mmHg, in order to reduce the risk of cardiovascular disease, providing they have no contraindications to aspirin.[18] One systematic review found insufficient evidence to define which patients with diabetes should be treated with aspirin.[19] Therefore the local protocol should be followed.

- Patients with a total cholesterol above 5 mmol/l should be offered lipid-lowering treatment.
- A care plan should be agreed with the patient.

Box 16.1   Sickness guidelines for diabetics

- Illness can increase the body's need for insulin so do not stop taking insulin or tablets
- Test blood glucose more often
- Test urine for ketones if using insulin
- Drink plenty of fluids
- Replace meals with drinks containing carbohydrates if unable to eat
- Contact your GP or diabetes nurse if not sure what to do or if the illness is getting worse

---

Procedure for a routine review

Blood and urine tests should be sent in advance of the appointment, so that the results are available for discussion. The following actions may be appropriate.

- Discuss the general health of the patient and any problems experienced, including psychological problems.
- Weigh the patient and encourage positive progress towards a normal BMI.
- Test urine for protein and ketones. Send an MSU if any proteinuria is present. Screen for microalbuminuria if applicable and not done already. Persistent microalbuminuria is a predictor for diabetic nephropathy.
- Take a blood sample of glycosylated haemoglobin to check the long-term blood sugar control (if not done already).
- Review the results of home blood or urine testing.
- Measure and record blood pressure. Levels of 130/80 mmHg or below are the ideal for people with diabetes. Aim for 120/80 if the patient has ischaemic heart disease or albuminuria. Treatment should be considered for patients with hypertension. The blood pressure should also be measured when the patient is standing, to detect orthostatic hypotension.
- Discuss any problems with the medication or diet.
- Check the feet.
- Discuss any sexual problems with male patients. Erectile dysfunction commonly occurs with diabetes.
- Assess the patient's understanding of diabetes and its management and review the care plan.
- Re-teach, as required, anything the patient is unsure about: the diet, blood glucose monitoring, urinalysis, foot care, insulin injections, hypoglycaemia or coping with illness.

Annual review

In addition to the routine review procedure, the annual review should cover the following.

- A full physical examination including any injection sites, neuropathy testing, peripheral pulses and fundi. Patients should be advised that they will be unable to drive for several hours after the pupils have been dilated for fundoscopy. The drops should not be used for patients who have glaucoma or a history of eye surgery. If fundoscopy is not undertaken in the practice, the patient can be examined free of charge by an ophthalmic optician.
- The diabetic control and treatment should be reviewed. (Blood tests for glucose, HbA$_1$c, lipids and creatinine can be taken beforehand, so that the results are ready for the review.)
- Assessment for complications. An early-morning urine specimen should be sent for albumin creatinine ratio (ACR) to test for diabetic nephropathy.

Records

The practice diabetes register must be kept up to date and the patients may also be entered in a district diabetes register. Patients should be encouraged to keep records of their home monitoring and treatment as well as a personal care plan. Patient-held shared care cards allow good communication between the hospital service and the practice. An entry should be made in the patient's records at each consultation.

Non-attenders need to be followed up and alternative arrangements suggested if the clinic times are unsuitable. The management of diabetes in teenagers can be challenging at times. Some teenagers need extra encouragement to take an active part in self-management. A chronic disease can lead to a degree of resistance at this age because the need for conformity with the peer group is so strong. Parents can feel torn between the need to protect their children and the need to allow them increasing independence, especially if the young people themselves are refusing to take a responsible attitude towards their disease. The natural anxiety for the welfare of their children can make some parents overprotective, thereby creating conflict in the home.

Assessing the success of the clinic

Statistics can be compiled about the patients with diabetes registered with the practice and be compared with the predicted number for the practice size. Details of clinic attendance, waiting times and non-attenders can be collated so that the service can be improved. Patient satisfaction surveys are carried out regularly as part of the nGMS Contract.

Clinical audit is undertaken in most practices, so that the attainment of quality points can be agreed. The National Diabetes Audit is one of the subjects supported by the National Clinical Audit Support Programme (NCASP) in order to help achieve the standards in the NSF for Diabetes.[20]

HYPERTENSION

High blood pressure increases the risk of heart disease and strokes and can cause particular problems for patients with diabetes. The pressure that the blood exerts on the artery walls is created in two main ways: by the cardiac output (the force of the blood expelled during systole) and the peripheral resistance (the calibre of the arterioles). The blood pressure is controlled centrally by the hypothalamus. Pressure receptors in the aorta and carotid arteries send stimuli to the vasomotor centre, which in turn controls the peripheral resistance via the autonomic nervous system. The cardiac centre controls the rate and contractility of the heart.

The kidneys, which require sufficient pressure for filtration, have their own system for raising the blood pressure if it is too low. Renin is secreted by cells near the glomeruli, which starts a chain reaction. As a result, angiotensin II increases the peripheral resistance by vasoconstriction and stimulates the adrenal cortex to secrete aldosterone, which increases the blood volume through the retention of sodium and water in the renal tubules.

No cause for the hypertension is usually found in 80% of patients with high blood pressure. This is known as primary or essential hypertension. There may be an inherited tendency but lifestyle factors also play a part. Secondary hypertension results from another medical condition – neurological, cardiac, renal or endocrine. Hypertension can be life threatening during pregnancy.

Diagnosis

Blood pressure increases naturally with age and in response to exercise or anxiety. The British Hypertension Society (BHS) has made recommendations for the treatment of patients with a persistently raised blood pressure.[21] The criteria are stricter for treating patients with diabetes or cardiovascular disease. No patient should be diagnosed as hypertensive on one isolated reading. The reading should usually be repeated on three separate occasions, after resting for at least ten minutes each time. Home monitoring or, preferably, 24-hour ambulatory blood pressure recording will be needed for patients with suspected 'white coat syndrome', where a patient's blood pressure is abnormally high when measured in the practice.

Treatment

Mild hypertension in patients without any cardiovascular system (CVS) or end-target disease might be managed by changes in lifestyle, such as increased exercise, reduced alcohol intake, healthy eating and weight loss if obese. Medical or surgical treatment may be possible for any condition causing secondary hypertension. Drug therapy is required to control more severe hypertension (see *BNF*). The drug treatments include the following.

- Thiazide diuretics, e.g. bendrofluazide 2.5 mg, may be used alone to control mild hypertension or in conjunction with other drugs.
- Beta blockers, e.g. atenolol or propranolol, lower blood pressure by reducing the cardiac activity and/or the peripheral resistance, depending on the selectivity of the drug used.
- Calcium channel blockers, e.g. nifedipine or diltiazem, prevent the influx of calcium ions across the membrane of smooth muscle and so reduce vasoconstriction. Some also affect the cardiac output by decreasing the myocardial contractility.
- Angiotensin-converting enzyme (ACE) inhibitors, e.g. captopril, enalapril or lisinopril, prevent the conversion of angiotensin I to angiotensin II in response to renin secretion, thus preventing peripheral vasoconstriction and aldosterone secretion.
- Angiotensin II receptor antagonists, e.g. losartan or valsartin, may be prescribed for patients who get a persistent dry cough with ACE inhibitors or for patients with type 2 diabetic nephropathy.
- Alpha blockers, e.g. doxazosin or terazocin, may be used to lower blood pressure in patients who also have benign prostatic enlargement.

Hypertension clinics

Nurse education

Training may be obtained through practice nurse courses or by distance learning. The British Hypertension Society has a distance-learning programme for nurses called Let's Do It Well. Details can be found on the BHS website. Heartsave, now part of Education for Health, runs one-day short courses and diploma-level courses on cardiovascular disease and heart failure. Completion of a course should equip the nurse with the necessary knowledge and skills to provide a high-quality service to patients, as well as providing evidence of the standard of learning achieved.

Equipment

Mercury sphygmomanometers are likely to be phased out in the near future because of the toxic effects of mercury. Replacement machines should meet and be maintained to the approved standards. Cuffs must be available in child, normal adult and large adult sizes. A thigh cuff is not suitable for an arm.

The following points should be considered while mercury sphygmomanometers are still being used.

- The rubber tubing and balloon should not be perished and the valve must be able to control the release of air at 2 mm a second
- The sphygmomanometer must be cleaned and maintained regularly
- Access to a mercury spillage kit is required in case of accidents (see Chapter 4).

Automatic digital blood pressure monitors are easy to use and can reduce observer bias, providing they are properly maintained. They are not likely to be reliable if the patient has a cardiac arrhythmia. The British Hypertension Society website has a list of validated blood pressure monitors. Many patients buy digital monitors for home use. This can be useful for encouraging them to take responsibility for their condition but the device used should be one validated by the BHS. Wrist devices are not recommended.

The hypertension protocol should be drawn up according to the knowledge and experience of the nurse.

Procedure for a first visit

The following information should be collected.

- Social history – including smoking, alcohol, diet, salt consumption, exercise, occupation and stress factors.
- Medical history – including asthma, diabetes, allergies, heart or kidney disease.
- Family history – including hypertension, CVS disease, diabetes and renal disease.

Make the following investigations.

- Blood pressure recordings – the patient should be seated and have rested for ten minutes. There should be no restrictive clothing around the arm.
- Height, weight and BMI – dietary advice is needed if the patient is overweight.
- Urinalysis – for protein.
- Blood tests:
  - Serum creatinine, urea and electrolytes for renal function
  - Fasting lipids to detect hyperlidaemia which increases risks for CVS disease
  - Fasting glucose to detect undiagnosed diabetes.
- Electrocardiogram to show any evidence of left ventricular hypertrophy.

Proceed according to the BP, investigation results and protocol. Discuss any lifestyle factors that can contribute to hypertension and negotiate any changes needed. These include:

- Weight reduction to achieve a normal BMI
- Increasing physical exercise

- Dietary changes – reducing salt and fat intake and eating at least five portions of fruit and vegetables a day
- Minimising alcohol consumption.

Smoking cessation is essential for patients with hypertension in order to reduce the risk of cardiovascular disease.

Patient education

The education of any patient with a medical condition requires good interpersonal skills. With hypertension in particular, dire warnings about strokes and heart attacks are more likely to be counterproductive. Anxiety about the reading can cause a significant rise in blood pressure; even a look of concentration on a nurse's face may alarm a patient. Patients with access to the internet may seek out their own information and wish to discuss it, but all patients will require suitable explanations and literature to back up any information given.

Agree a care plan with the patient and arrange a recall date.

Procedure for subsequent visits

Enquire about:

- Any changes in the patient's general health, lifestyle or social situation since the last visit. Review the patient's care plan
- Any side effects from the medication (if used), e.g. nausea, diarrhoea, giddiness, lassitude, faintness, erectile dysfunction, cold extremities
- Has the patient been taking the drugs (if prescribed)?

Investigations should include:

- Blood pressure – take two readings and calculate the mean pressure
- Blood tests according to the protocol and any medication used
- Weight and recalculation of the BMI
- Pulse rate (if beta blockers used).

The nurse must know the blood pressure levels at which he/she is expected to refer the patient back to the doctor.

Health promotion should include the following.

- Check the patient's understanding of hypertension and any treatment prescribed. Correct any misunderstandings and make sure that the patient is aware of the need to report any side effects and not to stop the medication suddenly.
- Encourage the continuation of appropriate lifestyle changes.

Records

Computer records are most commonly used. A patient-held card is useful if a patient is also being treated at a hospital. It can be infuriating when a patient with well-controlled hypertension has his/her treatment discontinued in hospital because the blood pressure is found to be normal.

Recall

The frequency of appointments will depend on the degree of hypertension and its control. The recall system should be able to identify non-attenders, so they do not slip through the net. All adults should have blood pressure measured at least once every five years and annual checks are recommended for those with any history of blood pressure outside the normal range or other risk factors for CVS disease. The hypertension guidelines include hypertension in the elderly, under Special Patient Groups. Hypertension is common in older people but several measurements are needed because they can show a greater BP variability. BP should be measured when the patient is seated and standing because orthostatic hypotension is common in this age group. Medical decisions on initiating treatment for hypertension in patients over 80 years should be based on the presence of other co-morbidities.[22]

Audit

In addition to the clinic statistics and QoF targets, an audit may cover:

- The amount by which patients' blood pressures are reduced. The BHS audit standards for BP levels in the surgery are <150/90 in non-diabetic patients and <140/85 in patients with diabetes. Targets for both systolic and diastolic readings should be reached. Lower target blood pressores should be reached wherever possible
- The incidence of heart attack and stroke in hypertensive patients, with a comparison between those who did and did not attend the hypertension clinic
- The incidence of side effects with antihypertensive drugs.

CORONARY HEART DISEASE (CHD)

The National Service Framework for Coronary Heart Disease sets out 12 standards for the prevention, diagnosis and treatment of CHD. Some of these standards apply to society in general and others to hospital and the emergency services. However, practice nurses should be aware of the specific standards that involve primary care, as follows.

- Reducing heart disease in the population by reducing risk factors and inequalities and by increasing the number of ex-smokers.
- Identifying people with established cardiovascular disease and offering secondary prevention measures.
- Primary prevention of CHD by targeting people at risk and offering appropriate advice and treatment.
- Aspirin to be given to people thought to be having a heart attack and thrombolysis within one hour of calling for professional help.
- People with symptoms of angina to receive appropriate investigations and treatment.
- Patients with suspected heart failure to receive appropriate investigations and treatment.
- Patients admitted with CHD to be offered cardiac rehabilitation and secondary prevention to reduce the risk of further cardiac problems and to help them return to a normal life.[23]

Practices are required to maintain a working CHD register and to work to a protocol for the assessment, treatment and follow-up of patients with cardiovascular disease. Annual audit data are required to demonstrate the achievement of the goals of the NSF and the QoF.

Cardiovascular disease is yet another field in which practice nurses are proving their ability. Specialist nurses have been employed by many primary care organisations to help general practices comply with the standards of the NSF. Many of these nurses organise teaching sessions for the practices and will provide support to practice nurses in setting up CVD clinics within their own surgeries.

Primary healthcare team members can undertake distance-learning courses. The DTC Primary Care Training Centre runs a programme accredited by Huddersfield University, which can be satellited if enough people wish to take the course within a locality. The British Heart Foundation Heartsave programme is another distance-learning course that gives an excellent education in all aspects of heart disease.

CONCLUSION

Whatever practice nurses undertake in the field of health promotion for patients with chronic diseases, the requirement to produce evidence of its worth remains the same. In fact, the greater the number of opportunities for nurse involvement, the greater the need to use the scarce resources most effectively. This means ensuring that the aims of the clinics are being fulfilled and being able to demonstrate their effectiveness. The practice nurse journals regularly feature inspirational articles by experienced practice nurses, which demonstrate how nurses have improved the health and welfare of their patients.

Traditional management of chronic diseases has changed with the advent of expert patients. The Department of Health has published its vision for the future of chronic disease management through the NICE guidance, NSFs and the quality indicators in the new General Medical Services contract. Yet the role of practice nurses working with patients with chronic conditions has always had this precise intention of helping patients to take control and to self-manage their diseases.

Suggestions for reflection on practice

- Are you able to provide a high-quality chronic disease management service in your practice?
- What further education or resources do you need?
- How do you know whether you are meeting the needs of your patients?

REFERENCES

1. NHS Expert Patient Programmes (2005) *Report on the EPP Pilot Course for Children.* www.expertpatients.nhs.uk/publications.aspx (accessed 27/1/06).
2. Asthma UK Factfile (2004) *The Asthma Audit.* www.asthma.org.uk/about/factsheet18.php (accessed 27/1/06).
3. BTS and SIGN (2005) *British Guideline on the Management of Asthma.* www.sign.ac.uk/pdf/sign63.pdf (accessed 27/1/06).
4. International Union Against Tuberculosis and Lung Disease (2005) *Management of Asthma: a guide to the essentials of good clinical practice,* 2nd edn. www.iuatld.org/pdf/final_asthma_guide_12-02-05.pdf.
5. Prodigy Guidance (2005) *Asthma.* www.prodigy.nhs.uk/guidance.asp?gt=Asthma (accessed 28/1/06).
6. Asthma UK (2004) *Where Do We Stand? Asthma in the UK today.* www.asthma.org.uk/about/pdf/wheredowestand.pdf (accessed 28/1/06).
7. Action on Smoking and Health (2004) *Factsheet No.5 Smoking and Respiratory Disease.* www.ash.org.uk/html/factsheets/html/fact05.html (accessed 28/1/06).
8. National Institute for Clinical Excellence (2004) *Chronic Obstructive Airways Disease. Management of chronic obstructive airways disease in adults in primary and secondary care.* Clinical Guideline No. 12. National Institute for Clinical Excellence, London.
9. Department of Health (2004) *Quality and Outcomes Framework Guidance – August 2004.* www.dh.gov.uk/assetRoot/04/08/86/94/04088694.pdf.
10. Donohoe, J.F. (2005) Combination therapy for chronic obstructive pulmonary disease: clinical aspects. *Proceedings of the American Thoracic Society,* **2** (4), 272–81.
11. Diabetes UK (2005) *Obesity Sends Type 2 Diabetes Rates in Children Soaring.* www.diabetes.org.uk/news/apr05/Type2.htm (accessed 28/1/06).
12. World Health Organisation (1999) *Definition, Diagnosis and Classification of Diabetes Mellitus and its Complications: report of a WHO consultation.* World Health Organisation, Department of Noncommunicable Disease Surveillance, Geneva.
13. National Institute for Clinical Excellence (2005) *Published Guidelines and Cancer Service Guidelines.* www.nice.org.uk/page.aspx?o=guidelines.completed (accessed 28/1/06).

14. National Institute for Clinical Excellence (2003) *Technology Appraisal No 63. Glitazones in the treatment of type 2 diabetes (review of current guidance no. 9 and no. 21).* www.nice.org.uk/page.aspx?0=83263 (accessed 28/1/06).

15. Diabetes UK (2006) *Blood Glucose Targets.* www.diabetes.org.uk/infocentre/inform/targets.htm (accessed 28/1/06).

16. Diabetes UK (2003) *Good Practice in Diabetes Care.* www.diabetes.org.uk/good_practice/index.html (accessed 29/1/06).

17. Lucas, S. (2005) *Structured Education. Factsheet No 39.* www.diabetes.org.uk/update/winter05/downloads/Factsheet.pdf (accessed 28/1/06).

18. Diabetes UK (2001) *Care Recommendation. Aspirin treatment in diabetes.* Diabetes UK, London.

19. Sigal, R., Malcolm, J. & Meggison, H. (2003) *Prevention of Cardiovascular Events in Diabetes. Prophylactic aspirin. Clinical Evidence.* www.clinicalevidence.com/ceweb/conditions/dia/0601/0601+15.jsp (accessed 29/1/06).

20. National Clinical Audit Support Programme (2006) *About National Clinical Audits.* www.icservices.nhs.uk/ncasp/ (accessed 29/1/06).

21. Wiliams, B., Poulter, T.M., Brown, M.J., Davis, M., McInnes, G.T., Potter, J.F., Sever, P.S. & Thom, S.McG. (2004) Guidelines for management of hypertension: report of the fourth working party of the British Hypertension Society. *Journal of Human Hypertension,* **18**, 139–85.

22. British Hypertension Society (2004) Guidelines for management of hypertension. Hypertension in the elderly. *Journal of Human Hypertension,* **18**, 161.

23. Department of Health (2000) *National Service Framework for Coronary Heart Disease – modern standards and service models.* Department of Health, London.

FURTHER READING

Department of Health (2000) *National Service Framework for Coronary Heart Disease – modern standards and service models.* Department of Health, London.

Department of Health (2001) *The Expert Patient: a new approach to chronic disease management for the 21st century.* Department of Health, London.

Department of Health (2005) *National Service Framework for Long-term Conditions.* Department of Health, London.

Price, D.B., Freeman, D., Foster, J. & Scullion, J. (2003) *Asthma and COPD (In Clinical Practice).* Churchill Livingstone, Edinburgh.

USEFUL ADDRESSES AND WEBSITES

Education for Health (Incorporating NRTC and Heartsave), The Athenaeum, 10 Church Street, Warwick CV34 4AB
Telephone: 01926 493313
Website: www.educationforhealth.org.uk

Asthma UK, 70 Wilton Street, London EC2A 2DB
Telephone: 020 7786 5000
Website: www.asthma.org.uk

British Thoracic Society
Website: www.brit-thoracic.org.uk

Diabetes UK (Central Office),
10 Queen Anne Street, London W1G 9LH
Telephone: 020 7323 1531
Website: www.diabetes.org.uk

British Hypertension Society
Website: www.bhsoc.org

British Heart Foundation,
14 Fitzhardinge Street, London W1H 6DH
Heart Information Line: 08450 70 80 70
Website: www.bhf.org.uk

DTC Primary Care Training Centre,
Crow Trees, 27 Town Lane, Idle, Bradford BD10 8NT
Telephone: 01274 617617
Website: www.primarycaretraining.co.uk

Appendix 1
Examples of the Clinical Equipment Needed in the Nurses' Rooms

EXAMINATION EQUIPMENT

Examination couch, paper rolls, pillow, waterproof protective pillow covers
Directable, heat-filtered lamp
Accurate weighing scales, height measure and body mass index chart
Sphygmomanometer
Stethoscope
Ear thermometer and disposable probe covers
Otoscope with disposable aural specula
Pen-torch and tongue depressors
Spare batteries and bulbs
Eye chart
Tissues
Examination gloves and jelly
Disposal bags and bins

CLINICAL TEST EQUIPMENT

Urinalysis test strips
Pregnancy tests
Sterile universal containers
Sterile paediatric urine collection bags (if used)
Tray with range of pathology blood tubes, alcohol wipes, swabs, tourniquet, needles and vacuum tube holders, small adhesive plasters
Pathology request forms
Blood glucose test strips, lancets and glucose meter with control solution
Sharps bins and yellow bags for clinical waste
Sterile bacterial, endocervical and viral swabs
Vaginal specula, cervical brooms, endocervical brushes, vials with preservative, request forms and transport bags
Adult and paediatric peak flow meters and disposable mouthpieces
Spirometer

Charts of normal values
Placebo inhaler devices and medication for reversibility tests
Carbon monoxide monitor
Electrocardiogram machine
Doppler ultrasound
Screening audiometer

EQUIPMENT FOR TREATMENT ROOM PROCEDURES

Dressings

Sterile dressing packs, sterile and unsterile gauze
Normal saline sachets/pods
Comprehensive range of dressings, bandages and adhesive tapes (see Chapter 5
    under dressings)
Skin closure strips and tissue adhesive
Plastic bowl for washing feet and legs, with disposable plastic liners
Emollient creams
Dressing scissors
Sterile stitch cutters and staple removers
Ring cutter
Cold-pack for soft tissue injuries
Disposable plastic aprons

Ear irrigation

Otoscope with disposable specula
Waterproof cape
Headlight or head mirror and lamp
Electric ear irrigator and disposable jet tips
Noots ear tank or receiver
Jobson Horne probe
Cotton wool
Tissues

Nasal examination/treatment

Thudicum nasal specula
Tilley nasal forceps

MINOR SURGERY EQUIPMENT

Trolley
Sterile CSSD packs or autoclave
Disposable plastic aprons
Surgical hand scrub
Sterile surgeons' gloves
Local anaesthetic injections, plain and with adrenaline
Ethyl chloride spray
Sterile minor surgery packs or dressing packs
Gallipots
Povidone iodine skin cleanser
Scalpel handles and blades or disposable scalpels
Toothed and non-toothed dissecting forceps
Straight and curved artery forceps
Curette
Needle holders
Straight and curved scissors
Splinter forceps
Sinus forceps
Nail elevator
Specimen containers and formaldehyde solution
Cautery
Silver nitrate applicators
Sterile suture materials
Liquid nitrogen or aerosol freezer spray
Disposal bags for clinical waste and bag/container for used instruments

If CSSD not used:
Washing up liquid and household gloves
Ultrasonic bath and enzymatic solution
Lubricant spray for instruments

GYNAECOLOGICAL EQUIPMENT AND FAMILY PLANNING

Vaginal specula – Cusco's small, medium and large and Winterton's (with
   longer blades)
Rampley sponge-holding forceps
Allis tissue forceps
Galabin uterine sound or disposable sounds
Hegar double-ended dilators in range of sizes
8" artery forceps
Sims uterine scissors

Emmett thread retriever
Sterile IUDs and IUSs
Sanitary towels and pantie liners
Diaphragms and caps in range of sizes
Range of condoms (if supplied to general practice)
Spermicides for demonstration
Injectables:
  Medroxyprogesterone acetate
  Norethisterone oenanthate (if needed)
Demonstration samples for teaching: contraceptive pills, condoms, diaphragms, IUDs and implants
Teaching models for IUD, diaphragm and condoms
Instruction leaflets for all methods

Appendix 2
Emergency equipment

Emergency box with syringes, needles and swabs
Drugs, depending on practice policy:

- Aspirin 300 mg chewable tablets
- Atropine sulphate 600 mg
- Benzylpenicillin 600 mg and water for injection
- Chlorpheniramine 10 mg
- Diazepam 2 mg and 5 mg (oral)
- Diazepam 5 mg (rectal)
- Diclofenac 75 mg
- Epinephrine (adrenaline) 1:1000
- Frusemide 20 mg
- Glucagon 1 mg in 1 ml
- Glyceryl trinitrate spray
- Glucose 50% solution 50 ml for IV use, follow by normal saline solution
- Hydrocortisone 100 mg
- Naloxone 400 mcg
- Prednisolone 5 mg tablets/dispersible tablets
- Procyclidine 10 mg
- Terbutaline 500 mcg

Adult and child resuscitation masks with one-way valves and Ambu bag
Oxygen cylinder and giving set
Suction
Intravenous needles, giving set and infusion solution
Adult and paediatric laryngoscopes and range of endotracheal tubes (if clinicians in the practice able to use safely)
Defibrillator (not commonly kept in urban practices, but essential in rural practices)

EMERGENCY ASTHMA TREATMENT

Large volume spacer and salbutamol inhaler
Nebuliser with supply of single-patient-use nebulising kits with mouthpieces
    and adult and child masks
Salbutamol 2.5 mg and 5 mg nebules
Budesonide 0.5 in 2 ml nebules
Ipratropium bromide nebules

EYE TREATMENT

Magnifying head lens (loup)
Normal saline for irrigation
Eye drops:

- Fluorescein 1%
- Amethocaine 1%
- Chloromycetin (chloramphenicol)

Blue/green light torch or ophthalmoscope to examine fluorescein-stained eyes
Tipped applicators
Tissues

Index

Page numbers in italic refer to tables.

A
abortions, 233–4
abrasions and lacerations, 125
abscess incisions, 74
accountability, 22
acne vulgaris, 151–2
Advance Nurse Practitioners, 19
advanced nursing practice, expansion of
    roles, 9–10
Agenda for Change (AfC), 20
aggression and violence, 279–80
air travel advice, 208–9
airway obstructions, foreign bodies,
    111–12
alcohol abuse, 286
alcohol advice, 173–5
allergies, 137–8
alternative medicines, 9
altitude sickness, 207–8
Alzheimer's disease, 285–6
amenorrhoea, 240–41
amphetamines, 287
anaphylaxis, 112–14, 187
anorexia nervosa, 288
antenatal care, 247
anticoagulation monitoring, 91–2
antihistamines, 138
appointments, 37–8
    Choose and Book schemes, 33
    triage systems, 19–20
appraisals, 6
arterial bleeds, 121
arterial ulcers, 66–7, *67*
asphyxia, 109–12

assessment of prior learning (APL), 24–5
assessment procedures
    asthma patients, 298
    diabetes patients, 308–9
    hypertensive patients, 314–15
    older persons, 167–9
asthma management, 294–300
    clinics, 297–300
    diagnosis, 295
    emergencies, 119–21, *120*
    incidence and causes, 294–5
    nurse training, 297–8
    treatments, 295–7
athlete's foot, 156
audiometry, 98–100
audit, 26
autoclaves, 51–2

B
babies, postnatal checks, 181–2
bacterial vaginosis, 146
bandages and strapping, 63
basic life support, 108, *109*, *110*
bee stings, 128
benign prostatic hyperplasia (BPH),
    264–6
bereavement support, 277
bipolar affective disorders, 283–4
blood glucose monitoring, 92, 307,
    310–11
blood pressure monitoring, 313–16
blood spills, 49, *50*
blood tests, 82, *83–4*, 91–3
'Blue Book', 4–5
boils and carbuncles, 155
breast awareness advice, 243–4

breast screening, 244
breastfeeding advice, 180–81
bronchodilators, 296, 302
bulimia nervosa, 289
burns and scalds, 126

C
CAGE questionnaires, 174
Caldicott Guardians, 34
candida albicans, 146
cannabis, 287–8
cardiovascular conditions, 317
    dietary advice, 170–71
care pathways, 36–7
Care Programme Approach (CPA),
    276–7
carers
    of mentally ill patients, 278–9
    registration, 6
case control studies, 27
catarrh, 137–8
CATS (credit accumulation and transfer),
    24
cerebrovascular accidents (CVAs), 115
    dietary advice, 170–71
cervical caps, 229–30
cervical screening, 79, 85–6, *87–8*,
    241–3
    targets, 241–2
CHAT (Checklist for Autism in Toddlers),
    182
chest compressions, 108, *109*, *110*
chickenpox, 147–8
    vaccines, 196
child abuse, 184–5
childbirth, 131, 180–81
children
    abuse concerns, 184–5
    consent to treatment, 185
    health promotion activities, 180–84
    immunisation schedules, 188–9, 191,
        191
    legislation, 185
    life support procedures, 107–8, *110*
    safety considerations, 183–4
    travel advice and checks, 209–10

children's nurses, 11
chlamydia, 146–7, 234–5
    tests, 89–90
choking, 111–12
cholera vaccinations, 216
chronic bronchitis, 300–1
chronic disease clinics, general
    considerations, 293–4
chronic obstructive pulmonary disease
    (COPD), 300–3
    clinics, 303
    diagnosis, 301–2
    nurse training, 300
    treatments, 302–3
vCJD (variant Creutzfeldt-Jakob disease),
    286
clinical equipment *see* equipment issues
clinical governance, 16
clinical investigations *see* tests and
    investigations
clinical pathways, 36–7
clinical supervision, 23
clinical waste, 53–4
clothing, protective wear, 47–8
clozapine, 285
cocaine, 287
Cochrane Collaboration, 25
cohort studies, 27
cold sores, 154–5, 235
collapsed patients, 105–8, *109*
colposcopies, 243
combined oral contraceptive (COC) pills,
    223, *224*
communication issues, 163–4
community matrons, 11
community mental health nurses
    (CMHNs), 11
complaints handling, 37
complementary therapies, 9
compression hosiery, 63
computer use, 33–4
condoms, 230–1, 236
confidentiality, 31–2
conjunctivitis, 129–30
constipation, 142–3
consulting rooms, 42–4

continuing professional development
GPs, 6
practice nurses, 22
contraceptive methods, 223–32
cervical caps and diaphragms, 229–30
condoms, 230–31, 236
depot hormones, 227–8
emergency treatments, 225–6
intrauterine devices/systems (IUD/Ss),
226–7
natural methods, 231
oral formulations, 223–6
postcoital IUDs, 236
progesterone implants, 228–9
sterilisation, 231–2
transdermal patches, 229
contracts of employment
GPs, 2, 4–6
practice nurses, 21
convulsions, 116–17, *116*, *117*
corneal abrasions, 130
coronary heart disease (CHD), 260–61,
316–17
corticosteroids, 296, 302
COSHH (control of substances hazardous
to health), 44–5
crab lice, 151
credit accumulation and transfer (CATS),
24
cultural diversity, 161
and sexual health, 219–20
Cumberlege Report (1986), 16–17
cystitis, 144–5

D
data protection, 34
deafness, 138–9
decongestants, 138–9
DEET (diethyltoluamide), 203–4
dementia, 285–6
dendritic ulcers, 130
depot contraceptives, 227–8
depressive disorders, 282–4
diabetes management
clinics, 307–12
diagnosis, 304–5

hypoglycaemic attacks, 118–19
monitoring blood glucose levels, 92,
307, 310–11
patient education, 305–6, 309–10
travel advice, 210–11
treatments, 306–7
diarrhoea, 140–41
travel advice, 203
dietary advice and monitoring, 170–73
diabetes management, 305
diphtheria vaccines
adults and travellers, 192, 213
children, 188
directed enhanced services, 5
disease registers, 34
disinfection regimes, 49–50, 52–3
district nurses, 10
Doppler assessment, 65–6
dressings, 61–2, 322
drug abuse, 287–8
drug storage, 45
dysmenorrhoea, 240
dyspepsia, 141–2

E
e-groups, 24
ear irrigation equipment, 52–3, 322
ear problems, 68–71, *70–71*
hearing tests, 98–100
swab tests, 89
temporary deafness, 138–9
eating disorders, 288–9
eczema, 153–4
education issues *see* training and
education
electrocardiography, 94–5, *95*
ELISA (enzyme-linked immunosorbent
assay) tests, 89–90
emergency situations
general principles and procedures,
104–8, *105*, *109*
equipment needs, 325–6
nurse training, 55–6
anaphylaxis, 112–14
asphyxia, 109–12
asthma attacks, 119–20, *120*

emergency situations (*cont'd*)
  cerebrovascular accidents (CVAs), 115
  choking, 111–12
  contraceptive measures, 225–6
  convulsions, 116–17, *116*, *117*
  delivering a baby, 131
  eye problems, 129–30
  fainting, 114
  foreign bodies, 130–31
  haemorrhages, 120–23, *123*
  head injuries, 117–18
  hyperventilation, 119
  hypoglycaemia, 118–19
  immunisation problems, 187
  myocardial infarctions, 114–15
  pain, 123–4
  poisonings, 123, *124*
  stings and bites, 127–8
  transient ischaemic attacks (TIAs), 115
  trauma and minor injuries, 124–7
emphysema, 301
encephalitis, immunisations, 215–16
endocervical swabs, 89–90
enhanced services, 5
environmental consideration, nurse work
    rooms, 42–4
epileptic seizures, 116, *116*
epistaxis, 122–3
equipment issues
  emergency drugs and supplies, 54–5,
    325–6
  general clinical items, 321–4
  minor surgery needs, 322–3
  ordering practices, 55
  role of practice nurse, 54
erectile dysfunction (ED), 269–71
erythema infectiosum, 149–50
ethnicity
  language issues, 32
  see also cultural diversity
evidence-based practice, 25
examination equipment, 321–3
exercise advice, 173
'expert patient', 292–3
eye care, 68, *68*
  acute glaucomas, 130
  conjunctivitis, 129–30

emergencies, 129–30
  foreign bodies, 130
  visual acuity tests, 100, *100*

F
faecal specimens, 90–91
fainting, 114
febrile convulsions, 116–17, *117*
fertility issues, 221–33, 244–6
  contraceptive choice and methods, 222,
    223–32
  education, 232
  IVF and embryo transfer, 245–6
  preconceptual care, 244–5
  reviews and administration, 232–3
fire precautions, 56
foreign bodies, 130–31
  airway obstruction, 111–12
  ear/eye/nose, 130–31
  vagina, 131
formularies, 135
fractures, 127
fungal infections, 155–6
furnishings, 43–4

G
gastrointestinal disorders, 140–44
  bleeds, 122
  constipation, 142–3
  diarrhoea, 140–41
  dyspepsia, 141–2
  worms, 143–4
general medical services (GMS), 4
  GP contract arrangements, 4–6
general practice nursing *see* nurses in
    general practice; practice nurses
genital herpes, 235
genital warts, 157, 235
German measles, 149
glaucomas, 130
Gleason scores, 267
gloves, 47, 50
GP fundholding, 2
GP practices
  healthcare team members, 7–9
  performance indicators, 5–6
  population profiles, 6

remuneration systems, 4–5
skill-mixes, 19
GPs
contract arrangements, 2, 4–6
education, 6
'Green Book' (*Immunisation against Infectious Disease*), 186, 201
guidelines, defined, 36
Gynefix, 227

H
haematemesis, 121–2
haemorrhages, 120–23, *123*
'Hall Report' (2003), 180
hallucinogens, 287–8
hand washing, 47, 81
hand, foot and mouth disease, 150
hangovers, 140
hay fever, 137–8
head injuries, 117–18
head lice, 150–51
headaches, 139–40
health checks, 164–7, 167–9, 262–3
'health education', 162–3
health inequalities, 160
health promotion activities
general considerations, 163–4
childhood concerns, 180–85
mental health issues, 277–8
new patient health checks, 164–7
older person's health checks, 167–9
terminology, 161–3
well-person checks, 167, 262–3
health and safety issues, 44–54
control of substances hazardous to health (COSHH), 44–5
infection control measures, 47–54
protocols and directives, 37
storage of drugs, 45–6
health visitors, 10, 181–2
healthcare assistants, 8, 17–18
Healthcare Commission, 3, 16
hearing tests, audiometry, 98–100
heatstroke, 205–7
hepatitis A vaccines, 196, 213–14
hepatitis B infections, 48, 235
vaccines 190, 195, 214

heroin use, 287
herpes simplex, 154–5, 235
herpes zoster, 148
'hierarchy of evidence', 26
HIV (human immunodeficiency virus), 48, 236
hormone replacement therapy (HRT), 250–51
hospital and community-based specialist nurses, 11
human parasites, 150–51
hypertension management, 312–16
clinics, 313–16
treatments, 312–13
hyperventilation, 119
hypoglycaemia, 118–19, 309
hysterectomies, 249

I
immunisations
contraindications, 189, 212, *212*
emergency situations, 187
GP payments, 185–6
injection sites, 187
medicolegal aspects, 186–7
nurse skills and training, 186–7
parent information, 189–90
private patients, 35–6
public health issues, 196
schedules for adults, 191–6
schedules for children, 188–9, 191, *191*
schedules for travellers, 211–16
special risks, 190–91
vaccine storage, 45–6, *46*
impetigo, 155
incontinence of urine, 253–4
indemnity insurance, 21
independent practice nurses, 7
independent prescribing, 135
infected wounds, 61
infection control measures, 37, 47–54
influenza vaccines
adults, 193–4
children, 190
information for patients
embarrassing topics, 254
leaflets (PILs), 59–60

information resources
practice libraries, 18
systematic reviews, 25
ingrowing toenails, 74
inhaler devices, 297
injection procedures, 59–60
insect bites, 127–8
insomnia, 140
insulin administration, 306–7
insurance arrangements, 21
integrated nursing teams, 9, 16–17
Internet
as information resource, 25, 254
as support tool, 24
intrauterine devices/systems (IUD/Ss),
75, *76*, 226–7
IVF (in vitro fertilisation), 245–6

J
Japanese B encephalitis, 215–16
job descriptions, practice nurses, 20–21

L
laboratory investigations, 81–91
blood tests, 82, *83–4*
urine tests, 82–5
language issues, use of interpreters,
32
League of Friends, 12
learning disabilities, detection and
recognition, 182–3
learning disability nurses, 11
leg ulcers, 65–7, *66, 67*
libraries, 18
life support procedures, 105–8, *109,
110*
lighting, 43
link workers, 32
lipid-lowering diets, 170–71
liquid-based cytology (LBC), 85–6
local enhanced services, 5
LSD (lysergic acid diethylamide), 288
lung function tests, 95–8, *99*, 301

M
Macmillan nurses, 11
malaria, 203–5, *206*

male morbidity/mortality, 258
male patients, 261–2
health checks, 262–3
mania, 283–4
Mantoux testing, 190
mast cell stabilisers, 138
measles, 148
medical history taking, 165–6
medical records *see* record systems
medical secretaries, 8
medications
nurse prescribing, 135–6
storage, 45
meetings, 39
melaena, 122
meningococcal meningitis, travel
vaccines, 214–15
menopause issues, 249–51
menorrhagia, 240
menstruation abnormalities, 239–41
mental health issues
development of services, 275–7
in general practice, 277–9
staff self-awareness, 289
mercury sphygmomanometers, 44–5,
313–14
microscopy, 93–4
midwives, 10–11
migraines, 139
minocycline, 152
minor surgery, 72–6
equipment needs, 322–3
miscarriages and stillbirths, 248
Misuse of Drugs Act (1971), 45
MMR vaccines, 148, 149, 188, 196–7
motivational interviewing, 164
MSU (mainstream specimen of urine)
tests, 82
mumps
adult vaccines, 193
child vaccines, 149, 188
see also MMR vaccines
myocardial infarctions (MIs), 114–15

N
NAATs (nucleic acid amplification tests),
85

nail and hair samples, 90
nasal swabs, 89
National Clinical Assessment
    Authority/Service (NCAA/S),
    3
national enhanced services, 5
National Health Service (NHS)
    background, 1
    organisational structures and changes,
    2–3, 4
National Institute for Clinical Excellence
    (NICE), 3, 25
National Service Frameworks (NSFs),
    2
    for mental health, 4, 275, 276–7
    for older people, 12, 115, 167–9
necrotic wounds, 60–61
needlestick injuries, 49
neighbourhood nursing, 16–17
networking, 22–3
New General Medical Services (GMS)
    contract, 4–6
new patient health checks, 164–7
NHS and Community Care Act (1990),
    3–4
NHS Direct, 134
NHS Improvement Plan (HM Government
    2004), 3
NHSNet, 33
nose bleeds, 122–3
nucleic acid amplification tests (NAATs),
    85
nurse practitioners, 7–8, 19
nurse prescribing, 135–6
nurse triage, 19–20, 134
nurse-led PMS schemes, 4
nurses in general practice
    background history, 16–20
    employment terms and conditions,
    20–22
    profession-led team structures, 9–11,
    16–17
    support measures, 22–4
    see also practice nurses
Nursing and Midwifery Council (NMC),
    standards of proficiency, 9–10
nutritional advice, 170–73

O
obesity, dietary advice, 170–73
occupational hazards, 260
older person's health checks, 167–9
opiate abuse, 287
osteoporosis, 251–2

P
pain, acute problems, 123–4, *124*
paramedical staff, 8–9
parasites, 150–51
Patient Advice and Liaison Services
    (PALS), 37
patient consent, 80
    children, 185, 187
Patient Group Directives (PGDs), on
    immunisations, 186
patient information leaflets (PILs), 59–60
patient participation, 12, 39
patient records *see* record systems
patient satisfaction questionnaires, 39
pelvic examinations, 242
pensions, 21
performance indicators, nGMS quality
    frameworks, 5–6
personal indemnity insurance, 21
Personal Medical Services (PMS), 4
pharmacists, 8–9
    diagnostic testing, 92–3
phlebotomists, 9, 19
pneumococcal disease vaccines
    adults, 194–5
    children, 191
poisonings, 123, *124*
poliomyelitis immunisations
    adults and travellers, 192, 213
    children, 188
postnatal care, 181–2, 247–8
postpartum affective disorders, 283
practice managers, 8
practice nurses
    background history, 16–18
    employment contracts, 21
    information resources, 18
    job descriptions, 20–21
    roles, 7–8, 18
    training and education, 17, 24–5

pregnancy advice, 180–81
  antenatal care, 247
  miscarriages and stillbirths, 248
  postnatal care, 247–8
  preconceptual care, 244–5
  terminations, 233–4
  travel considerations, 209
pregnancy tests, 93
premenstrual syndrome (PMS), 241
prescribing protocols, 135–6
Primary Care Act (1997), 4
Primary Care Organisations (PCOs), 3
primary healthcare teams (PHCTs), 9
private patients
  medical records, 35–6
  walk-in centres, 134
Prodigy Guidance, 136, 174, 189
professional registration, 22
progesterone implants, 228–9
progesterone-only pills (POPs), 223–4,
  224
Project 2000, 17
prostate cancer, 266–9
prostate diseases, 264–9
PSA (prostate-specific antigen) tests,
  266–7
psoriasis, 152–3
psychotic disorders, 284–5
public involvement initiatives, 12, 39
puerperal psychosis, 283
pulmonary rehabilitation, 302–3

Q
qualitative studies, 27
Quality and Outcomes Framework (QOF),
  5–6, 26, 292
quantitative studies, 26–7

R
rabies, 215
receptionists, 8
record systems, 32–4
  access and confidentiality, 31–2, 35
  computerised systems, 33–4
  manual systems, 32
  nursing notes, 35

private patients, 35–6
  transferral methods, 32
rectal bleeds, 122
rectal swabs, 90
Red Book (Statement of Fees and
  Allowances), 4
reflections on practice, 25
rescue breathing procedures, 107, *109*, *110*
research, 26–7
respiratory function tests, 95–8, *99*, 301
respiratory tract infections, 136–8
resuscitation procedures, 55, 105–8, *109*,
  110
revalidation, GPs, 6
rhinitis, 137–8
ringworm, 156
Royal College of Nursing (RCN), 24
rubella, 149
  adult vaccines, 192–3
  child vaccines, 188
  see also MMR vaccines

S
scabies, 150
schizophrenia, 284–5
school nurses, 11
screening, 162
  clinical guidelines, 79–80, 244
  patient consent and information, 80
  records management, 80–81
  targets, 241–2
sebaceous cyst removal, 74
semen samples, 91
sensible drinking, 173–5
sexual identity, 219–20, 261
  relationship issues, 220
sexually transmitted diseases, 146–7, 207,
  234–6, 263
sharps
  disposal, 54
  injuries, 49
shingles, 148
skill-mix systems, 19
skin samples, 90
skin tags, 74
slapped cheek syndrome, 149–50

sleep problems, 140
smoking cessation advice, 175–6, 302
Snellen charts, *100*
social services, 12
soft tissue injuries, 126–7
solvent abuse, 288
specialist nurses, 9–11
spillages, 50, *53*
spirometry, 96–8, *99*
sports injuries, 259–60
sputum samples, 91
staff meetings, 39
staff support *see* support measures
sterilisation and disinfection regimes,
    49–52
sterilisation methods, 231–2
steroids
    oral, 138
    topical, 154
stings and bites, 127–8
stool specimens, 90–91
storage, drugs and vaccines, 45–6
stress disorders, 280–82
stress incontinence, 253
strokes, 115
    dietary advice, 170–71
substance abuse, 286–8
suicide, 258–9
sun exposure, 205
supplementary prescribing, 136
supplies procurement, 54–5
    equipment types, 321–6
support measures
    clinical supervision, 23
    national associations and e-groups, 24
    networking and practice nurse groups,
      22–3
Sure Start, 183
surgery *see* minor surgery
Suzy Lamplugh Trust, 279
swabs, 86, 89–90
systematic reviews, 25

T
teamwork, 7–12
teenage health problems, 184

telephone use, 38
tension headaches, 131
testicular cancer, 263–4
tests and investigations, 79–101
    equipment needs, 321–2
    laboratory tests, 81–91
    result protocols, 38
    within-practice tests, 91–100
tetanus immunisations
    adults and travellers, 192, 212–13
    children, 188
threadworms, 90
throat swabs, 89
thrush, 146
ticks, 128, 216
training and education
    GPs, 6
    healthcare assistants, 18
    practice managers, 8
    practice nurses, 17, 24–5
    receptionists, 8
    for asthma management, 297–8
    for chronic disease management, 292
    for COPD, 300
    for diabetes management, 307
    for emergency procedures, 55–6
    for health promotion, 161
    for hypertension management, 313
    for screening and diagnostic tests,
      79
    for travel health, 200–1
transdermal contraceptive patches (Evra),
    229
transient ischaemic attacks (TIAs), 115
trauma and minor injuries, 124–7
travel advice
    blood-borne diseases, 207
    food and water, 202–3
    information sources, 201
    malaria, 203–5, *206*
    sun and heat exposure, 205–7
travel immunisations, 211–16
triage, 19–20, 134
Trichomonas vaginalis, 146
tuberculosis, BCG immunisations, 190
typhoid vaccines, 213

U
unconscious patients, 105–8, *109*
upper respiratory tract infections,
     136–8
urge incontinence, 254
urinary problems, 144–5, 253–4
urine tests, 82–5, 93

V
vaginal discharge, 145–7
vaginal swabs, 89
  and foreign bodies, 131
varicose veins, 121
vasectomies, 231–2
venous ulcers, 65–6, *66*
violent patients, 279–80
vision testing, 100, *100*
vitamin K, 181
voluntary services, 12
vomiting, 140–41
  blood loss, 120–21

W
waiting rooms, 42–3
walk-in centres, 134
warfarin, blood tests, 92
warts and verrucae, 74–5, 156
wasp stings, 128
waste disposal, 53–4
weight loss advice, 171–3
well-person checks, 167, 262–3
workplace considerations, design and
     furnishings, 43–4
worms, 143–4
wound care, 60–68
  dressings, 61–2
  healing phases, 60–61
  patient assessment, 64–5
  strapping and bandages, 63
  ulcers, 65–8

Y
Yellow Fever Centres, 35
yellow fever vaccines, 35, 214